THEORY OF
Bakery AND Patisserie

Parvinder S. Bali

Corporate Chef, Learning and Development
The Oberoi Centre of Learning and Development
New Delhi

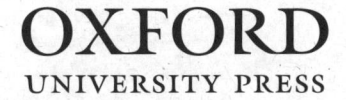

OXFORD
UNIVERSITY PRESS

OXFORD
UNIVERSITY PRESS

Oxford University Press is a department of the University of Oxford.
It furthers the University's objective of excellence in research, scholarship,
and education by publishing worldwide. Oxford is a registered trade mark of
Oxford University Press in the UK and in certain other countries.

Published in India by
Oxford University Press
Ground Floor, 2/11, Ansari Road, Daryaganj, New Delhi 110002, India

© Oxford University Press 2018

The moral rights of the author/s have been asserted.

First published in 2018

All rights reserved. No part of this publication may be reproduced, stored in
a retrieval system, or transmitted, in any form or by any means, without the
prior permission in writing of Oxford University Press, or as expressly permitted
by law, by licence, or under terms agreed with the appropriate reprographics
rights organization. Enquiries concerning reproduction outside the scope of the
above should be sent to the Rights Department, Oxford University Press, at the
address above.

You must not circulate this work in any other form
and you must impose this same condition on any acquirer.

ISBN-13: 978-0-19-948879-7
ISBN-10: 0-19-948879-7

Typeset in Adobe GaramondPro
by E-Edit Infotech Private Limited (Santype), Chennai
Printed in India by Repro India Ltd, Surat

Cover image: mixform design / Shutterstock

Third-party website addresses mentioned in this book are provided
by Oxford University Press in good faith and for information only.
Oxford University Press disclaims any responsibility for the material contained therein.

I dedicate this book

to

my two lovely children, *Ojas* and *Amora*,
my nephew and nieces, *Guranjan, Jaijeet, Harshita, Kanan, Vriti,* and *Dhwani*,
my parents, *Late Major Ranjit Singh Bali* and *Gominder Kaur Bali*,
and my wife, *Shalini Bali*.

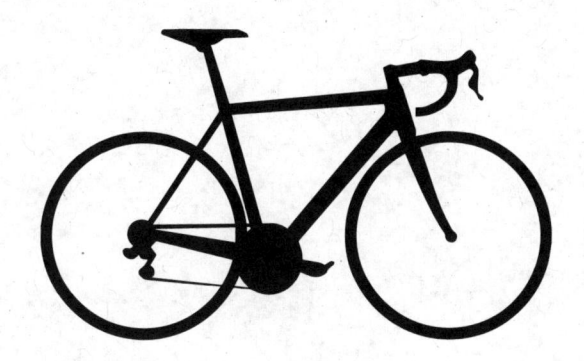

My two favourite things in life are –'Libraries and Bicycles'. They both move people forward without wasting anything.

—Chef Bali

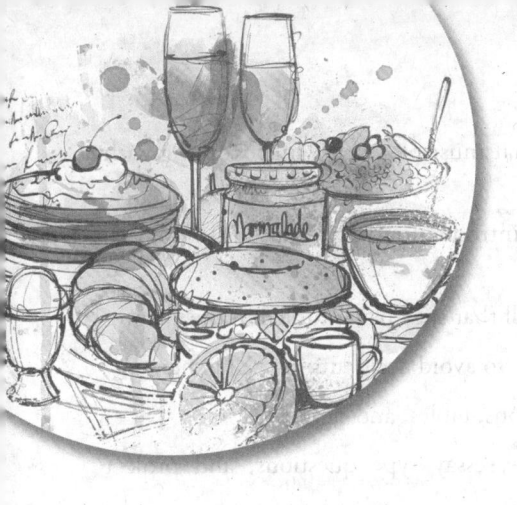

Preface

Is baking an art or a science? *Bakery and Patisserie* are two aspects of a pastry kitchen that make a perfect blend of art and science. The art in *Bakery and Patisserie* is mostly limited to the presentation skills and arrangement of the product on display. The science part involves identifying correct ingredients, understanding their chemical reaction on any given product, and following the right process to make an ideal recipe. Due to constant awareness of health and eating organic food, many professionals and home bakers have started excelling in producing high fibre and gluten free bakery and pastry products for the discerning customers.

Globalization has changed the mind-set of many youngsters in India who wish to pursue careers in hospitality. Today, *Bakery and Patisserie* has become one of the most pursued careers in the hospitality sector. With many international chains coming to India, more and more job opportunities are seen to have been created in the kitchen. A lot of skilled bakers and patissiers also find jobs in large bakery production centres, high end hotels, and on ships. In fact with this surge of good hotels in the country, it has become fundamental for students to develop a keen interest in understanding the subject; hence making it a much-sought after course.

ABOUT THE BOOK

The book is intended for students of Diploma and Food Craft courses in hotel management, catering to the syllabus of National Council for Hotel Management and Catering Technology. It has been designed to give an introduction to bakery and pastry, layout of a pastry kitchen, basic culinary terms, and associated methods of production. It will help students to gain technical knowledge and skills of pastry making as well as familiarize themselves with the day-to-day working atmosphere of the department.

It has been developed keeping in mind the changing trends in modern pastry kitchen across the world. As there is a myriad of differences in the commodities and technology used across the world, it is important that one should be aware of the dynamics of pastry kitchen operations. The book also brings in my 26 years of experience with Oberoi Hotels and Resorts. This professional knowledge percolates down through chapters in the form of 'chef tips' which have been handed and circulated by chefs down the generations.

PEDAGOGICAL FEATURES

- Discusses roles of various commodities used in bakery and pastry along with different techniques used in preparation of bakery and pastry products
- Explains in detail the methods of incorporating air by chemical, physical, and biological methods in creating a range of pastry and bakery products
- Describes in detail the structure of the wheat and its milling process that determines the final quality of the baked product

- Explains the art of sugar work and lists all the precautions that must be taken whilst working with sugar
- Begins every chapter with learning objectives which give an introduction to the various topics discussed in the chapter
- Concludes chapters with a summary to help students gather all that they have studied in the chapter
- Provides important points (chef's tips) interspersed in the text to avoid accidents in the kitchen
- Explains practical aspects of bakery and pastry with photographs, tables, and figures
- Includes assessment tools such as objective type questions, essay type questions, and project assignments

STRUCTURE AND COVERAGE

The book is divided into 11 chapters.

Chapter 1, *Introduction to Pastry and Bakery* defines various sections of a professional pastry kitchen and provides an overview of the hierarchy and layout of the same. It discusses different kinds of weights, measurements, and oven temperatures (in Celsius and Fahrenheit) to be used while baking. Discussion on large and small equipment used in bakery and pastry along with pictures have also been provided for easy understanding.

Chapter 2, *Commodities in Bakery and Pastry* discusses in detail commodities such as fats and oils, types of dairy products, eggs, sweeteners, raising agents, chocolate, and various types of cheese used and their impact while baking. It also explains the structure of wheat and the milling process that determines the final product.

Chapter 3, *Techniques in Bakery and Pastry* covers different types of techniques used in bakery such as sifting, autolysis, kneading, proofing, shaping, panning, and baking as well as storing of breads. Other techniques used such as aerating, docking, whisking, whipping, folding, shortening, blind baking, rubbing, pinning, piping, icing, creaming, and lamination have also been explained in detail along with examples.

Chapter 4, *Bread Fabrication* explains the principles of basic dough making, role of ingredients such as flour, yeast, sugar, and salt on breads and how these are mixed to create variations. Various steps involved in production of breads with regards to temperature and timings have also been included. Popular international breads along with rich and laminated dough such as croissant, danish, brioche and more are discussed too.

Chapter 5, *Basic Pastes in Bakery and Pastry* discusses short crust, puff pastry, choux paste, sweet paste, *pate brise*, and *pate sable*. Precautions that need to be kept in mind whilst making them and different types of products made with these pastes are listed in tabular form along with pictures.

Chapter 6, *Basic Creams and Sauces* explains types of creams such as crème chantilly, caprice cream, buttercream, lemon cream, ganache, almond paste, touille paste, and pastry cream along with sauces, and coulis that are used in pastry kitchen. Various kinds of meringues, their preparation and storage and a few classical desserts made by using these common creams and bases have also been covered.

Chapter 7, *Basic Sponges and Cakes* elaborates on the composition and types of basic cakes, sponges, and icings. It also discusses various kinds of faults that can occur in cake making. Different kinds of cakes and pastries that are served during afternoon tea are also listed in tabular form for student's benefit.

Chapter 8, *Cookies and Biscuits* discusses the difference between a cookie and a biscuit, types of cookies and various methods of preparing them. Various kinds of faults that can occur whilst making cookies are also discussed in this chapter.

Chapter 9, *Hot and Cold Desserts* classifies desserts under categories—hot, cold, and frozen. Under each category a few classical desserts that are commonly made internationally in pastry kitchen have been discussed. This chapter also talks about frozen desserts such as ice creams, sorbets, bombes, coupes, and gelatos.

Chapter 10, *Sugar Confections* covers types of sugar used for sugar confections. Products such as marshmallows, fudges, toffees, and candies made from sugar are discussed in detail along with their recipes for better understanding. Apart from this, the process of creating a sugar sculpture and precautions related to its preparation have been covered in detail.

Chapter 11, *Indian Sweets* explains the stages of sugar syrups with regards to the Indian cuisine. This chapter discusses in detail the regional influences on sweets from all parts of India. It also talks about various equipment used in making Indian sweets and desserts.

ACKNOWLEDGEMENTS

I want to mention certain people and organizations who have either directly or indirectly contributed towards this book. First and foremost, I would like to mention Mr Prithvi Raj Singh Oberoi, Executive Chairman and Mr Vikram Oberoi, Managing Director and CEO, under whose able guidance I have been able to collect all the knowledge pertaining to this book. I also want to thank Oberoi Centre of Learning and Development for letting me use the resources for research. I would like a special mention of all my colleagues and friends who have lent their encouragement and support in this venture of mine. I would like to thank the whole Oberoi Group for their support as well.

My thanks would be incomplete, if I did not mention the academicians and reviewers who reviewed the book and gave corrective feedback that helped frame the contents of the book. I also thank the editors and the team at Oxford University Press India for their constant follow-ups and support that motivated me to accomplish this project.

I extend my special thanks to all my near and dear ones and the professionals in the industry who have in some ways influenced the development of this book.

Last but not the least, I am grateful to my wife Shalini and my children Ojas and Amora, for their immense patience while developing this book.

Parvinder S. Bali

Features of

Chef's tips
Important points that should be kept in mind appear as tips throughout the text for quick recapitulation.

CHEF'S TIPS
- Get to know your oven as it is an important factor in successful baking.
- Have the accuracy of your thermostat checked regularly.
- Do not open the oven door during the early baking stages and avoid opening it too frequently as some products may collapse. If you often open the oven door, the moisture tends to escape from it by dropping the pressure and temperature inside it, resulting in collapse of products.
- Place items to be baked on a tray in an interlocking manner to allow free passage of air through them so that they bake evenly.
- Close the oven door slowly.

Activities
Activities have been interspersed in the chapters to aid students in understanding the practical side of the subject.

ACTIVITY

1. In groups of five, conduct a market survey of hotels and speciality restaurants and make a list of various kinds of frozen desserts served by them. Further, make a note of commercially available and home-churned ice creams and share with the rest of the group.
2. In groups of three or four, make at least two sundaes or coupes with sauces, garnish, and accompaniments. Present the dishes to other groups and get your product evaluated and critiqued. Make standard recipes of the same and distribute to everybody.
3. In groups of five, undertake a market survey of hotels and speciality restaurants and note the components of a dessert buffet. Observe how the desserts are balanced with regard to textures, temperatures, etc. Record your observations and share your findings with other groups.
4. Divide the class into groups and prepare a range of hot puddings using different bases as explained in Table 9.1. Compare the taste, textures, and flavours and observe what desserts can be served hot or cold. Share your learnings with other groups and record them.

Exercises
A series of objective type and essay type questions highlight the major topics covered in the chapter. The questions enhance learning and can be used for review and classroom discussion.

OBJECTIVE TYPE QUESTIONS

1. Define a sponge and how is it different from a cake and bread.
2. List down the role of ingredients used in sponge making.

   mousse cake, and dark and white chocolate mousse cake?
10. How is chiffon cake different from angel cake?
11. What is the difference between Victoria sponge

ESSAY TYPE QUESTIONS

1. Define icing and what equipment is used for making it.
2. Explain different types of icings used on cakes and pastries.
3. Write down the procedure of making joconde sponge.
5. Differentiate between chilled cheesecake and baked cheesecake.
6. Why are Yule logs popular during Christmas?
7. Briefly describe at least five types of hi tea cakes and pastries.

the Book

Figures and Tables
All chapters contain figures and tables to illustrate the topics discussed in the chapters.

- Endosperm (85%)
- Bran (12%)
- Seed coat
- Pericarp
- Germ/Embryo (3%)

Fig. 2.1 Structure of wheat grain

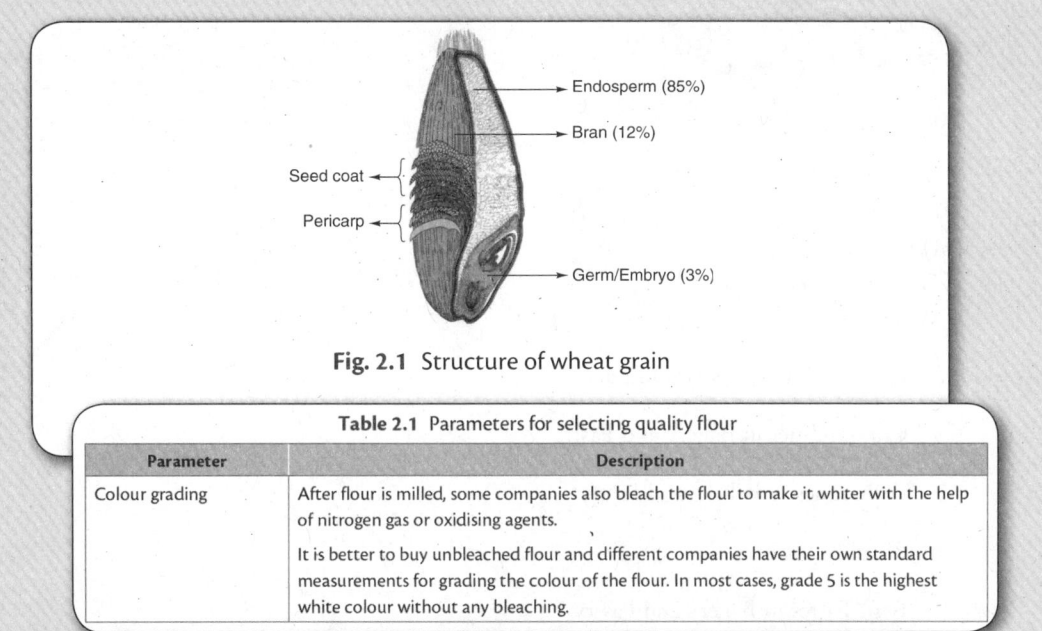

Table 2.1 Parameters for selecting quality flour

Parameter	Description
Colour grading	After flour is milled, some companies also bleach the flour to make it whiter with the help of nitrogen gas or oxidising agents.
	It is better to buy unbleached flour and different companies have their own standard measurements for grading the colour of the flour. In most cases, grade 5 is the highest white colour without any bleaching.

Photographs
Photographs have been added in the chapters to help readers understand concepts better.

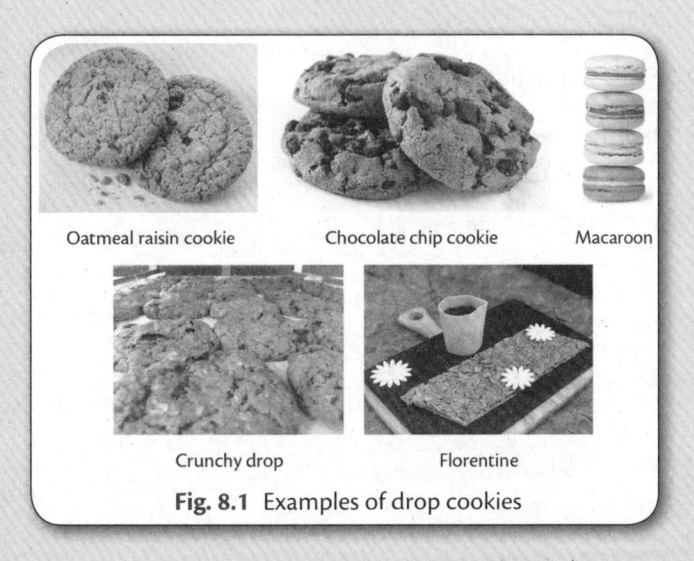

Oatmeal raisin cookie   Chocolate chip cookie   Macaroon

Crunchy drop   Florentine

Fig. 8.1 Examples of drop cookies

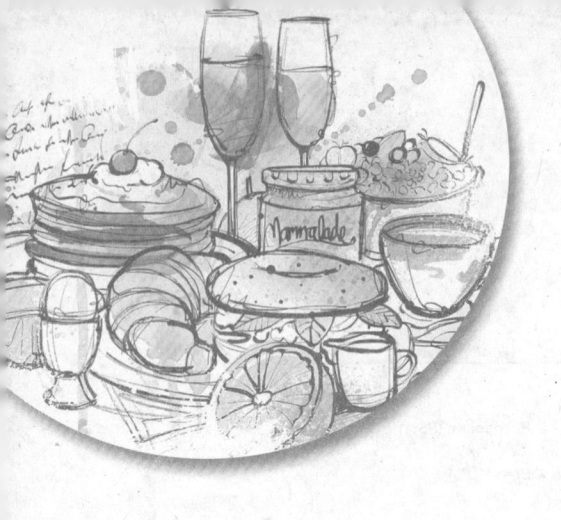

Brief Contents

Preface v
Features of the Book viii
Detailed Contents xi

1	Introduction to Pastry and Bakery	1
2	Commodities in Bakery and Pastry	21
3	Techniques in Bakery and Pastry	49
4	Bread Fabrication	61
5	Basic Pastes in Bakery and Pastry	94
6	Basic Creams and Sauces	103
7	Basic Sponges and Cakes	125
8	Cookies and Biscuits	150
9	Hot and Cold Desserts	166
10	Sugar Confections	198
11	Indian Sweets	219

Index 243
About the Author 249

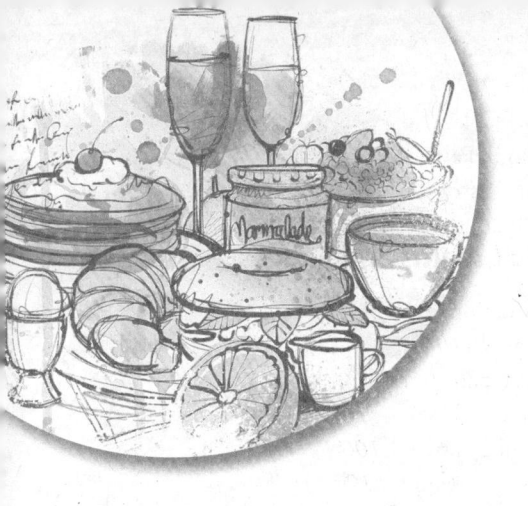

Detailed Contents

Preface   *v*
Features of the Book   *viii*
Brief Contents   *x*

1 Introduction to Pastry and Bakery   1

Introduction   *1*
Sections of Patisserie   *5*
Hierarchy in Kitchen   *6*
Weights and Measurement   *7*
   Sweet Paste Recipe   *7*
   Types of Measuring Systems   *8*
   Oven Temperature Comparisions   *8*
Layout and Workflow   *9*
Large Machinery Used in Bakery and Pastry   *11*

2 Commodities in Bakery and Pastry   21

Introduction   *21*
Flour   *22*
   Structure of Wheat Grain   *22*
   Milling of Flour   *23*
   Selection Criteria of Good Flour   *24*
Types of Flour   *25*
   Flours Obtained from Wheat   *25*
   Flours from Various Grains   *25*
   Gluten-free Flour   *27*
Fats and Oils   *27*
   Usage of Fats and Oils in Baking   *27*

Milk and Dairy Products   *29*
   Types of Milk   *29*
   Cream   *29*
Cheese   *30*
   Kinds of Cheese   *30*
   Cheese in Pastry and Bakery   *30*
Eggs   *31*
   Structure of an Egg   *31*
   Selection and Storage of Eggs   *32*
   Uses of Eggs   *32*
Sweeteners   *36*
Raising Agents   *36*
   Chemical Raising Agents   *38*
   Biological Raising Agents   *38*
   Mechanical Raising Agents   *40*
Chocolate   *41*
   Processing of Chocolate   *41*
   Types of Chocolate and its Uses   *43*
   Uses of Chocolate   *45*

3 Techniques in Bakery and Pastry   49

Introduction   *49*
Techniques of Preparing Bread   *50*
   Sifting   *50*
   Autolysis   *50*
   Kneading   *50*

    Prooving   *51*
    Shaping   *51*
    Baking   *53*
    Scoring   *54*
  Techniques Related to Pastry Making   *55*
    Creaming   *55*
    Whisking   *55*
    Rubbing-in   *55*
    Folding-in   *56*
    Docking   *56*
    Blind Baking   *57*
    Pinning or Rolling   *57*
    Piping   *57*
    Laminating   *58*
    Icing   *58*

4 Bread Fabrication   61

Introduction   *61*
Understanding Baking   *62*
Role of Ingredients in Bread Making   *63*
Bread Making Methods   *67*
Basic Faults in Bread Making   *73*
Common Bread Diseases   *75*
Equipment Used in Bread Making   *75*
Basic Shapes of Breads   *78*
International Breads   *79*
  France   *79*
  Italy   *80*
  Germany   *82*
  Great Britain   *83*
  Jewish Breads   *84*
  Middle East   *84*
  America   *86*
Enriched Dough   *86*
Laminated Dough   *87*
  Danish and Croissant   *87*
Storage and Service of Bread   *90*

5 Basic Pastes in Bakery and Pastry   94

Introduction   *94*
Pastes   *95*
  Short Crust Paste   *95*
  Sweet Paste   *97*
  Choux Paste   *98*
  Puff Pastry   *101*

6 Basic Creams and Sauces   103

Introduction   *103*
Creams   *104*
  Marzipan   *104*
  Almond Paste   *105*
  Touille Paste   *106*
  Pastry Cream   *107*
  Chantilly Cream   *108*
  Caprice Cream   *109*
  Buttercream   *109*
  Lemon Curd Cream   *110*
  Ganache   *111*
Sauces   *112*
  Types of Sauces   *114*
  Components of Sauce   *115*
  Uses of Sauces   *118*
  Classical and Contemporary Sauces   *119*
  Storage and Service of Sauces   *121*
  Common Faults in Sauce Making   *122*

7 Basic Sponges and Cakes   125

Introduction   *125*
Basic Sponge Cake   *126*
  Ingredients Used in Cake Making   *126*
  Principles of Sponge Making   *127*
  Baking and Cooling of Sponges   *129*
  Important Points for Making Sponges and Cakes   *130*
  Types of Basic Sponges   *130*
Classical Cakes and Pastries   *136*
Cakes Served During Hi Tea   *142*
Common Faults in Cake Making   *143*
Icing   *144*
  Kinds of Icing and its Classical Types   *145*

8 Cookies and Biscuits   150

Introduction   *150*
Preparation of Simple Cookies   *151*
Types of Cookies   *152*
  Drop Cookies   *152*
  Piped Cookies   *154*

Hand-rolled Cookies　*155*
　　　Cutter-cut Cookies　*156*
　　　Bar Cookies　*157*
　　　Sheet Cookies　*158*
　　　Frozen and Cut Cookies　*159*
　　　Festive Cookies　*159*
　　Uses of Cookies　*161*
　　Common Faults in Cookie Preparation　*162*

9　Hot and Cold Desserts　166

　　Introduction　*166*
　　Hot and Cold Desserts　*167*
　　　Hot Desserts　*167*
　　　Cold Desserts　*173*
　　Presentation of Desserts　*179*
　　　Salient Features of Presenting
　　　　Desserts　*179*
　　　Tips for Presenting Pre-plated
　　　　Desserts　*180*
　　Buffet Desserts　*180*
　　Frozen Desserts　*181*
　　　Churn-frozen Desserts　*182*
　　　Still-frozen Desserts　*187*
　　　Other Types of Frozen Desserts　*188*
　　　Classical Frozen Desserts　*189*
　　　Ingredients Used in Frozen
　　　　Desserts　*191*
　　　Equipment Used in the Production of
　　　　Frozen Desserts　*192*
　　　Storage and Service of Frozen
　　　　Desserts　*193*

10　Sugar Confections　198

　　Introduction　*198*
　　Stages of Sugar and its Uses　*199*
　　Products Made from Sugar　*201*
　　　Sugar Syrup　*201*
　　　Marshmallows　*201*
　　　Caramels, Fudges, and Toffee　*202*
　　　Candies　*203*
　　　Fondant　*203*
　　　Gum Paste　*204*
　　　Nougatine　*204*
　　　Rock Sugar　*205*
　　　Honeycomb　*206*
　　　Jam　*206*
　　　Spun Sugar　*206*
　　　Pate De Fruits　*207*
　　Art of Sugar Work　*207*
　　　Preparation Prior to Commencing
　　　　Sugar Work　*208*
　　　Ingredients for Sugar Work　*209*
　　　Cooking Sugar　*210*

11　Indian Sweets　219

　　Introduction　*219*
　　Origin and History of Indian Sweets　*220*
　　Ingredients Used in Indian Sweets　*220*
　　Regional Influenece on Indian Sweets　*227*
　　Equipment Used in Halwai　*237*
　　Religious Importance of Sweets　*238*

Index　*243*
About the Author　*249*

Introduction to Pastry and Bakery

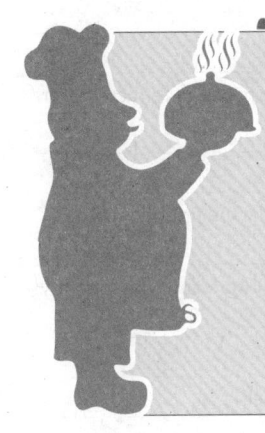

LEARNING OBJECTIVES

After reading this chapter, you should be able to
- understand the pastry and bakery department
- differentiate between the various sections of the pastry kitchen
- remember the terms associated with day to day pastry and bakery operations
- memorise the hierarchy of the department and reporting structure
- know the basic layout of the pastry kitchen and understand the importance of the same
- weigh and scale ingredients as per the required recipe
- identify the large equipment and machinery used in the pastry department

INTRODUCTION

Though the term bakery is related to baking, the bakery department is not restricted to only making and baking of breads. Breads are one of the earliest products that were made by the Egyptians and Romans around 5,000 years ago. Some of the world's oldest breads can be found in Switzerland, and since they might be as old as 5,000 years, their baking technique and who started the same is not very clear and certain.

The first premier baker's guild was established in Rome in 14 AD in the reign of Emperor Augustine and breads were one of the most important commodities for armies and peasants. The grain was offered to people for free by the government, which led to opening of professional bakeries that in turn would make breads for the people by charging a small amount of money. Since many homes did not have ovens to make their own bread, they usually bought it from bakeries. The earlier ovens were huge and wood fired. The enormous size ovens were hence restricted to professional bakeries and in 14th century there were close to 2,500 bakeries that had been set up to meet the needs and demands of people wanting a loaf of bread.

The modern bakery produces all kinds of products such as breads, cakes, pastries, cookies, desserts and hence, is commonly referred to as bakery and confectionary. In olden times, bakeries were restricted to the production of breads and biscuits but the advent of technology and introduction of new ingredients such as chocolate, sugar, and dairy products, created yet another array of sweet products that got associated with baking. Since then this department in hotels came to be known as pastry kitchen or *patisserie* in French. Bakery and confectionary is one of the most important sections in a large hotel as it produces goods that are used during all meal periods whether breakfast, lunch, dinner, or snacks. It is because of this reason that the department has to work round the clock and is one of the busiest sections in any given hotel.

Since several terms are related to bakery and confectionary, therefore, before we start to read this book, let us get acquainted with the bakery and pastry terminologies to better familiarise ourselves with the subject.

Table 1.1 Terms related to bakery and confectionary

Term	Description
Agar Agar	Dried purified stems of seaweed that swell with water to form gel. It is also used as a substitute as vegetarian gelatin and also known as china grass
Batter	Flour and liquid mixture of flowing consistency
Baume	Unit or scale of measuring the density of sugar syrup through a saccharometer or refractometer
Blind bake	Baking of a tart or flan without any filling inside
Bouchée	Small bite size pastry cases usually filled with savoury fillings
Brûlée	Literally translates to burnt. Applied to dishes such as crème custards that are finished with caramelized or burnt sugar
Candied	Preservation of fruit or vegetable by cooking in super saturated sugar solution and subsequently drying, which results in coating of sugar crystals
Caramelize	To heat the sugar until it melts to a golden brown colour
Chemiser	To line a mould as for ice cream bombe mould or to coat an item with jelly
Coagulate	Partial or complete hardening of protein with application of heat
Comfiture	A mixture of fruits and sugar cooked to a jelly consistency, for example, jams and marmalades
Congeal	To change a liquid into solid by lowering the temperature whilst cooking. It also refers to formation of gelatin or gelling of a product
Coulis	A liquid fruit puree cooked with sugar and usually strained to a smooth sauce consistency
Coverture	Covering chocolate with a minimum cocoa butter content of 32%
Creaming	Process of mixing butter and sugar together to a fluffy stage
Crimping	Giving a decorative edge to various doughs and pastes with the help of pinching tools
Croquant	Caramelized sugar and nut mixture that is crushed to form a granular mixture
Crust	The top most layer of a baked product, usually a bread which gives the name to the bread such as soft roll or crusty roll
Crystalize	A property of sugar to get back into solid stage from liquid stage either with agitation or temperature change
Curdle	Separation of emulsion formed when fat, sugar, eggs, etc., are beaten together. Usually, caused by adding liquids too quickly or are at cold temperature. Curdling can also happen when a diary product is heated with acid
Dariole	A deep round mould with sloping sides
Dead dough	A bread dough that is made without any addition of yeast or other leavening agents. These doughs are used to prepare breads for displays and not consumption
Dessert	Last course of the meal. Also, commonly used word for sweet dishes

Table 1.1 (Contd)

Term	Description
Dextrin	A soluble gummy substance formed from starch by the action of heat
Docking	Making holes in a rolled dough or paste, which allows the pastry to bake without rising
Dough	A mixture of flour and liquid and other products. Dough can be fermented or non-fermented
Doyle	Fancy lace mat on which goods are presented
Dredge	To sprinkle or coat with flour or sugar
Emulsifying agents	Substances such as gums, agar, lecithin that aid in mixing two immiscible liquids such as oil and water
Enrobe	Coating chocolate with melted chocolate or icing
Entremets	Sweet course in French classical menu
Essences	Aromatic compounds used for flavouring pastry products
Fermentation	The action of yeast with sugar that produces carbon dioxide and alcohol. The CO_2 is responsible for expansion of the dough
Filigree	Piped laces of chocolate or royal icing used for decoration purpose
Folding	Method of gently combining fragile ingredients
Fondant	Icing made from boiled sugar and liquid glucose and then agitated to form a homogeneous mass of minute crystals
Frosting	To coat a cake with icing, usually of whipped cream or cheese
Ganache	Paste made from a mixture of fresh cream and chocolate
Gelatin	Transparent protein made from animal bones and tissues that melt with hot liquids and form a jelly when cold
Glace	Ice or ice cream in French
Glazed	Coating with a gel or sugar to give a smooth and shiny surface
Gliadanin	One of the proteins present in flour
Glutenin	One of the proteins present in flour
Glycerin	Sweet, odourless, and colourless liquid syrup used in cake mixtures to extend shelf life
GMS	Glycerol mono stearate, an emulsifier that helps to distribute fat evenly through a product and helps to stabilise an emulsion
Gum Arabica	Sticky substance obtained from the acacia tree that hardens on exposure to air
Gum Tragacanth	Gum obtained from tragacanth plant, used as an ice cream stabiliser, for thickening of creams, jellies, and pastes and for stiff royal icings
Hulling	A process of removing calyx from strawberries, raspberries, etc.
Humidity	The amount of moisture present in air and crucial to making of breads, production of chocolate, and sugar work
Hydrogenated fats	Oil hardened with addition of hydrogen, for example, margarine
Hygroscopic	Property of attracting moisture
Kneading	Mechanical action applied for formation of dough
Leavening	Addition of yeast or aerating agent to dough to help it to rise in favourable conditions

(Contd)

Table 1.1 (Contd)

Term	Description
Macerate	To flavour foods by steeping them in aromatic liquids such as liquors
Marinate	To place food into oil, liquid, herbs, and spices to flavour it or tenderise it
Marsala	Fortified wine made from grapes grown near Marsala (Sicily)
Marshmallow	Elastic spongy sweet made from sugar, egg whites, gelatin, and liquid glucose
Marzipan	A paste made from ground almonds and sugar
Masking	Act of covering with icing, cream, marzipan, fondant, etc.
Nappe	To coat foods evenly with sauce
Overrun	The increase in the volume of an ice cream resulting from incorporation of air
Panada	A thick roux or sauce for basis of soufflé
Patisserie	The department which makes pastry preparations. Also applies to the art of pastry cook and the place where the pastry goods are prepared or even displayed
Pectin	A substance obtained from fruits and used in setting jellies and jams
Persipan	Paste made from stone fruit kernels and sugar. A cheaper substitute to marzipan
Pinning	Rolling out a pastry or dough with a rolling pin
Pith	The whitish cellular lining under the skin of citrus fruits
Plaiting	Weaving a rope of dough, paste, boiled sugar, etc., into orderly shapes
Praline	Caramelized mixture of almonds and sugar that is either crushed or ground into a paste. Since these pastes are used as fillings in moulded chocolates, it is a common word also used for small moulded chocolates
Prove	A term used to describe the fermentation of dough with action of yeast which results in doubling the volume of the dough
Prover	A temperature and humidity controlled equipment that is used for proving the dough
Puree	A smooth thick pulp or paste prepared from soft fruits or vegetables
Royal icing	Icing made from egg whites and icing sugar, often used for filigree work
Sabayon	A mixture of egg yolks, sugar, and liquid whipped together to a ribbon consistency over a double boiler
Salpicon	A mixture of diced fruits
Sorbet	Frozen and churned dessert of fruit and juice
Sorbetiere	An ice cream machine used for churning ice creams or sorbets
Steep	To immerse the food item in hot or cold liquid and leave it to stand in it for considerable amount of time either to infuse flavours, extract colour or soften a product
Syneresis	Also known as weeping of proteins. This happens when the protein is over heated and starts to loose water
Syrup	A syrupy sweet liquid made by boiling sugar and water
Texture	The mouth feel of a product when eaten
Viscosity	The degree to which a liquid resists flow under applied force
Vol au vent	A puff pastry case, usually open in centre, which is filled with savoury mixtures
Zest	Outer skin of citrus fruits that is used for flavouring

SECTIONS OF PATISSERIE

The size of a pastry kitchen can vary from one hotel to another and its sections will depend upon the kind of operations and the magnitude of business. For example, there is no requirement of a separate chocolate room, if there is no pastry shop or requirement of chocolate products is limited on the menu.

The pastry kitchen like the main kitchen is divided into two broad sections namely bakery and pastry. The bakery usually is limited to production of breads and contains an oven where all baking activities are carried out. The pastry section on the other hand is temperature controlled as this section largely deals with eggs, dairy products, chocolates, and other high risk food items that need to be protected from bacterial contamination.

Various sections of bakery include:

Breads section All types of dough and breads are made and baked here. The laminated breakfast rolls such as croissant and Danish may be prepared in the pastry section, but are eventually baked in the bakery section. The ovens are usually placed in this area, so that the heat does not affect the temperature of the pastry kitchen. The breads made here are supplied to restaurants, other kitchens as well as for selling through pastry shops.

Pastry section As discussed earlier, this section of the department is air conditioned to maintain cooler temperatures. This is done not only for protecting food from getting spoilt, but certain products in pastry kitchen such as whipped cream and chocolates need a specific temperature for correct applications.

This section makes various types of bases and fillings for cakes and pastries and makes cakes, pastries, and other products related to these for restaurants, buffets, banquets as well as pastry shops.

Puff section This section does all the laminated doughs such as puff, croissant and makes basic pastes such as sweet paste. This section also makes various products such as vol au vents, savoury quiches, and pies. This part of the pastry kitchen is a highly skilled job and croissants are one of the most important products of any hotel. Many guests judge the stature of the hotel from the quality of croissants produced by that hotel. This section produces laminated products, related dough, and pastes for all sections of pastry. Whether the pastry section requires a puff pastry base for its cakes or the dessert section needs something for making desserts, this section will make products for them.

Dessert section This section produces desserts for both banquets and restaurant buffets as well as à la carte. However, this section gets supported by the pastry section as well, which produces cakes and pastries for buffets. As we can see that all the sections of bakery and pastry are interdependent therefore, a close coordination is required between all the sections of this kitchen. The person in charge of the dessert section may need bread from the bakery section to make desserts such as summer pudding, bread and butter pudding, or may need sponges and fillings that are made by the pastry section.

Chocolate room This is a very specialised section in the pastry kitchen. All the work related to chocolates such as making chocolate garnishes, room amenities, and showpieces for display is done here. This area is usually a separate area as it has to be maintained at a temperature of 18-20°C with relative humidity at around 50%. This environment is most suitable for producing good quality chocolates. All the sections of the kitchen such as the dessert section or the pastry section rely on this area for chocolate products and garnishes. This section also has sophisticated machinery depending upon the size of the operations.

HIERARCHY IN KITCHEN

Figure 1.1 depicts the typical hierarchy of a large hotel which has well defined sections. However in many smaller scale hotels, there could be one pastry chef and few other multiskilled people who would be rotated in the department on rota basis. Pastry is a highly technical and specialised field, and getting the right talent for this section of the kitchen has always been a challenge for both the HR department and the executive chef.

Let us now discuss about the roles of these positions in the pastry kitchen.

Pastry chef As the name suggests, he/she is a person who is in charge of the bakery and pastry kitchen. As this department is a highly specialised department with regards to its production schedules and modern and sophisticated machinery, the pastry chef has a crucial role to play in managing his/her department effectively. He/she is responsible for all hot and cold desserts.

It may be cakes, pastries, ice creams, creams, etc. In most of the hotels, the pastry chef reports directly to the executive chef and is one of the most senior persons in the kitchen hierarchy. His job is to ensure that the department operates smoothly delivering consistent high quality products all through the year. No festivity is complete without desserts and that is the reason why this department is very busy throughout the year. Festivities such as new year's, Christmas, Valentine's, and Easter are the busiest seasons for the pastry department, and the pastry chef is responsible for planning the festive menus, staffing and even the budgets of the department.

Boulanger He is the baker who works under the pastry chef and is responsible for all the baked products such as breads and breakfast rolls for the restaurant outlets, pastry shops and even banquet parties. Baking breads is an art and high quality breads are the most important part of any meal starting from breakfast early in the morning. The bakery section being a hot kitchen is usually a separate room from the main pastry kitchen as it contains ovens that produce heat.

Dessert chef A dessert chef prepares basic creams such as whipped creams, pastry cream, bases such as sponges, short crust, and sable, and fillings such as ganache and mousses for various desserts. He/she

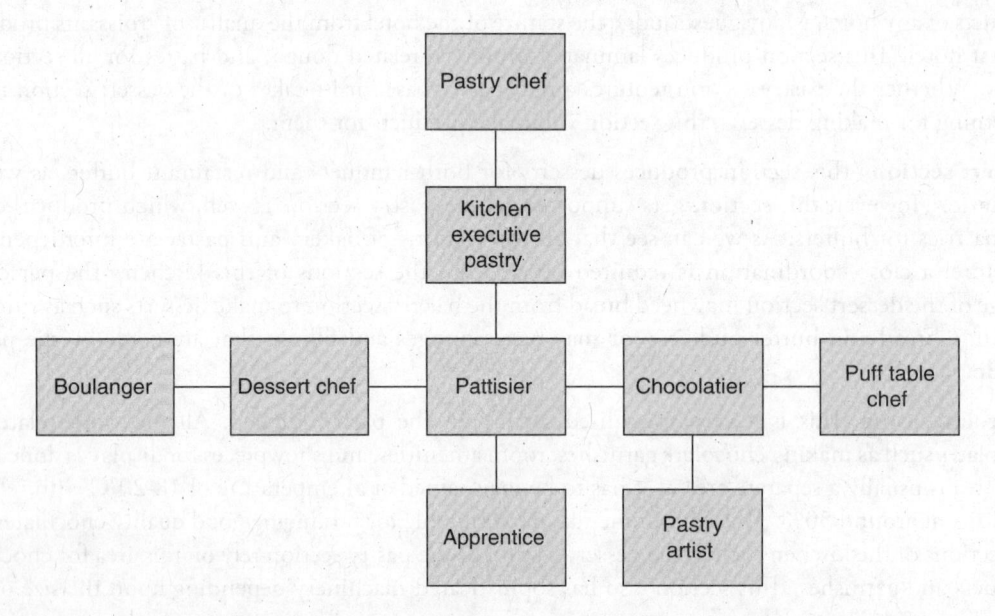

Fig. 1.1 Hierarchy of pastry kitchen

is also responsible for making ice creams and sorbets that are used in various outlets. The dessert chef works in close co-ordination with the cake and pastry chef as they both are interdependent upon each other. In smaller hotels, both these sections are usually taken care of by a single chef, who is responsible for preparing desserts for buffet, banquets and even à la carte.

Pattisier This is a French word for cake and pastry person. The modern style cakes are known as entremets but this word should not be confused with a chef called *entremetier*, who is responsible for preparing vegetables in the hot kitchen. The person in-charge of the patisserie section is responsible for preparing various cakes and pastries for guest orders, dessert buffets for restaurant and banquets and even for à la carte portions.

Chocolatier The chocolatier of the kitchen makes all products related to chocolates. This section is also one of the busiest sections in festive season as all kinds of chocolate bons bons, chocolate garnishes and figurines, etc., are in high demand during this season. This section also usually has a kitchen artist, who makes sculptures and showpieces with chocolates and sugar.

Puff table chef This person is usually a part of boulanger or the baker and is responsible for preparing laminated pastries such as croissant, Danish, puff pastry, and the dough for breakfast rolls such as doughnuts and brioches. We will discuss more about these products in the forthcoming chapters.

WEIGHTS AND MEASUREMENT

Weights and measurements are one of the most important aspects of the pastry kitchen. Unlike other areas of kitchen where recipes are used as inspiration and not really measured to the last gram, in pastry it is the other way around. A few grams of ingredients can change a product's texture and appearance completely.

In any given recipe, you would need either weight or mass of a solid ingredient or the volume of a liquid. Gas is rarely measured and used in cooking, therefore, we will leave this part out and discuss largely weights and volume.

Sweet Paste Recipe

Refer to the following basic recipe of a basic pastry product called sweet paste for a better understanding of weights and measures.

Table 1.2 Ingredients for the recipe and their measurement

Name of ingredients	Metric	Imperial	Volumetric
Flour	400 g	1 lb	3 cups and 2 tbsp
Butter	200 g	8 oz	1 and half cup
Caster sugar	100 g	4 oz	1/2 cup
Eggs	100 ml	4 fl oz	2 numbers

Method

1. Cream butter and sugar until pale white in colour, in a bowl fitted with flat beater attachment. Add eggs little by little allowing them to emulsify.
2. Remove from the machine and incorporate flour with spatula taking care not to over mix the paste.
3. Flatten the paste onto a clean tray lined with a plastic film.
4. Cover the paste with a plastic wrap and chill it in refrigerator for a couple of hours.
5. Use as required.

As you can see in the aforementioned recipe, there are three types of measuring systems—Metric, Imperial, and Volumetric. In India, we usually follow the Metric system of weights however in most of the Europe, Imperial system of weights is more prominent. Americans usually follow the Volumetric system of measurement, where the ingredients are measured in cups and spoons.

It is also important to know the degree of temperature required for baking and we shall also discuss the conversions of Fahrenheit to Celsius and vice versa. But first let us discuss the weights.

Types of Measuring Systems

In this section, we will discuss the Metric and Imperial measuring systems in detail.

Metric System

Table 1.3 Weights

Name	Abbreviation used
Gram	g
Kilogram	kg

1 kg = 1000 g; 1/2 kg = 500 g; 1/4 kg = 250 g

Table 1.4 Capacities

Name	Abbreviation used
Millilitre	ml
Decilitre	dl
Centilitre	cl
Litre	lt

1 lt = 1000 ml; 1/2 lt = 500 ml; 1/4 lt = 250 ml; 1 dl = 100 ml; 1 cl = 10 ml

Imperial System

Table 1.5 Weights

Name	Abbreviation used
Ounce	oz
Pound	lb

16 oz = 1 lb; 8 oz = 1/2 lb; 4 oz = 1/4 lb
The ounce can be further divided into 3/4 oz, 1/2 oz, and 1/4 oz.

Table 1.6 Capacities

Name	Abbreviation used
Fluid ounce	fl oz
Gill	gill
Pint	pt
Quart	qt
Gallon	gal

1 gal = 8 pt or 4 qt or 160 fl oz; 1/2 gal = 4 pt or 2 qt or 80 fl oz; 1 qt = 2 pt or 40 fl oz; 1 pt = 20 fl oz; 3/4 pt = 15 fl oz or 3 gill; 1/2 pt = 10 fl oz or 2 gill; 1/4 pt = 5 fl oz or 1 gill

Oven Temperature Comparisions

The temperature of the oven is either used in Fahrenheit also written as F or in Celsius written as C. To convert C into F, multiply by 9, divide by 5 and add 32. For example, to change 204°C into °F, we will use the following formula.

$$204 \times \frac{9}{5} + 32 = 399\,(400°F)$$

To convert F into C, subtract 32, multiply by 5 and then divide by 9. So now to convert 400°F in C, we will use the following formula.

$$400 - 32 \times \frac{5}{9} = 204.44°C$$

In few ovens, the knobs are set to various markings such as 1/8, 1/4, 1/2, 1 and so on. These settings correspond to a particular temperature as listed in Table 1.7.

Let us see the following table to understand the various degrees of temperature and its uses.

Table 1.7 Degrees of temperature and its uses

Gas mark	Centigrade	Heat range	Uses
1/8	80–90	Very cool	Meringues and dehydrating
1/4	115–116	Cool	Dry roasting of nuts and spices
1/2	130–131	Slow cooking	Nut and meringue based sponges like japonaise
1	142–144	Slow cooking	Baked custards and creams
2	155–156	Moderate cooking	Macaroons
3	165–168	Moderate cooking	Biscuits, sponges, and cookies
4	178–181	Medium	Choux pastries
5	190–193	Medium hot	Flans, tarts, and pies
6	200–204	Hot	Soufflé
7	218–220	Hot	Cones, yeast goods, puff paste
8	228–230	Very hot	Swiss rolls
9	240–244	Very hot	Breads and rolls
10	258–260	Extremely hot	Breads and rolls

LAYOUT AND WORKFLOW

As we have read before that this is one of the busiest kitchens in a large hotel, it is important to have the layout and organisation of equipment in the most thoughtful manner, so that the department works efficiently and produces products of high quality. All the sections such as bakery, pastry and their sub sections such as dessert table, puff table, and à la carte are carefully planned and laid out. There is a separate chocolate room which produces chocolates and garnishes and a separate artist room that can be used for making artistic showpieces like sugar sculptures that do not need a temperature controlled environment.

Figure 1.2 depicts the layout of a bakery and confectionary of a large hotel. The areas are well laid out in a way that there is not much of walking around and the operations can be carried out smoothly, with sections of the pastry kitchen coordinating with each other.

The bakery area is separated from the confectionary, as the latter is air conditioned and the bakery area could be warm due to the heat expelled from the ovens. However, some modern oven ranges like combination ovens have sorted this problem, whereby the heat is not spread around too much. But still in case of bakery, the yeast leavened products need a certain kind of temperature, between 25-30°C, in order to ferment and double in volume.

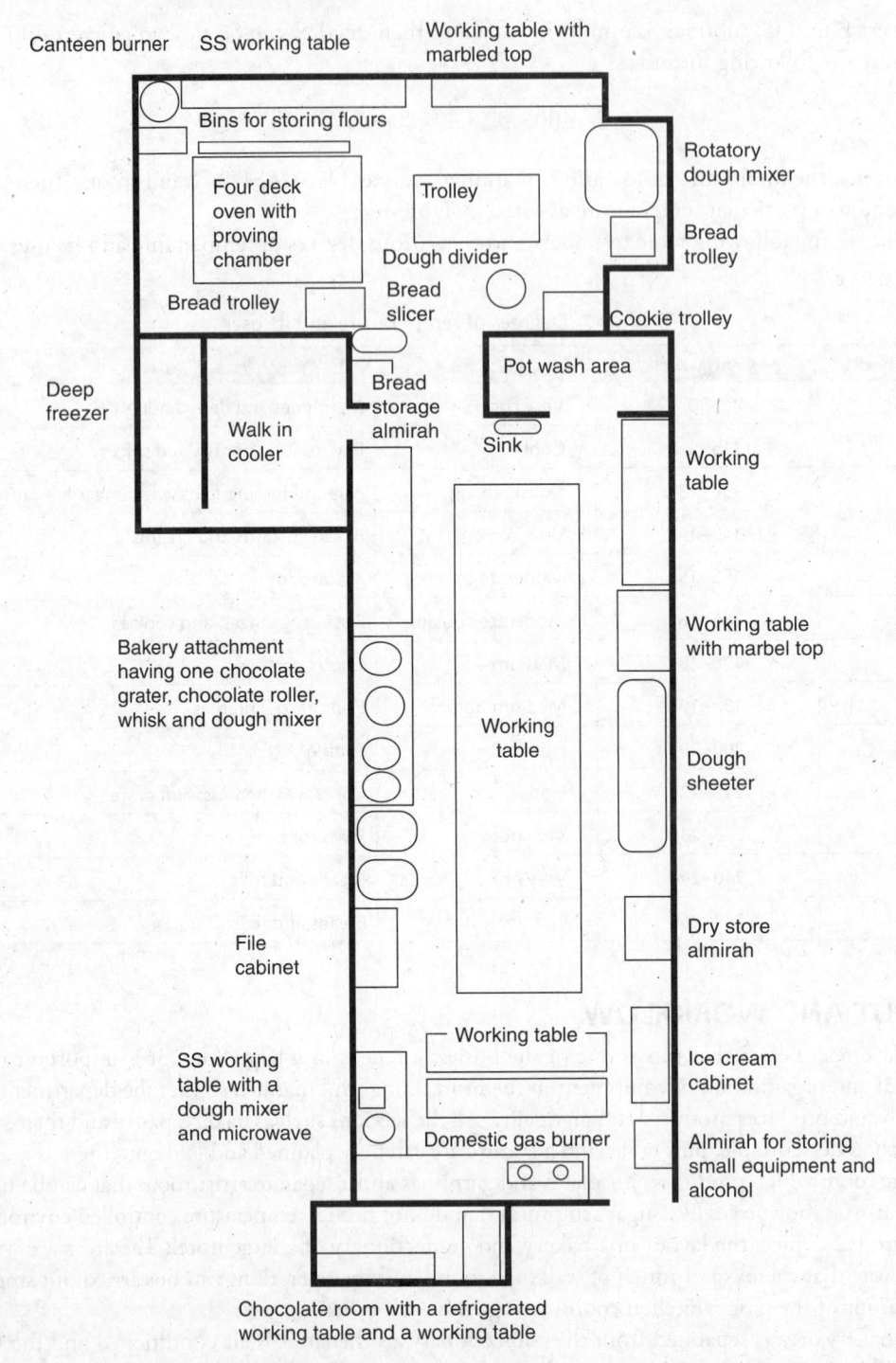

Fig. 1.2 Layout of a bakery and confectionary of a large hotel

Introduction to Pastry and Bakery

The chocolate room is also a separate area as the temperature needs to be maintained between 18-20°C with a relative humidity of 50%. In some regions where humidity levels are high, equipment such as dehumidifiers are installed to maintain the humidity levels at a required setting.

Areas such as puff table are also part of the pastry kitchen, as the laminating of dough requires butter to be layered between the layers of dough and hence, the lower temperatures are essential to lock the butter in the dough and prevent it from softening and oozing out whilst laminating.

LARGE MACHINERY USED IN BAKERY AND PASTRY

Bakery and confectionary host a range of sophisticated equipment as it is a specialised area of kitchen. Though much smaller equipment is used for doing daily jobs, from Table 1.8, we will get to know some of the large machineries and equipment used in bakery and confectionary.

Table 1.8 Large machinery used in bakery and confectionary

Machinery	Description
Ovens **Other names:** Batch ovens, rotator ovens	Ovens are traditionally used for baking purposes and they come in various shapes and sizes. The type of the oven largely depends upon the kind of operations. In large operations, where the baked products are required to be made in bulk, large rotator ovens are a good choice. There are also large ovens with automatic feeding belts, where entire batches of products are loaded and removed from the oven with the help of an automatic feeder. Such an oven is known as batch oven as big batches of products are baked in it.
Convection ovens **Other names:** Combi ovens	These ovens come in various sizes and work on the principle of circulation of hot air. Some models are also available with roll-in trolleys that can be loaded and rolled inside the cabinet. This equipment comes very handy in cooking as well as reheating of food. They are called combi ovens as they have the facilities of moist as well as dry heat.
Pizza ovens	These ovens are different from regular ovens as they are used mostly for baking pizzas only. These are available in various sizes. The height of the deck of these ovens is as low as eight inches so that a pizza can be slipped into it by using a long shovel known as pizza bat. The floor of this oven is usually made of stone so that it gives a rustic look to the pizza.
Walk-in **Other names**: Cold storage room	Walk-ins are refrigerated compact areas where one could walk inside and hence the name walk-in. They can be custom made to any size to be suited for an operation. One could have walk-in refrigerators or freezers depending upon the requirement. Certain companies are now specialising in modular shelving so that the storage of food can be as per the food safety norms and Hazard Analysis and Critical Control Points (HACCP).
Freezers **Other names:** Deeps	Freezers are a very important part of any bulk cooking operation. As quantity cooking involves planning and advance *mise en place*, we need ample refrigerated space to store the same until it is ready for cooking. These are available in various sizes depending upon the requirement. You could have roll-in trolley style or the ones which have shelving. The deep freezers are used in pastry kitchen for storage and also many products need prior freezing before any other application is carried out. For example, an entremet has to be frozen, before it can be glazed or sprayed with cocoa butter.

(Contd)

Table 1.8 (Contd)

Machinery	Description
Blast chillers/Freezer **Other names:** Blast chilling units	Blast chillers and freezers are one of the most important equipment used in pastry operations for modern cakes and pastries. Blast freezers allow the cakes and pastries to freeze quickly so that they can be glazed or sprayed depending upon the finish required.
Deep fat fryers **Other names:** Deep frying unit	Deep fat fryers are safer in bulk cooking for deep frying as they are available from small table top models to large ones that can hold up to 30 litres of oil. It is always safe to use deep fat fryers rather than open pots and *kadhai* whilst frying in large quantities. Deep fat fryers are commonly used for frying doughnuts and other fried products used in bakery and confectionary.
Flour sieves **Other names:** Sifter	As the name suggests, this equipment is used for sifting flour. It is electrically operated and can sift large quantities of flour in less than a minute. It comes in very handy as it saves time and avoids too much handling of the raw commodity.
Dough mixers **Other names:** Planetary dough mixer/Spiral dough mixer	Dough mixers are available in various sizes and one could chose depending upon the size of operation. Some dough mixers can easily knead up to 100 kg of flour and even more. This machine comes in handy when one has to produce breads in bulk.
Table top mixers **Other names:** Universal dough mixer	Some table top models are very important to do mixing and whipping of meringues for smaller batches as well. These small dough mixers come with attachments such as beater, paddle, and balloon whisks and can be used for kneading small quantities of dough, batters or whipping creams and meringues.
Dough divider **Other names:** Dough cutter	As the name suggests this equipment is used to divide the dough. Some models also help to shape the rolls. Usually, a standard model divides the dough into 36 pieces. So if we want each roll to be of 50 g we would scale the dough of 1800 g. This when divided into 36 pieces will yield a roll of 50 g and so on. This saves time and also helps to maintain the costs as the yield is same every time.
Proving cabinets	It is a cabinet with water being heated with an element. Electric, gas, and pressure steam models are available. It maintains the temperature of 25°C and humidity of 90% and is used for proving breads.
Retarder proofer	Retarder proofer is a very helpful equipment used in bakery operations involving yeast leavened products. It can be timed for around 24 hours, where the products will freeze, thaw, and proof as per the programme set. This is quite a helpful equipment in bulk production.
Dough sheeter **Other names:** Sheeting machine	Dough sheeter is commonly used in bakery kitchen and helps to roll out the dough for fabricating breads. It comes in various sizes and one can choose depending upon the kind of operation.
Ice cream machine **Other names:** Sorbetiere	These can be table top models or floor mounted depending upon the volume of business. The ice cream mix is poured in the machine and it churns the mixture whilst continuously freezing it, thereby preventing crystal formation and hence, preparing a smooth ice cream or sorbet.
Chocolate tempering machine **Other names:** Tempering machine	These are commercially available machines that work on temperature control. The machine automatically melts the couverture to 40°C and then cools it down to 28°C until all the good crystals are formed. The machine then brings the temperature to the working temperature, which is different for each kind of couverture. This machine can be programmed according to the specific requirement of the chocolate. The paddle in the chocolate tempering machine keeps stirring the chocolate constantly and this ensures that each particle of chocolate has been evenly melted.

Table 1.8 (Contd)

Machinery	Description
Chocolate guitar **Other names:** Guitar	This equipment is used for cutting a square piece of set ganache into equal and neat pieces. As this equipment uses stainless steel chords of a guitar hence the name.
Bread slicing machine **Other names:** Bread slicer	This is an important equipment in bakery and is used for slicing bread loaves for toasts and sandwich preparations. This equipment saves time whilst slicing breads and gives uniform slices.
Chocolate shaving machine	This machine is used in places where there is a large requirement of chocolate flakes. In this machine, a block of chocolate is secured in a place that moves to and fro over a sharp blade to scrape the chocolate very thinly to make chocolate flakes. These flakes should be hardened in the fridge and should be handled very carefully as they will melt from the heat of the palm if handled for too long.
Chocolate spray gun	This is an atomiser kind of an apparatus attached to a compressor. The jar holds melted chocolate mixed with melted cocoa butter and is sprayed onto chocolate figures to give a matte kind of finish.

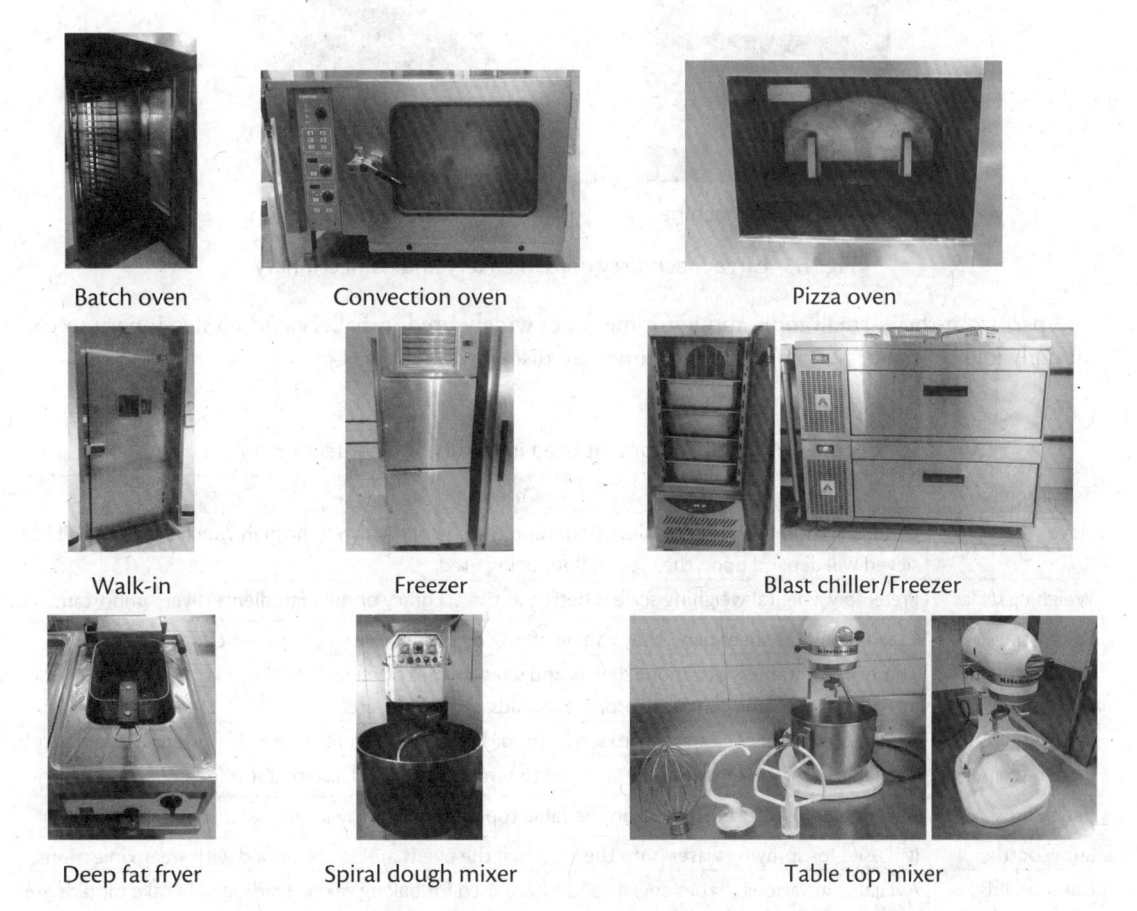

Batch oven   Convection oven   Pizza oven

Walk-in   Freezer   Blast chiller/Freezer

Deep fat fryer   Spiral dough mixer   Table top mixer

Fig. 1.3 Large machinery used in bakery and confectionary (Contd)

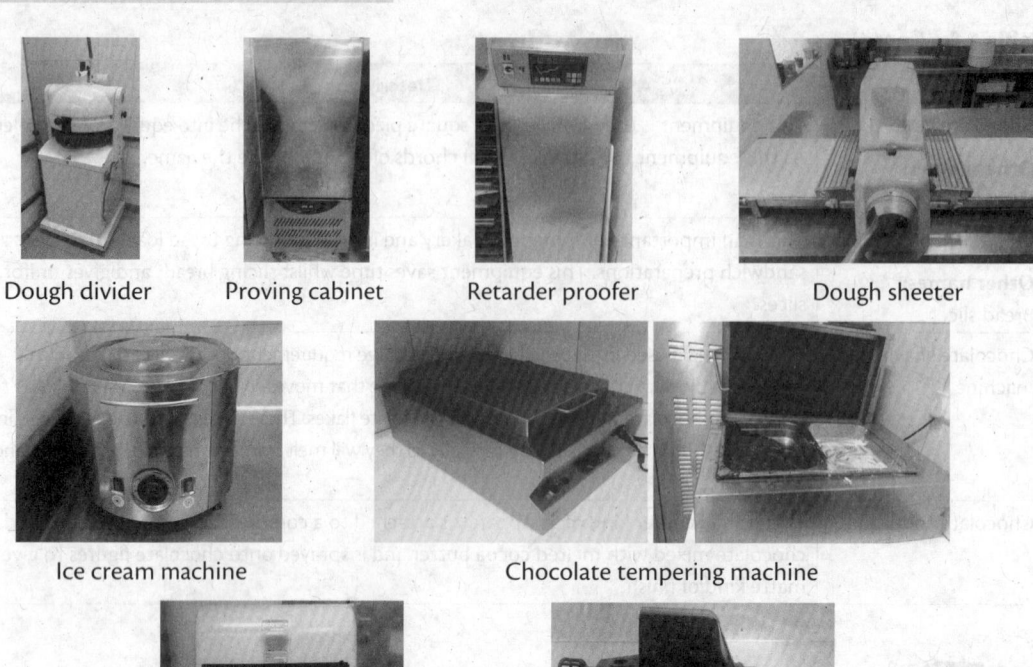

Dough divider   Proving cabinet   Retarder proofer   Dough sheeter

Ice cream machine   Chocolate tempering machine

Bread slicing machine   Chocolate spray gun

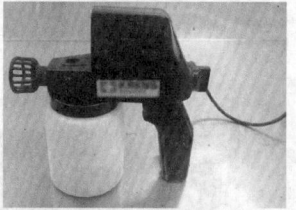

Fig. 1.3 Large machinery used in bakery and confectionary

Apart from these, small tools and equipment are widely used in bakery and confectionary to carry out daily jobs. Some of the most common ones are discussed in Table 1.9.

Table 1.9 Small equipment used in bakery and confectionary

Small equipment	Description
Sieve	Drum sieve is mostly used to sieve flours and the size of the mesh through which the flour will be sieved will depend upon the type of flour being used.
Weighing scale	Preferably a digital weighing scale is better, as the accuracy of the ingredients is very important.
Baking trays	Often known as sheet pans, they can be of iron or Teflon, coated for non-stick.
Bread moulds	These are containers of various shapes and sizes and are often sold by the volume they are intended for. So one can easily procure moulds of 1 lb, 2 lb, etc.
Dough scorers	A piece of equipment having a sharp surgical blade in the end, to score the breads at an angle before baking.
Dough scrapers	Available in plastic or steel, they are used to scrape dough and also to cut it for scaling.
Bench brush	A large hard bristle brush to clean the table top and to brush away excess flour.
Spray bottle	It is used for spraying water onto the breads, if the ovens are not equipped with steam injections.
Cake moulds	Available in various shapes and sizes, they are used for baking cakes. Traditionally cake moulds are round, but now a day's various shapes such as triangles, ovals and even pyramids are available.

Table 1.9 (Contd)

Small equipment	Description
Tart and flan moulds	These are available in various shapes and sizes such as boat shapes, square, round, and fluted. These moulds are used for preparing tart, pies, and flans.
Cutters	Various types of cutters are used in bakery and pastry. They can be of various shapes and sizes and are used for making cookies and biscuits. Few cutters such as doughnut cutter is typically used for cutting doughnuts.
Savarin mould	A mould used for making Baba au rhum. The hole in the centre of the cake is filled with fresh fruits after baking.
Tube shaped round mould	It is used for baking angel food cakes and chiffon cakes. The mould is seldom greased for a better finish and hence, it will be advisable to use non-stick moulds.
Serrated knife	It is used for slicing sponges into layers, which can then be layered with assorted fillings to create cakes and gateaux.
Palette knives	A flat knife used for icing the sponges. They can be straight or angular and are available in various sizes.
Piping bags and nozzles	Made from material similar to that of shower curtain, piping bags are used to pipe designs on top of cakes to decorate them.
Turn table	Also called Lazy Suzanne or cake turn table, it is used for icing and finishing the cakes. It rotates on an axis thereby allowing the chef to evenly spread the cream and other fillings with ease. It is available in metal and plastic as well. Today many manufacturers are making motorised cake turn tables.
Flat paddle	An attachment of a dough mixer, it is used for creaming butter and sugar to make sponges by creaming method.
Balloon whisk	A balloon shape wire whisk used for whipping the ingredients.
Wire racks	A piece of equipment used for cooling the baked goods.
Silpat	These are non-stick silicone baking sheets used for baking things that tend to stick on other surfaces.
Zesters	Various kinds of graters are used in pastry and bakery kitchen to extract the zest from citrus fruits. Some of the common ones used are: **Micro plane grater**: Micro plane graters have a sharp tooth and their sleek shape helps to maintain a grip whilst grating spices such as nutmeg. **Zester**: As the name suggests, this tool is used for removing zest from citrus fruits such as lemons and oranges. This has a slightly curved tip with sharp holes in it, which removes the zest without any bitter pith attached to it. **Channeller**: Channel knife is a kind of small peeler that has a curved V shape at the tip or sometimes on the side. It helps to remove a thick strip from the sides of the citrus fruit. The fruit is then sliced and this yields decorative slices.
Utility tools	These are a range of tools used in pastry kitchen for various kinds of jobs. These tools not only help to do the job efficiently but also help to get a consistent product. Some of such tools used are: **Can and bottle opener**: Pastry kitchen uses lots of canned and bottled items and this piece of equipment is very handy to open cans and tins. These are available in various shapes and sizes. **Corers**: As the name suggests, these tools are used for coring the central part of a fruit without cutting it open. This tool is used when we need the fruit intact or it needs to be cut into slices. Corers are used mainly for coring apples and pears and some large corers are also used for coring pineapples. **Pitters**: These small tools are the most important small tools used in pastry kitchen. They can be used for removing pits from stone fruits such as cherries and olives.

(Contd)

Table 1.9 (Contd)

Small equipment	Description
Silicone moulds	Various companies around the world are manufacturing moulds in silicone that can withstand high temperatures. There are various benefits of using silicone moulds. They do not require greasing and the product does not get stuck to the base. Silicone moulds can be of various designs and shapes and they give a very modern look to the cakes and pastries. Silicone moulds can also be used for preparing garnishes such as caramel and chocolates.
Butane torches	These are small torch burners that get attached to a butane canister. They come in very handy to spot caramelize products. This tool has various uses, it can be used to extract chilled cakes out of the metallic moulds by heating the sides of the cake with the torch burner. It can be used for caramelizing sugar on many desserts such as crème brûlée.
Modelling tools	These are also known as marzipan tools as they are used mostly for making decorations from marzipan. They come in a set of various shapes and each tool has a specific usage. The tools are used for making flowers, figures, faces of living things, etc.
Combs	Various kinds of combs are used for creating designs on the sides or top of the cake. Combs are available in various materials such as metal, plastic or high grade silicon rubber. These combs are used for preparing various garnishes for cakes and pastries.
Printing apparatus	This is a fairly new piece of equipment added to the confectionary world. It is a normal inkjet printer to print computerised images on a special edible paper made from rice. Edible food coloured cartridges are used for this purpose. Any design can be printed on these sheets and the same can be placed on top of cakes or pastries.
Confectionary funnel	This piece of equipment is commonly used in confectionary to fill liquid ganache into moulded chocolates whilst making pralines and truffles.
Expandable trellis cutter	Small steel discs with sharp edges are mounted on metal bars that can be stretched and closed to arrange the distance between the rollers. This equipment is used for cutting dough and marking the lines for cutting rectangular blocks of pastries.
Chocolate thermometer	A chocolate thermometer is available in various shapes and materials. The grading on this thermometer corresponds to the various degrees required by a particular kind of chocolate. It also has markings which display the correct working temperature of a chocolate. It is also available in digital mode.
Moulds	These are poly carbonate plastic moulds available in various shapes and designs, commonly used for making moulded chocolates. Some moulds such as eggs and spheres are moulded and stuck together, whereas some moulds of figures, when joined together have an opening from where the excess chocolate can be poured out, when making moulded chocolates.
Scrapers and spatulas	The most important tool that a pastry chef cannot do without is a flexible plastic scraper or a spatula. These are used for mixing and removing items from one bowl to another.

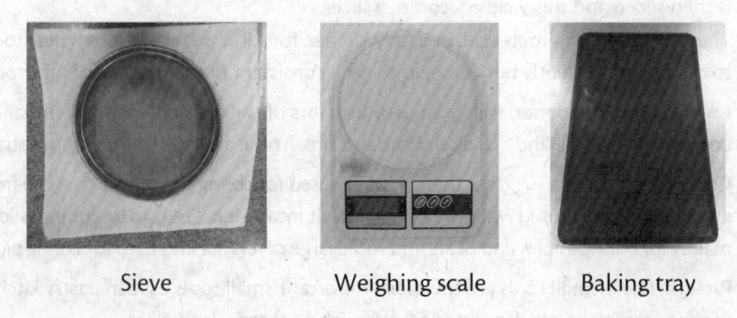

Sieve   Weighing scale   Baking tray

Fig. 1.4 Small equipment used in bakery and confectionary

Introduction to Pastry and Bakery   17

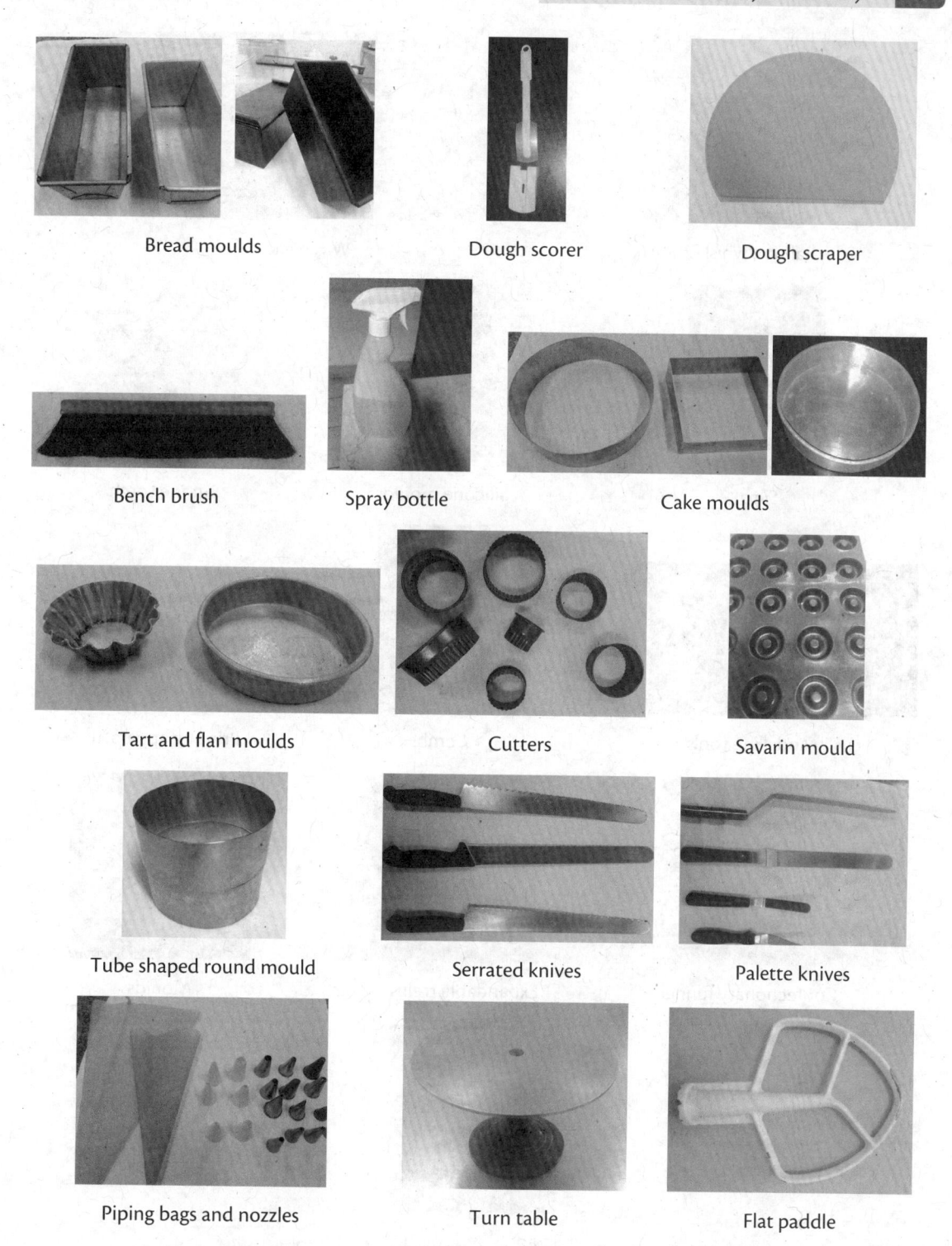

Bread moulds	Dough scorer	Dough scraper
Bench brush	Spray bottle	Cake moulds
Tart and flan moulds	Cutters	Savarin mould
Tube shaped round mould	Serrated knives	Palette knives
Piping bags and nozzles	Turn table	Flat paddle

Fig. 1.4 Small equipment used in bakery and confectionary (Contd)

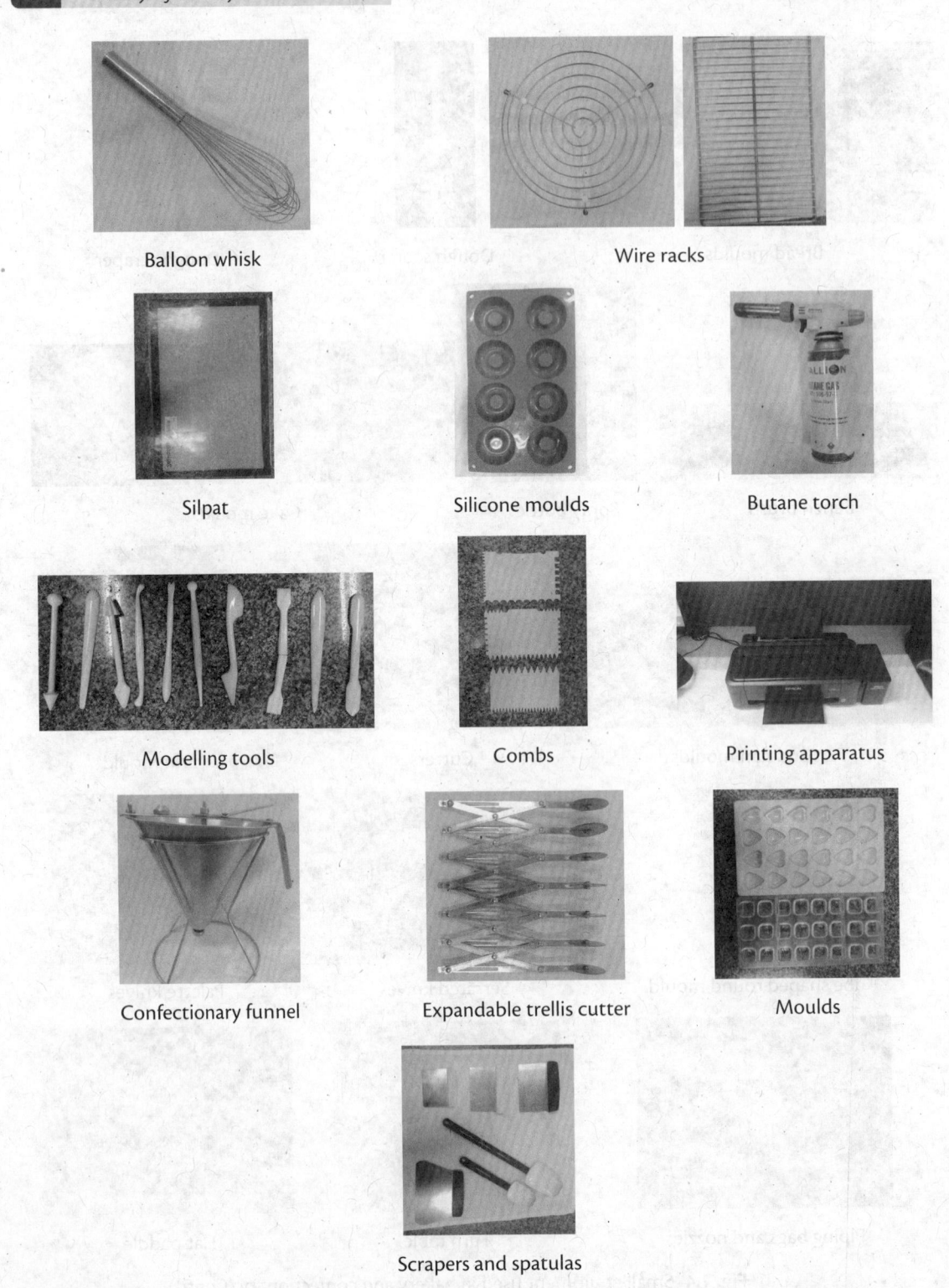

Fig. 1.4 Small equipment used in bakery and confectionary

These are some of the most common tools and equipment used in bakery and pastry and the list is endless. Modernisation has created many choices of unique tools and equipment for pastry chefs that make their work easier and more efficient.

SUMMARY

This chapter dealt in basic introduction to the pastry and bakery department. It largely discusses the ideal set up of a pastry kitchen in a large hotel with full-fledged pastry operations, which include a pastry shop outlet attached to it where the pastry goods are sold and also supplying to various restaurants and banquets of the hotel. Before we started to dwell into this department, it was important to know the key terms associated with bakery and pastry department and its operations, so that it will be easier to comprehend what will follow in this book. So we have discussed a range of key terms that will be very helpful for the students to understand the nitty-gritties of this department and its work.

Then we discussed various sections of the department as a whole and understood what is the role and function of the in charge of that particular section. We also discussed the coordination between the various sections in the kitchen and how they are interdependent on each other for a smooth functioning of the department.

We also discussed the hierarchy of the department and reporting structures. The students will benefit from knowing the individual responsibilities of each position and the jobs that they are responsible for. This section also explains some French terms associated with the positions in the kitchen which are commonly used internationally.

We also threw light on the various systems of weights and measurements such as metric and imperial systems and how to convert them from one to another. In this chapter, we also discussed about the oven temperatures and how to convert from Fahrenheit to Celsius and vice versa.

We also discussed the layout of the kitchen, the large equipment and machinery as well as the small tools and equipment used in the pastry department.

KEY TERMS

A la carte A bill of fare, where dishes are mentioned along with their price

American system System of measurement where units such as cups and teaspoons are used

Baba au rhum French dessert made with yeast leavened dough that is baked in a savarin mould and then soaked in rum flavoured sugar syrup

Banquets Large gathering of people in a designated function area, where meals are served

Bon bon Small bite size chocolate preparations, usually round in shape

Bread and butter pudding Dessert made by soaking left over bread, butter, and custard and then baked

Buffet Arrangement of food for self service

Croissant Laminated breakfast pastry

Danish Laminated breakfast pastry glazed with jam

Dehumidifier Equipment used for controlling humidity in an area

HACCP Short form of Hazard Analysis and Critical Control Points, which is a food safety management system

Imperial system System of measurement where units such as pound, ounce, and pints are used

Lamination Layering of fat and dough in such a manner that there are alternate layers of fat and dough

Metric system System of measurement where units such as kilograms, grams, and litres are used

Mise en place French word for pre preparation required before the actual cooking of the meal

Quiche Custard based, baked preparation of meats or vegetables, in a tart or a pie shell

Savoury Salted products made in kitchen that are eaten as snacks

Summer pudding Dessert made with stale bread and berries

OBJECTIVE TYPE QUESTIONS

1. What is entremets?
2. Define blind baking.
3. What is a coverture?
4. Differentiate between caramelization and crystallization.
5. What are emulsifying agents?
6. Define frosting.
7. What is proving?
8. Define synerisis.
9. What is a vol au vent?
10. Who is a Boulanger?
11. What are the two systems of measurement?
12. What are the two units in which temperature is often measured?
13. What is an oz?
14. How much would one decilitre be with regards to millilitres?
15. How much is 1 gallon with regards to quart?
16. What is a Sorbetiere?
17. Define retarder prover.
18. What is a chocolate guitar?
19. Name two types of ovens used in bakery.
20. Name the equipment that is used for portioning the dough into small portions.

ESSAY TYPE QUESTIONS

1. What do you understand by kitchen layout? Describe various sections of pastry kitchen.
2. What is the importance of a chocolate room and why is it a separate area?
3. Describe the puff section and the work carried out there.
4. Describe the hierarchy of the pastry kitchen and its reporting structure.
5. What is the importance of using machinery in pastry kitchen? List any five large machineries and two small tools and describe their uses and how they will help to do the job efficiently.

ACTIVITY

1. In a group of 4 to 5 students, visit a hotel and study the layout of its pastry kitchen with regards to its food style and service. Critique the layout and offer necessary solutions.
2. Visit at least 3-4 pastry shops and list down the names of products. Now in groups identify which product was made in which section of the kitchen.
3. Make a chart of conversions for weights and measures and prepare a table depicting conversions from metric to imperial system. Laminate and put up in your kitchen for future reference.
4. In groups of 3-4, measure the most commonly used ingredients in pastry kitchen such as flour, sugar, milk, and cream, and weigh them in cup measures. Then weigh each one to prepare a chart of cup to metric conversion. This will help you to identify what is the weight of one cup of sugar to one cup of flour.

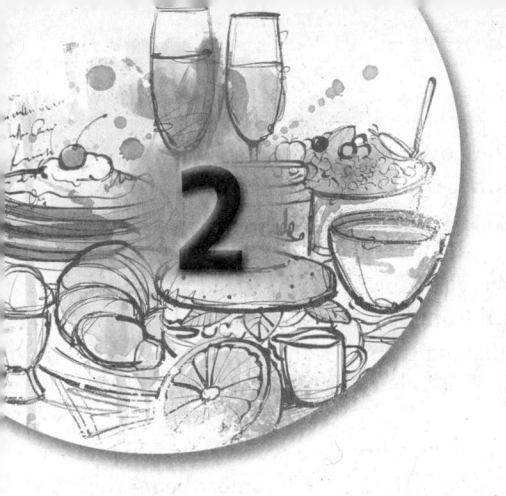

2 Commodities in Bakery and Pastry

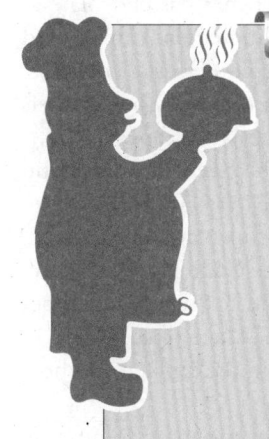

LEARNING OBJECTIVES

After reading this chapter, you should be able to

- understand the different types of flour and their uses
- know the various types of gluten free flours and their importance in modern baking
- identify the various types of oils and fats and know their characteristics
- recognize the importance of raising agents in bakery and their functions
- understand the various types of sugars and sweeteners that affect the quality of baked products
- appreciate the usage of various dairy products used in cooking as well as baking and confectionary to produce various types of desserts
- analyse the structure of egg and its usage in bakery and pastry
- know the selection of chocolate for various uses
- identify the cheeses that are used commonly in bakery and pastry

INTRODUCTION

In the previous chapter, we read about the various key terms that are associated with pastry kitchen, which will help us to understand the forthcoming chapters in a better manner. In any cuisine, the basic requirement for a chef is to understand commodities such as fruits and vegetables, meats and eggs, various kinds of seeds, for example, cereals, pulses, and nuts and spices. It is only after understanding these commodities can one relate them to the principles of cooking and start to create dishes or at least cook the classical dishes in a more structured manner. Similarly, before we go on creating those delicious pastry and bakery products, it is important for us to know about the basic commodities that are used in bakery and pastry. Though these commodities are also used extensively in other principles of cooking, we will be discussing them as a foundation to the section on bakery and pastry. Since this is a much specialised field in cooking, most hotels have a separate pastry and bakery department which supplies desserts and breads to the entire hotel.

Cooking is an art combined with science and this is 100% true for bakery and pastry as well. The understanding of ingredients is the most important for the chef, because today there are many guests who have various kinds of allergies to food, the most common ones being egg, nuts, and flour. Since flour is the most widely used commodity in bakery and pastry, it is our moral obligation to provide the customers with gluten free breads; but this would be possible only once we are aware of gluten free flours or otherwise we can harm the guests more rather than satisfy them. Similarly, the knowledge of various types of sugars will help us to produce pastry goods of different textures and mouth feel.

Eggs are the most common ingredient used in pastry and bakery products. We shall read about the various uses of eggs and how they are used creatively in most of the applications of pastry and bakery, ranging from an ingredient in breads, sponges, cookies, etc., to making garnishes and creams. It is also important to know the use of dairy products such as milk, cream, and cheese as these are used extensively in pastry kitchens.

Not to forget the chocolate, for chefs working in the pastry kitchen, chocolate is the most sought after and used ingredient in the department for various reasons. The first and the foremost being the divine taste of the chocolate. Chefs believe one can never go wrong in a dessert that has chocolate as an ingredient. The second reason is the variety of ways in which this wonderful ingredient can be used in the confectionary world. One can create beverages, cakes, pastries, hot and cold desserts, chocolate confections and also showpieces. Chocolate is commonly used for garnishing and decorating as chefs conjure up showpieces that are commonly displayed in restaurants, buffets, and pastry shops.

In this chapter, we would discuss the origin and history of chocolates so that we can understand how this unique ingredient got transformed into something that almost each one of us in the world got introduced to at an early age of 2 years or even younger. Today, various kinds of chocolates are available in the market. A layman would classify a chocolate on the basis of brands such as Cadbury and Nestle, but a professional pastry chef knows it much differently. We will introduce you to the various types and kinds of chocolate in this chapter, and also take you through the process of usage of each type of chocolate. We would also talk about the various ways in which chocolate is used in the kitchen and how does one go about creating garnishes and showpieces for decorative purposes.

But first let us discuss the ingredients used in bakery and talk in detail about the most commonly used ingredient—*Flour*. Flour is the base of almost all products made in bakery and pastry. For a professional chef, it is important to understand the quality aspects of flour and its chemical composition and properties such as pH values, water absorption capacity, and different grades.

FLOUR

Flour is obtained when we mill grains and pulses. The milling can be of various degrees to give a particular structure to the product and the usage of each milled product will be different from one another. For example, the milling of wheat grain can produce bulgur, cous cous, semolina, and flour. When in bakery we refer to flour we always mean the refined flour, unless specified as wholemeal flour or any other name for reference. The shelf life of milled grain is shorter than that of unmilled grain, therefore, care should be taken whilst storing the flour.

Wheat is among the most extensively cultivated cereal crops in the world; it is a member of grass family and is botanically named *triticum*. It is an annual or biennial crop which grows in the temperate regions of the world.

Structure of Wheat Grain

Wheat grain can be divided into three major parts—the bran, the embryo or the germ, and the endosperm; wherein bran is 12%, germ is 3% and the endosperm constitutes almost 85% of the total wheat grain and has starch cells, soluble and insoluble protein, oil, moisture, sugar, and minerals. The white flour or the refined flour is milled out of the endosperm whereas the wholewheat grain is milled for the wholemeal flour, which is the healthier option.

When the flour is milled, the only wastage is the outer layer husk, which is an insoluble fibre and is often sold as cattle feed. When milling refined flours, the wastage is bran, which is also sold as cattle feed but these days people have realised the health benefits of bran and it is being used in many food products, which are sold as health foods.

Flour is one of the structural ingredients used in pastry and bakery kitchen. There are many different kinds of flours used in the pastry kitchen and each flour has a different role to play in the final outcome of the product. Therefore, it becomes important to choose the right type of flour for the right type of product. You would commonly hear chefs using the words such as strong flour and weak flour. These words merely indicate the amount of *gluten* present in the flour. There are two types of non-soluble proteins in the flour—*glutenin* and *gliadin*. When the dough is kneaded, these two proteins combine to produce gluten in the dough. Gluten provides elasticity to the dough, which in turn traps the air and gas released by yeast and forms a sponge like texture in baked breads.

Milling of Flour

Flour can be milled at home by traditional stone grinding machines but for industrial usage, it is milled in flour mills, which have to follow stringent quality checks and norms to produce a consistent product each year. The flour mills purchase the wheat grains from farmers and after purchasing, they check the moisture content and density of the grain. Before the grain is milled, it needs to undergo a few steps of processing to be ready for milling. Let us discuss these steps in detail.

Processing

Pre-cleaning The wheat sacks obtained are first weighed and classified. Then they are opened and put into the pre-cleaning process where the wheat grain is made to pass through a drum sieve and a series of separators and rollers to separate all the rough impurities such as stones and straws. The entire cleaning system consists of vertical and horizontal belts of conveyer.

Main cleaning After the pre-cleaning, the wheat is again passed through different separators and rollers to remove impurities. Different sieves with different mesh sizes are used in order to differentiate the cleaned wheat. For instance, sieve of 8 mm is used to remove smaller straws and other impurities while that of 13 mm is used to remove bigger straws and so on. It also consists of magnetic plates, separator, destoner, scourer (to remove the top layer of grease), etc.

Combinator This is a machine that separates stones from the grain, throwing away the stones forward and the wheat backward. It works on the principle of *specific gravity* segregating the lighter and heavier grains. This machine is also called *Destoner*.

Cockle cylinder It is a pitted cylinder that separates the broken wheat from the whole grains.

Emery scorer It is a special kind of machine which cleans the surface of the raw wheat kernel.

Tempering Tempering is the process of increasing the moisture content in the grain. The moisture content present in the grain is usually 9-10%. It is taken up to 14-15% by adding measured quantity of water through water wheel dampener. There are two stages in tempering after each of which the grain is rested for a certain duration of time depending on the climate, relative humidity, etc. For instance, in winters the resting period is for about 24 hours and in summers 4-6 hours. Water is required to separate bran and endosperm.

Acquatron It is a machine which is used to check and regulate the flow and the quantity of water to be used for second tempering. This uses a unique mechanism which ensures that the quantity of water matches the quantity of wheat.

Horizontal scorer Once the process of tempering is over, the wheat is cleaned with a horizontal scorer, which cleans mud in the crevice of wheat kernels. Here actually the bran softens and is made ready for the next process, that is, milling.

Milling is done in different rolls—grooved rolls and polished rolls. The kernels are broken and sifted in sieves with different mesh sizes to obtain semolina, refined flour, and wholewheat flour. Refined flour is obtained at 132 microns and the grinding loss is generally about 8%. The final moisture content in the flour is maintained between 13.5-14%.

When food establishments purchase flour, they must obtain certification of the flour with regards to its quality standards. Though some hotels do have their own food labs to check the parameters, but establishments which do not have such an arrangement, can procure these from the flour producers.

The parameters that we should check for flour are given in Table 2.1.

Selection Criteria of Good Flour

Flour is usually milled industrially these days and most millers do a fantastic job of producing good quality flour. The entire grain is milled to produce a variety of flours and its by-products such as wholewheat flour, coarse flour, refined flour, and semolina.

The basic criteria of a flour is that it should be clean and free from any foreign particles. It should smell pleasant and should be free from any particular odour. For a pastry chef, the quality of flour is measured in its gluten content. It does not mean that the flour with low gluten, which is often referred to as weak flour is not good, the only thing it means is that this flour will not be suitable for products such as breads, which need higher amounts of gluten. Similarly, the high gluten flour will not be suitable for making biscuits or cakes, as these products need weak flour.

Apart from this, the parameters listed in Table 2.1 determine the selection of quality flour.

Table 2.1 Parameters for selecting quality flour

Parameter	Description
Colour grading	After flour is milled, some companies also bleach the flour to make it whiter with the help of nitrogen gas or oxidising agents.
	It is better to buy unbleached flour and different companies have their own standard measurements for grading the colour of the flour. In most cases, grade 5 is the highest white colour without any bleaching.
Moisture	A good quality flour has a moisture content between 13-14% by its volume. To check the same a sample of flour is provided a temperature of around 45–50°C for at least 20 minutes, which leads to evaporation of water; the loss of weight is the quantity of moisture in the grain.
Gluten content	An equipment called extensometer is used to check the gluten content and extensibility of the flour. It has graphs to measure the resistance and the extensibility. Each flour is produced with a certain gluten content suitable for the purpose. Generally, the gluten content can range between 10-28%, where the 10% is used for products such as biscuits and cakes, and the 28% is usually used in bread making.
pH	In Chemistry, pH is a measure of alkalinity or acidity of any given solution. On a pH scale, 7 is the basic and anything less than 7 is acidic and anything more than 7 is alkaline. A good quality flour is slightly acidic with a reading of 6-6.8 on the pH scale.

Table 2.1 (Contd)

Parameter	Description
Ash content	Ash content is the amount of minerals that still remain in the flour after it has been milled. A wholewheat flour in which the entire grain is milled will have higher mineral content and the ash content can be as high as 1.50. This number is calculated on the basis of the amount of residual ash that remains after 100 g of flour is burnt in controlled environment.
	Lower ash content means that the flour is milled from germ and endosperm and in case of refined flours, lower the ash content, more pure the flour is but in case of wholewheat flours, higher ash content means that the flour is more pure.
Diastatic quality of flour	This is an industrial process and in this case a small percentage of flour is allowed to germinate for a few days. It is then dried and finally added to the remaining grains to produce flour. The diastataic flour is considered best for bread making. The enzymes developed during the germination process help convert complex sugars into simple sugars, which are needed by the yeast to produce high quality bread. This process is also known as malting and usually, wheat grain or barley grain is used for this purpose.
Water absorption	Water absorption or water hydration is the term used for the property of flour as to how much of water it can absorb to form a smooth dough. It is also abbreviated as WAC, which stands for *Water Absorption Capacity*. Normally, a good quality flour has a WAC of 65-70%, but for slack doughs such as ciabatta, the WAC is preferred at 85-90%.

TYPES OF FLOUR

Apart from wheat flour, any grain can be milled into a flour of varied coarseness. People who are allergic to gluten in flour have varied options from other grains such as corn or lentils, which do not contain gluten and are safe for consumption. In this part of the chapter, we will discuss about various kinds of flour obtained from the wheat kernel and later we will also read more about flours obtained from other grains.

Let us discuss about the various types of flour obtained from wheat and other grains.

Flours Obtained from Wheat

The wholewheat grain consists of various components as discussed in Fig. 2.1. Each component is milled in various proportions to yield different types of flours from the same plant and each type of flour has a particular usage in the bakery kitchen. Let us discuss some of these flours in Table 2.2.

Flours from Various Grains

Apart from the various flours that are derived from wheat, there are other grains and seeds from which many other flours are obtained. It is very important for chefs to have knowledge of such flours as we can make different products with the range of the flours, which will be healthier. Moreover, since many people are suffering from gluten allergies, it is important that we have products that are gluten free. Many types of grains are available in market but few of the popular flours obtained from them are discussed in Table 2.3.

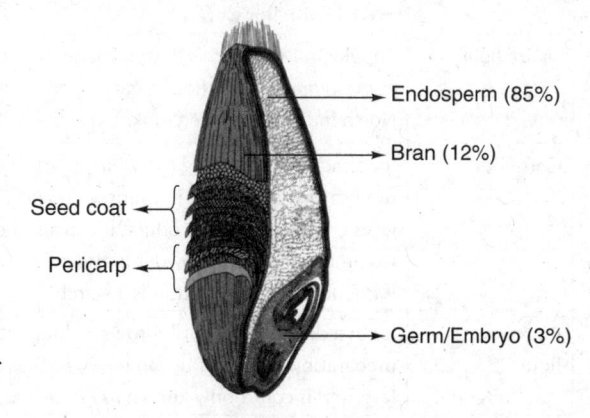

Fig. 2.1 Structure of wheat grain

Table 2.2 Various flours from wheat

Type of flour	Description
Wholemeal flour	Also called as *atta* in India, it is the whole milled wheat kernel. The flour is cream to brown in colour as it has the bran grounded with it. It is not advisable to sift the wholewheat flour as you will lose most of the bran, which is an important dietary component.
Brown flour	This is almost 85% of the grain millet, where some amount of bran has been extracted. It is nutritious as it has high percentage of germ.
Strong flour	This is milled from hard flour, in other words from high protein flours. Strong flours absorb more water than weak flours, as gluten can absorb twice its own weight of water. This flour is used for products that will have a high rise in the oven such as yeast breads, choux pastry, and puff pastry. Strong flour is also known as *baker's flour*.
Weak flour	Weak flour is also known as *soft flour* or *cake flour*. As the name suggests, this flour has less gluten and hence, it is used for products that need a softer texture such as cookies, cakes, and sponges.
All-purpose flour	The all-purpose flour is a blend of flours and has medium strength. In India, the refined flour that we get is all-purpose flour only.
Cake flour	Refer to weak flour
Pastry flour	This flour consists of very finely ground polished soft wheat kernels usually enriched and bleached.
Self-rising flour	This flour is usually of medium strength and contains baking powder in a proportion. Since the flour contains moisture, it can react with the baking powder and lessen its effect. Hence, it is not advisable to buy the commercial self-rising flour. It is advisable to use 60 g of baking powder to 1 kg flour to make it rise. This flour is commonly used to make afternoon cookies called *scones*.

Table 2.3 Types of flours from various grains

Type of flour	Description
Rye flour	Rye flour does not have so much amount of gluten as the flour and hence, it is sometimes mixed in proportions with flour for the production of breads. Breads that use only rye flour are more dense and chewy. It is majorly used in Russian and Scandinavian breads. Rye flour dough is quite heavy and sticky.
Rice flour	These are the finely ground polished rice with a texture similar to that of corn starch, usually used as thickening agent. Rice flour is free of gluten and if its dough has to be made, one would have to make it with hot water.
Maize flour	Popular in Mexico, this flour is made from cooked maize corn and then grounded. It is also known as *masa harina*. This flour has also been used in India since time immemorial and a very popular North Indian dish called *makke ki roti* is made from it. The flour is also free from gluten.
Cornflour	It is made by grounding the white heart or the germ of the corn kernel, and is one of the widely used thickening agents in Chinese cooking. This is also free of gluten, and its usage in products gives crispness to the product. It can also be added to strong flour to make it into weak flour. Commercial custard powder is also made with cornflour with colour and flavour added. Cornflour is not actually a flour but it is a starch.
Buckwheat flour	It has a distinctive greyish brown colour with an earthy bitter taste. It is used to make classical preparations such as Russian blinis, pancakes, and French galettes. In India, it is widely eaten during fasts and is commonly known as *kuttu ka atta*.

Gluten-free Flour

Apart from the aforementioned types of flours, it is also very important for chefs to know about gluten free flours, as the demand of the same is increasing constantly. Some of the gluten free flours mentioned in Table 2.3 are most commonly used in hotels. However, India has some unique ingredients that can be ground to produce flour substitutes thereby offering a guest a wide selection of bakery goods. Seeds of many edible legumes can be ground into flours for usage in gluten free breads. Chick pea flour is very commonly used in India and Mediterranean countries. Many other seeds such as amaranth, soya bean, millets, and quinoa can also be used in gluten free products.

FATS AND OILS

The scientific term *lipid* comprises of a group of substances that include natural fats and oils. Both these lipids consist of fatty acids and glycerol. The only difference between fats and oils is that oils are liquid at room temperature whereas fats are solid as they contain saturated fatty acids. The exception to this rule is coconut oil and palm oil, which are solid at room temperature. When talking about fats and oils you will come across many terms such as MUFA (monounsaturated fatty acids) and PUFA (polyunsaturated fatty acids). Saturation means the density of fat; in other words it is the molecular structure of the fat where the carbon atoms are bonded with oxygen and hydrogen.

Saturation is increased artificially by adding hydrogen into the fat through a process known as *saturation* or *hydrogenation* of oil. The oil is converted into margarine by passing hydrogen into it to make it saturated. This is done to stabilise the fats and oils which in turn increases the shelf life of the product as it does not oxidise easily. Fats are naturally saturated with hydrogen whereas some fats are artificially transformed from oils like margarine and are known as *trans fats*. They are unhealthier in comparison to other fats as they are the prime cause of cardiac disorders.

Fats and oils do not dissolve in water, but they can be emulsified with water to produce salad dressings and sauces. Fats along with carbohydrates and proteins make up the major components of food. Fats and oils are extracted from animals, and seeds of nuts, spices, etc. Animal fats such as suet and lard come naturally from animal meat of beef and pork respectively, and products such as butter are churned out mostly from cow's milk.

Usage of Fats and Oils in Baking

Fats and oils are the prime ingredient in any dish around the world. They give richness, variety of textures, and smoothness to the foods that otherwise may be too dry to eat. The melting points of oils and fats are very important for chefs, as it is this property that decides the usage of the particular lipid in a dish. One cannot deep fry in butter as it will burn to black, when it reaches the temperature of frying.

Fats and oils are used in cake-making to moisten the batter and improve the keeping qualities of the cake. The fats have the ability to retain a certain amount of air during the preparation stage. Butter is used in laminated dough such as puff pastry and croissants, during the baking process, the fat melts and produces steam which in turn aerates and lightens the product.

Let us discuss the types of fats and oils used in bakery and confectionary in Table 2.4.

Table 2.4 Fats and oils used in pastry and bakery

Type of fat and oil	Description
Lard	This fat is from pork and is commonly used in cooking and baking. Though with more awareness of health, the use of lards and other natural animal fats is restricted to special dishes only. Animal fats are rendered before using. Rendering is a process where the fats are heated on a low heat to remove the non-fatty membrane. The non-rendered fat has more pronounced flavour and hence, it is commonly used to line pates, etc., in *charcuterie*.
Suet	Fat from beef is called suet. Due to its stability, it used to be a very common ingredient for short crust pies, etc., but butter has majorly replaced all the natural saturated animal fats.
Margarine	This is an emulsion of water and oil. It is mainly a vegetable oil but at times it may contain a mixture of both animal and vegetable oils. These oils are then saturated by addition of hydrogen, which makes the oils more stable and increases their melting point. The handling of this fat becomes very easy in warmer conditions and it can cream very well to give more structure and volume to the baked product. Margarine is used mainly in pastry work and is hardly used in cooking.
Butter	Dairy butter consists of about 80% fat and 20% water and whey. It is the milk protein in the whey that makes butter spoil quickly and together with milk sugar (lactose), causes it to scorch when overheated. In the West, most butter is made from cow's milk, but elsewhere butter made from the milk of water buffalo, yak, goats, and sheep is also available. The quality of butter is affected by the cream used for it, which in turn is influenced by the season and the feed of the animal. Colour varies from very pale to deep yellow, but producers may add colouring to butter, particularly salted butter, so that it looks uniform throughout the year. Sometimes the cream is allowed to ripen, or lactic yeast is added to give the butter a pleasant acidity and nutty aroma. For health reasons, most butter is pasteurized, which means that the milk used to make it has been sterilised by heating it briefly to destroy any harmful bacteria. In some countries, raw butter is also available; it has a better taste, but does not keep well. Butter is also graded according to quality in many countries. Unsalted butter is made from fresh cream. It is especially appropriate for delicate pastries, cakes, and icings, where even a pinch of salt would easily stand out. In most European countries, most of the butter sold is unsalted and made from ripened cream, while in Britain and the United States, the reverse is true. However, both salted and unsalted kinds are usually available. Butter may be clarified to separate the fat from the water and milk solids, so that the remaining fat will not scorch or turn bitter. Clarified butter may be heated to a much higher temperature than regular butter and is good for sautéing. Creamed butter can be mixed with various flavourings to form compound butters. Savoury butters are popular accompaniments to meats, fish, and vegetables; sweet butters include sugar and flavourings such as vanilla, grated citrus rind or liqueur.
Oils	The usage of oil in pastry kitchen is restricted to frying certain bakery and pastry products such as doughnuts and sweet fritters. Oil is also used for addition to bread dough to soften the gluten and produce soft textured bread. In some traditional recipes like focaccia, olive oil is poured over the bread before baking. In addition, oil is used mainly for greasing the baking trays.

MILK AND DAIRY PRODUCTS

Milk represents a major ingredient in our diet—poured over cereals, drunk in glasses, in tea and coffee—but it also enters the composition of many dishes especially desserts such as ice cream, custard, pancakes, and rice puddings. It is particularly high in calcium, but it is also fairly good in fat too. Milk is mainly made up of water and has many nutritional contents such as proteins, fats, and carbohydrates. Milk also has sugar called lactose and this is the reason why it changes colour if heated for a long time. In bakery, it is used as a liquid in place of water to enrich the dough or used as a liquid in making creams and pastes. In pastry products, milk improves the texture, flavour, nutrition value, and the quality of the product.

Types of Milk

It is important to know various kinds of milk used in cooking and especially in pastry the type of milk plays a very important role. Whole milk will give a different product from milk powder or milk solids and so on. Let us see the various types of milk in Table 2.5.

Table 2.5 Types of milk

Type of milk	Description
Whole milk	It can be cow's milk or milk from buffalo, sheep or even goat. This milk contains at least 3.5% of butterfat, which gives it that wholesome taste.
Homogenised milk	It is whole, pasteurized, and treated so that its fat globules are broken to the extent that there is no separation of fat from the milk. It is a mechanical process which reduces the size of the fat and then mixes them together.
Skimmed milk	The fat from the whole milk is removed by a centrifugal force. The fat from the milk is sold separately as cream. The skimmed milk has a trace amount of fat present which can be lower than 1%.
Buttermilk	It is a by-product obtained whilst making butter. When the butter is churned, the whey that is left behind is known as buttermilk. Today buttermilk is made from pasteurized milk with an addition of lactic acid bacteria. This milk can be used for making sorbets and ice creams.
Dehydrated milk	This is whole milk from which the water is removed by either spray drying or roll drying processes. Milk powder is used in breads or cookie dough to provide enrichment.
Condensed milk	This is reduced milk, in which sugar and stabilisers have been added to produce a thick and viscous creamy liquid. Condensed milk is used to make various cakes and pastries.

Cream

Cream is the butterfat content of whole cow's milk, separated from the water. The principal difference between the various types of cream—single cream, double cream, whipping cream, clotted cream, and soured cream—is the balance between water and butterfat. This will make them liquid or of a very thick consistency. Other differences are in the way they have been made and their time for maturing which results in different tastes. Some of the common types of creams used in cooking and confectionary are given in Table 2.6.

Table 2.6 Types of creams used in cooking

Type of cream	Description
Single cream	This cream contains not less than 18% butterfat. It cannot be whipped due to their being too little butterfat. This cream is also known as cooking cream as it is commonly used in cooking for making sauces or used in dressings and soups as well. Single cream in pastry is used for custards, etc., which will eventually be baked and cooked.
Double cream	This cream contains not less than 45% butterfat. It can be whipped but not too much as it will turn into butter. It can be used to enrich sauces, but may curdle if boiled along with acid ingredients.
Whipping cream	This cream contains not less than 38% butterfat. It is perfect for whipping as its name indicates. After whipping you will find a difference in texture and a change in volume. Sweetened or unsweetened cream can be used in desserts or can be used as an accompaniment, and is incorporated in mousses to lighten them.
Imitation cream	As the name suggests, this is not a real cream. The butterfat in the milk is replaced by vegetable oils. This cream is prepared commercially and is commonly used in kitchen because of its stability and keeping quality.

> **CHEF'S TIP**
> Cream should be whipped at a temperature of around 4°C. It will be also helpful to chill the bowl to allow the little dissipation of heat. Whisking of cream over a bowl of ice will help the cream to whip faster and reduce its chances of curdling into butter.

CHEESE

Cheese has always been the basic dish on every table of European continent. The French, Italians, Swizz, and Dutch boast of a large selection of cheese and this is undoubtedly true. The manufacturers prepare cheese that reflects the region and the place of its origin. Many of the cheeses are DOP (*Denominazione di Origine Protetta*) which is a classification given to a food item that denotes the origin of the product from that particular region. There are so many varieties of cheeses available.

The legend is that the first cheese was made accidentally by an Arab traveller who was carrying goat milk in a leather saddlebag. The jolts on the camel ride caused the milk to split into curds which were the first origins of cheese. Even today, cheese is prepared by separating the coagulated milk proteins known as curd through an enzymatic activity.

Kinds of Cheese

There are innumerable kinds of cheeses made around the world. Each country boasts about their speciality cheese and these cheeses are commonly made from milk of various animals such as cow, buffalo, sheep, goat and even yak, which lends a typical taste to the particular cheese.

Cheese in Pastry and Bakery

Cheeses have a unique place in Western cuisines and are served during breakfast, lunch, and dinner elegantly decorated on cheese boards or eaten in sandwiches. In bakery and pastry, various kinds of cheese are used in bread making to make cheese loaves, focaccia and other breads that can use a range of cheeses available around the world. However in pastry kitchen, cream cheese is the most desired as it is used for preparing some classical desserts and pastries.

Let us discuss some of the famous cheeses used in pastry in Table 2.7.

Table 2.7 Popular cheeses used in pastry and bakery

Type of cheese	Description
Philadelphia cheese	This cream cheese from United States of America is a creamy cheese that is classically used in making baked cheesecake. The cake is also known as New York baked cheesecake and when it is named as this, it must only use Philadelphia cheese.
Yoghurt cheese	In this case, the yoghurt is placed in a muslin/cheese cloth and hanged with a support to drain away the whey. The resulting thick creamy mass often known as yoghurt cheese is used for preparing chilled cheesecakes.
Quark cheese	This is a cream cheese from Germany and is also used in preparing baked and chilled cheesecakes. Some theories say that Quark cheese was the first cheese to be used in baked cheesecake.
Ricotta	It is a soft creamy cheese made from ewe's milk. The unique thing about this cheese is that it is made from the whey which is low in fat content. Ricotta cheese is drained in special baskets and the marks of the basket can be easily seen on the surface of the cheese. Ricotta cheese is often used as stuffing for Italian desserts such as cannoli and Sicilian cassata.
Mascarpone	This creamy cheese comes from the Lombardy region of Italy and is made from cow's milk. It is prepared by adding tartaric acid to warm milk and allowing it to curdle. It is then drained in cheese cloth and allowed to ripen for a few days. Mascarpone is commonly used for preparing a famous Italian dessert called Tiramisu.

EGGS

Many varieties of eggs are found around the world, but only a few are used for human consumption due to various reasons. The eggs can be of fish, poultry, game birds, or even reptiles, but in cooking when we refer to eggs, we are always talking about poultry and eggs of birds that are reared for consumption of meat. But then eggs from ducks and even quails have a very special place on gourmet tables. Eggs can be of various colours, patterns, and sizes; the only thing common among eggs is their natural oval shape. An egg is a rich source of protein as it has two types of proteins. Egg white contains *albumen* and yolk contains *lecithin*.

Eggs can be put through many uses. Apart from being relished in the breakfast as omelettes, poached, or boiled, it has a special place in bakery and pastry as it is not only used as an ingredient to add nutrition value to the product, but has a very distinct role to play with regards to texture, colour, and look of the product. They can be whipped up for delicate desserts and cakes. Eggs can be used for thickening or simply paired with milk to create sauces. Eggs and oil or butter emulsion also form sauces such as mayonnaise and hollandaise. Egg is a versatile commodity and chefs can put it to numerous uses.

Structure of an Egg

Let us discuss the structure of an egg (refer to Fig. 2.2) and then we shall discuss the different types of eggs and their uses.

Shell It is the outer covering of the egg and is composed of calcium carbonate. It may be white or brown depending upon the breed of the chicken.

Yolk This is the yellow portion of an egg.

Vitelline It is a clear seal that holds the egg yolk.

Chalazae These are the twisted cord-like strands of the egg white. They anchor the yolk in the centre of the egg. Prominent chalazae indicate high quality.

Shell membranes Two shell membranes, inner and outer membrane, surround the albumen. They form a protective barrier against bacteria. Air cell forms between these membranes.

Air cell It is the pocket of air formed at the large end of the egg. This is caused by the contraction of the contents on cooling after the egg is laid. The air cell increases with the age of the egg as there is considerable amount of moisture loss.

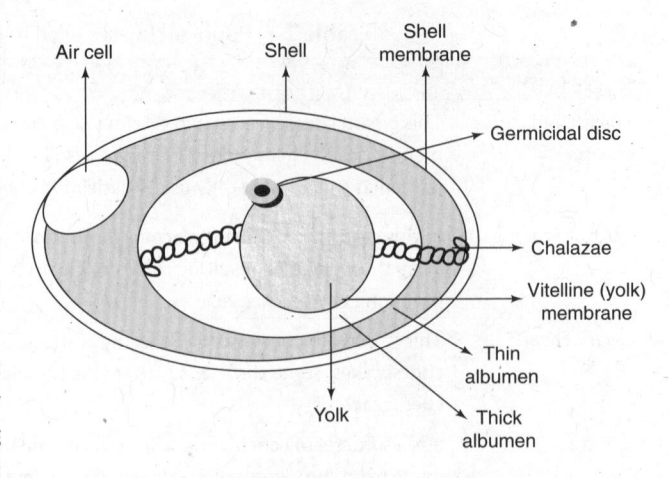

Fig. 2.2 Structure of an egg

Thin albumen It is nearest to the shell. When the egg is broken there will be a clear demarcation of the thin and thick albumen. As the egg gets older, these two albumens tend to mix into one another.

Thick albumen It stands high and spreads less than the thin white in a high quality egg. It is an excellent source of riboflavin and protein.

Selection and Storage of Eggs

When referring to eggs in the recipes of pastry, the standard egg weight for reference is taken at 50 g for a whole egg. This holds true when the recipe calls for eggs in numbers or pieces. Many recipes also have eggs mentioned in kilograms and grams, in which case the eggs must be broken, mixed and then weighed for the recipe.

When separating yolk from the egg white, one must be very careful as even a drop of yolk in a large number of egg whites can hamper the whipping of egg whites for purposes such as making meringues.

Ideally, the eggs should be refrigerated, but when they need to be separated and stored, the egg whites must be put in a clean container with a food grade plastic film touching the surface of the eggs.

The eggs and the whites should be refrigerated for a period of minimum three days and maximum six days. This way the moisture in the egg white gets evaporated making it more suitable for whipping for meringues and other uses.

> **CHEF'S TIP**
> Cold eggs and whites do not whip well, so before whipping allow the eggs to come to room temperature. If eggs of the best quality are desired, medium-sized ones that are uniform in size and colour should be selected. With regards to shape, they should have a comparatively long oval shell, one end of which should be blunt and the other, a sharp curve.

Uses of Eggs

Most of the eggs are enjoyed on their own, or are served boiled or fried. They add colour and taste to several dishes. So, before discussing the uses, it is important to know the three major cooking functions performed by eggs. These are as follows:

- Coagulation
- Leavening
- Emulsification

Apart from these three major functions, the eggs can be used for binding, making batters, adding colour, flavour, and texture to the products by being added to the dough, and creating a base for coating goods with other ingredients, for example, fried fish coated with bread crumbs or vermicelli.

Coagulation

We can vary the coagulation to our taste, and have the egg as soft boiled, hard boiled, fried, or scrambled. When too intense heat is used, the eggs become over-coagulated. Eggs coagulate at 65°C and continue to thicken till 70°C.

If other ingredients, such as milk and cream, are added to the eggs, it may raise the coagulation point. This helps to get a softer scrambled egg as eggs never over-coagulate to a hard texture. Uses of eggs based upon coagulation are:

- The process of coagulation thickens custard and sauce.
- Coagulated egg protein helps support cream puffs, cakes, and breads. It binds together foods as in meat loaves and burgers.
- It also coats foods in the form of egg-based batters.
- To clarify a consommé, a chef beats in egg whites into the soup.
- In pastry, egg yolks are whisked and hot sugar syrup at a temperature of 118-120°C also known as soft ball stage, is added whilst continuously whisking. This results in a thick sauce like product also known as *Baum* in French. *Baum* can be used as a base for many desserts such as soufflé and mousse.

Leavening

The effectiveness of the leavening depends on the amount of air trapped within the egg. Yolks when beaten transform into thick light yellow foam. A little acid in the form of cream of tartar or a squeeze of lemon juice helps stabilise the foam and the yolks as even a small trace of yolk will prevent the whites from rising properly.

Use of eggs based upon leavening are:

- Eggs are used for making baked goods such as sponges and cakes. Leavening of eggs gives these products a lighter texture that is desirable.
- Egg whites are whipped with sugar to make meringues.

Meringue is a type of dessert commonly made in French, Swiss, and Italian cuisines. In its most basic form, meringue is prepared by whipping egg whites with a pinch of salt and sugar. Heavy or light meringue can be made by addition of more or less sugar. Meringues can be baked to form a variety of pastry confections such as cookies, garnishes for cakes and pastries or used as a dessert by itself. Meringues can also be used with whipped cream and other flavouring agents to make the base for a variety of chilled desserts such as soufflé and mousse. In some cases, nut powders are combined with meringues to make special sponges for cakes. So in other words, the meringue can have various applications.

Meringues can be divided into three categories or types as follows:

French meringue Also known as cold meringue, it is prepared by whipping egg whites until they are frothy and adding castor sugar in small amounts, whilst whipping continuously. This meringue is supposed to be used instantly as it can separate if it is left outside for a longer period of time.

Swiss meringue This is a warm meringue. Egg whites are whipped on a warm water bath until frothy, sugar is added in smaller amounts and the mixture is whisked over the hot water bath until creamy and stands in peaks or when it reaches around 40°C. It is then transferred to a machine and whisked until it becomes stable and creamy.

Italian meringue This is the most stable meringue of all. For this, the egg whites are whipped with small amount of sugar until frothy and then hot melted sugar boiled to 118°C is added whilst continuously whisking the mixture until a thick meringue is obtained.

Meringues can be cooked in a variety of ways depending upon their uses and final desired texture. The meringue can be baked to a crisp cookie by allowing it to bake for a very long time such as 2–3 hours at a low temperature of 80°C, or it can be cooked for 40–45 minutes at 100°C to create a crisp outer layer and a chewy interior, much desired for a dessert called pavlova. Meringues can be gratinated under a salamander or with a blow torch for creating the burnt colour as in case of baked Alaska and lemon meringue pie.

Uses of meringue A meringue can be used in several ways. It can be used as a dessert by itself or as a base for cakes and pastries and even for garnishes and decorations.

Each type of meringue has its own unique use. French meringue is preferred for preparing soufflés and French macaroons. Whereas for fillings in cakes and mousses, Italian meringue is preferred more due to its stability.

Swiss meringue is commonly used for preparing garnishes such as meringue mushrooms or meringue sticks as it gives a pleasant creamy colour, and the garnishes are long lasting and also do not contain an egg odour as the egg whites are cooked over double boiler. Meringues are commonly used in desserts. Some common desserts made by using meringue are discussed in Table 2.8.

Table 2.8 Meringue-based desserts

Dessert	Description
Vacherin	Vacherins are made by piping meringue from a round tube one on top of another to resemble a shell. The shells are then baked dried and filled with whipped cream or pastry cream and decorated with fruits, berries, whipped cream, ice cream, etc.
Pavlova	Another of the meringue favourites, it is made by combining meringue with cornflour, vinegar, and vanilla essence. It is mainly served with sweetened whipped cream filling and fresh fruits. Coulis or tropical fruit salsas go well with pavlova.
Marshmallows	Marshmallows are sweet confections that are usually served for children's parties or on festive occasions. They can be flavoured with essence and colours.
Floating islands	This is a classical dessert, where quenelles of French meringue are poached in a vanilla sauce and served as a dessert. The name of the dessert is associated with floating meringue on sauce.
French macaroons	All high end pastry shops in most hotels are adorned with colourful French macaroons, which can contain a range of fillings. Macaroon is a dessert, where the meringue is mixed with almond powder and baked into flat shells. The two shells are joined together with the help of filling, which eventually lends its name to the macaroon. For example, pistachio macaroon, chocolate macaroon, etc.

| Vacherin | Pavlova | Marshmallows | French macaroons |

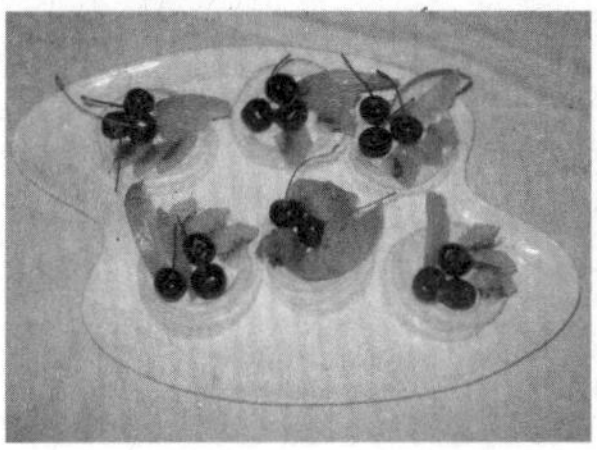

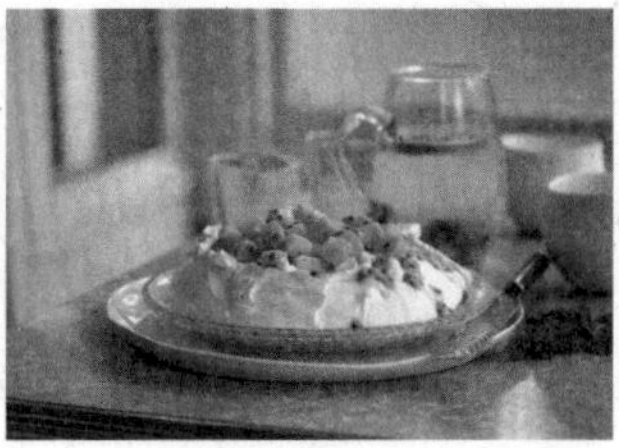

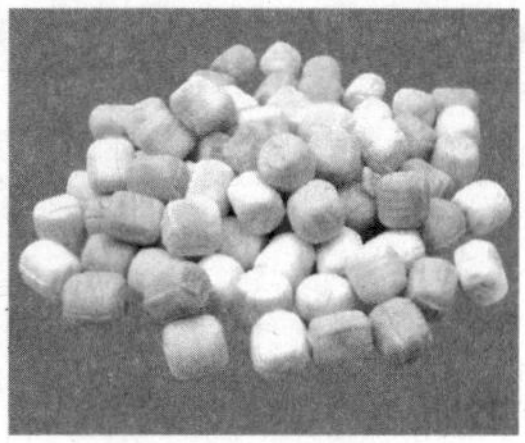

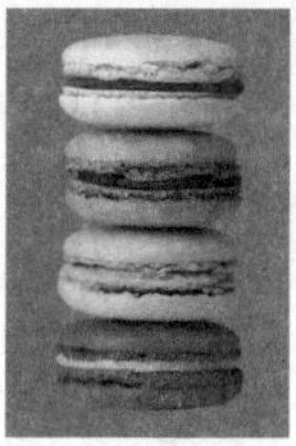

Fig. 2.3 Meringue-based desserts

Storage of meringue Meringues are made with egg whites and hence, one has to be extremely careful in storing them. They are supposed to be kept crisp and therefore, one cannot store them in refrigerated conditions.

The best way to store a meringue is in a cool and dry environment, preferably in an airtight box, so that it does not become soggy.

Not all meringues are kept for storage unless it is a baked meringue that will be used for desserts or garnishes. The French meringue is immediately used and if kept for even a short time, it can collapse and loose its volume.

Italian meringue on the other hand is a more stable meringue and if needed to be stored, it can be packed into a plastic bag and stored for up to 15 days under -20°C temperature.

Factors to be considered when preparing meringue Making a meringue is very simple. However, one has to take a lot of precautions whilst preparing this simple product. For most chefs an unsuccessful attempt in meringue making is very frustrating. There are many factors that affect the making of meringue. Apart from the equipment, even the environment plays a big role.

However, if the following precautions are taken, then you will enjoy making meringues.

- Choose a dry and not so humid day to prepare your meringues as humidity in air can cause meringues to go limp and soft.
- Choose a clean bowl and a whisk. Fat and water are the biggest enemies of meringues. Make sure that the bowl and whisk are dry, clean and free from any presence of fat or oil.
- The size of the bowl is also important. Choose a large size bowl as the meringue will whip up to 6–8 times its volume. The large bowl will be able to hold the expanded meringue and also the gradual whipping will not allow the egg whites to fall out of the bowl.
- Whilst separating yolks from the whites, ensure that the whites do not have a single drop of yolk as it can hamper the whipping of the meringue.
- Try and use glass or stainless steel bowls for preparing meringues, as plastic can have an invisible film of grease that is not visible to the naked eye.
- The meringue has a better volume when the egg whites are kept under refrigeration for at least 3–4 days. This helps to evaporate extra moisture present in them resulting in better volume.

- Never whip cold egg whites, take them out of the fridge and allow them to rest at room temperature for at least 30 minutes before whipping.

- Adding a pinch of tartaric acid/citric acid helps to stabilise the egg whites and results in better volume.

- Add sugar gradually and always use castor sugar. Start adding the sugar only when the egg whites have frothed up a little.

- Do not over whip the meringue. The meringues are usually whipped up to soft peaks. When the whisk is lifted off from the meringue and the peak curls at the tip and the appearance is glossy, then it is considered to be at soft peak.

- When making meringue in a whipping machine, never switch off the machine until you are ready to take the meringue out. In case you are not ready with other things, then keep mixing the meringue at the lowest speed of the machine.

> **CHEF'S TIP**
> It is always easier to separate whites from egg yolk when the egg is chilled.

Emulsification

Egg yolk acts as an emulsifying agent, because its protein can wrap itself around tiny globules of oil. Yolk also contains lecithin, which is an emulsifying agent. Uses of eggs based upon emulsification are:

- Oil is added to the yolks to form mayonnaise.

- The emulsifying power of egg yolks also contributes to the crumbly quality of a rich cake.

SWEETENERS

Sweeteners as the name suggests, are the soul of all desserts. When we refer to desserts, they have to be sweet. Sugar is one of the most important ingredients used in confectionary and its usage is not only limited to providing the sweetness, but it has various other uses such as altering the texture of products, and giving colour to the baked goods. Sugar also delays the coagulation of proteins in eggs and promotes aeration in a product. It is available in various forms such as grain sugar, icing sugar, breakfast sugar, and this categorization is basically done on the basis of the shape and size of the sugar crystal. Apart from these, there are still various other types of sweeteners used in cooking, especially confectionary. Honey, corn syrup, treacle, etc., are other very commonly used sweeteners in cooking and the choice would depend upon what kind of texture the final product is aimed at. For example, whilst making meringue the sugar crystals will not dissolve by the time meringue is completed. And usage of any other sugar apart from icing sugar in buttercream will form small crystals, which will give a grainy finish to the cake. Let us discuss the various types of sweeteners commonly used in bakery and pastry in Table 2.9.

> **CHEF'S TIP**
> Before removing the liquid glucose with bare hands, always wet your hands with water or else it will stick to your hands.

RAISING AGENTS

Some ingredients play a very vital role in baking. Raising agents are those ingredients which are responsible for the (inside) chemical changes in baking. They are also known as leavening agents. Some of these are available naturally like yeasts, whereas some of these are produced by chemicals such as

Table 2.9 Types of sweeteners used in cooking

Type of sweetener	Description
Granulated sugar	It is the sugar crystals usually obtained from sugar cane and is the regular white sugar that is used in homes. Commonly used for preparing sugar syrups.
Castor sugar/Breakfast sugar	It is commonly used in breakfast for tea and coffee and hence the name. It is small evenly graded sugar crystals that dissolve quickly and are easier to dissolve in creaming methods. Breakfast sugar is used in various pastry products, for making meringues, pastry creams, whipped creams, sable, etc.
Icing sugar	Granulated sugar is crushed into fine powder and has a small percentage of corn starch added to keep it smooth and free flowing. Icing sugar is used for creaming methods where it would be used as icing for cakes and pastries and hence the name icing sugar. Icing sugar can also be sifted on top of dry baked sweet products as a garnish. Commonly used for preparing buttercream or for dusting on top of dry cakes.
Brown sugar	This is granulated sugar which is available in a variety of shades of brown. The darker brown sugar is also known as Demerara sugar and the darker the colour, the more pronounced is the flavour. Brown sugar is the residual sugar obtained during the process of refining sugar. Used in cookies and other products where a pronounced colour and flavour is required.
Golden syrup	It is a thick amber coloured liquid obtained from sugar during the refining process. It is used in preparing festive Xmas cakes and candies.
Corn syrup	It is chemically refined syrup made from corn kernels. It is usually obtained as a clear liquid and the coloured corn syrup is artificially coloured. It is very sweet and contains high amount of fructose. It is combined with chocolate to make plastic chocolate also known as modelling chocolate.
Treacle	When sugar cane juice undergoes refining, it undergoes through many stages. The first stage comes where the white sugar or the raw sugar is removed. The remaining sugar syrup is used to make treacle which is stronger than golden syrup but less strong than molasses. It is used in festive cakes and breads.
Honey	Honey is a natural sugar obtained from the bee hives. The colour and flavour of honey will vary with its source. Some commercial honey farms allow bees to suck the nectar from only one particular flower to produce the honey of that flavour. One can use honey in most of the baked products but care has to be taken as honey can caramelise even at lower temperatures. Honey can be used as an invert sugar as well and is used in cookies, cakes, and festive preparations.
Molasses	Molasses is the by-product of sugar from sugar cane. There are three stages of refining of sugar and with every stage a residual sweetener is left behind that is known as molasses. As the stages increase, the colour and the flavour of molasses becomes stronger and darker. Molasses is used in making dark Xmas cakes or wedding cakes and other festive breads, cakes, and pastries.
Invert sugars	These are sucrose based syrups that are treated with acids or chemicals. The acid breaks the sucrose molecule into glucose and fructose. Since there are now two molecules of sugar, it will be sweeter than sucrose. Corn syrup is a type of invert sugar and this property of inverting sugar does not let the sugar to crystallize easily and hence the product stays moist.

(Contd)

Table 2.9 (Contd)

Type of sweetener	Description
Liquid glucose	Liquid glucose is obtained by treating the corn slurry by acid—a process known as hydrolysis. This is chemically made and results in a thick viscous liquid that is used to produce candies by not allowing the sugar to crystallize and also acts as a preservative. When added to products, it makes them pliable and hence is very commonly used to prepare garnishes and decoration pieces with sugar. It is also used in preparing ganache and filling for chocolates.
Isomalt	It is a natural sugar substitute and in reality it is a sugar alcohol. It is available in crystalline forms and is used for preparing sugar garnishes as it is more stable than sugar and does not caramelise. Modern day artistic sugar showpieces are prepared with isomalt. It is also used commonly to make garnishes and one has to be careful to buy only food grade isomalt for edible purpose.
Sugar substitutes	These are chemically produced and have no nutrition value at all. Saccharin and cyclamates are best known and more commonly used in food items especially for people who are diabetic. They have a slightly bitter taste and are used as sweetener in low calorie or diet soft drinks.

baking soda. They are added to batters and doughs to help them rise. The action of moisture, heat or acidity (or a combination of the three) triggers a reaction with the raising agent to produce carbon dioxide gas, which gets trapped as it bubbles through the dough. When you put the particular product for cooking or when the dough cooks, the bubbles become set in the mixture, as the protein in the flour coagulates upon coming in contact with heat thus giving breads, cakes, scones, etc., a soft sponge like texture.

Raising agents can be classified into three categories:

- Chemical
- Biological
- Mechanical

Let us discuss these individually.

Chemical Raising Agents

Though the name is chemical, they exist in natural forms in nature and are a result of chemical reactions in a laboratory and hence, termed as chemical raising agents. Some of the common chemical raising agents used in bakery are given in Table 2.10.

Biological Raising Agents

It will be unfair to call them natural, as even the chemical raising agents occur in nature and are only combined to produce chemical raising agents. The biological raising agents occur naturally and are most commonly used in bakery and pastry. Let us discuss some of the common biological raising agents in Table 2.11.

Table 2.10 Common chemical raising agents

Name	Description	Storage
Baking powder	Baking powder is used as a raising agent for a number of doughs and batters such as cakes, scones, puddings, and biscuits. Baking powder is made from a combination of alkaline and acid substances. The composition of baking powder is usually of cream of tartar and bicarbonate of soda that react when they come in contact with moisture and warmth to produce carbon dioxide gas in the form of small bubbles. Baking powder is usually a single acting agent, which means that it reacts as soon as it comes in contact with any liquid. Hence, it is extremely important to work quickly once milk or water comes in contact with the dry ingredients so that the resulting carbon dioxide does not get a chance to escape.	One should always store baking powder in airtight containers free from any moisture because even a slight presence of moisture will start the reaction in it. We can also make our own baking powder by mixing half the quantity of bicarbonate of soda to cream of tartar.
Bicarbonate of soda	Also known as baking soda or cooking soda, it is used in a variety of dishes such as biscuits, batters, and pudding. As mentioned earlier, it can be mixed with cream of tartar to produce baking powder. It usually reacts in the presence of any acidic medium such as sour milk, buttermilk or orange juice, which causes carbon dioxide to release leading to the desired result in baked goods.	The shelf life of baking soda can easily be around 3 years if stored in a cool dry place. However, if it gets damp or moist it will lose its effectiveness. The best way of testing baking soda is to take a little powder and add lemon juice to it; it will immediately start to fizz which indicates that the powder has been stored properly as stale powder will not give you the desired result.
Ammonia bicarbonate	In olden times, it was extracted from the antlers of reindeers and was commonly known as *salt of the horn halts*. In Scandinavian countries, it is still used for preparing gingerbread and a few Christmas cookies. Though this compound produces crisp and light cookies, it also leaves an unpleasant aroma of ammonia, which is not preferred by everyone.	This must be stored in airtight containers with silica gel as this has affinity towards water and can turn moist and give an unpleasant smell.

Table 2.11 Common biological raising agents

Name	Description	Storage
Yeasts	It is a single cell fungus that feeds on simple sugars to produce carbon dioxide gas and alcohol. It is used to ferment fruits, grains, etc., to produce wine, beer, and other spirits. It is also used as a **leavening agent to produce a** wide range of bakery products. There are two major types of food yeasts which are commonly available, one is non-leavening yeast known as brewer's yeast while the other is leavening yeast known as baker's yeast.	Baker's yeast is sold in fresh blocks, which must be used within a few weeks of purchase, or as dried granules which can be stored up to a year. Fresh leavening yeast may also be sold as starter yeast, which is traditionally used to make sour dough or sweet breads known as starter breads.

(Contd)

Table 2.11 (Contd)

Name	Description	Storage
	Yeast is available in three forms: • Fresh yeast also known as compressed yeast • Dry yeast which is available in the form of granular dry powder • Instant yeast, which looks very similar to dry yeast	
Cream of tartar	Cream of tartar is fine white powder that is extracted from tartaric acid, which crystallizes in wine casks during the fermentation process of grapes. It is also known as potassium salt and has a number of uses such as: • It may be combined with bicarbonate of soda to produce baking powder. • It can also be added to increase stability and volume of whisked egg whites when making meringues or folded into cake batters. Adding a small amount to sugar syrups will prevent them from crystallising and hence, it is used in sugar work and decorations.	It should be stored in airtight containers, as it has the ability to absorb moisture.

Mechanical Raising Agents

As the name suggests, the act of introducing air into a product to make it light and have a good volume is called mechanical aeration. For example, whisking of cream or beating of butter in a machine will cause air to get trapped inside the product, which will eventually help in making the product light and fluffy. Let us discuss a few mechanical ways of raising bakery and pastry goods in Table 2.12.

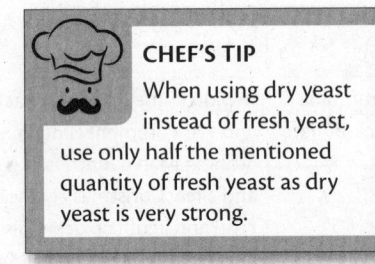

> **CHEF'S TIP**
> When using dry yeast instead of fresh yeast, use only half the mentioned quantity of fresh yeast as dry yeast is very strong.

Table 2.12 Mechanical ways of raising bakery and pastry goods

Name of way	Description	Examples
Sifting	Passing dry ingredients through a series of coarse or fine meshes to incorporate air.	Sifting of flour for cakes and biscuits, passing of boiled potatoes to prepare fluffy mashed potatoes
Rubbing-in	Using fingertips to mix fat into dry ingredients to incorporate air and help in creating a short texture in a baked good.	Rubbing of butter and flour to prepare short crust pastry
Creaming/Beating	Mixing fat with sugar to make a smooth paste, thereby creating bubbles of air, which help in raising the product. Creaming can be done with the help of palms of one's hands or it can be done mechanically in a machine fitted with a flat beater, in which case it can also be known as beating.	Creaming butter and sugar for muffins and tea cakes

Table 2.12 (Contd)

Name of way	Description	Examples
Steaming	Turning of the liquid in the product into gaseous state whilst steaming and thereby, raising the product making it light and airy.	Choux pastry is a good example of steaming where the liquid present in the choux paste makes the product rise
Whisking	Mixing of liquid ingredients such as cream or eggs causes the air to get trapped and create an increase in volume.	Whipping of cream or eggs to make cakes and sponges

CHOCOLATE

The origins of chocolate however were never consumed in the way that we do today. The plant was revered and prayed as Aztecs worshipped the tree *Theobroma Cacao* and the cocoa beans were only used for preparing a bitter beverage that was drunk as nectar of the holy plant.

For chefs working in the pastry kitchen, chocolate is the most sought after and used ingredient in the department. There are various reasons for it. The first and the foremost is the divine taste of the chocolate. Chefs believe one can never go wrong in a dessert that has chocolate as an ingredient. The second reason is the variety of ways in which this wonderful ingredient can be used in the confectionary world. One can create beverages, cakes, pastries, hot and cold desserts, chocolate confections, and also showpieces. Chocolate is commonly used for garnishing and decorating as chefs conjure up showpieces that are commonly displayed in restaurants, buffets, and pastry shops.

Processing of Chocolate

Cocoa beans, sugar, and vanilla are the three most essential ingredients that have always survived the tradition of chocolate making. Even with the advent of machines, the techniques of making chocolate still remain unchanged even after hundreds of years, when Spanish first made their sweet chocolate. The most suitable ingredient in pastry kitchen today is the chocolate and this is obtained from the magical cocoa beans that are obtained from the cocoa tree. The plantations of cocoa from Africa around the regions of Ivory Coast and Ghana are more popular with chocolate lovers. Let us read about the processing of this unique bean and see how it gets transformed into a chocolate. Processing of chocolate involves eight steps which are as follows:

1. Harvesting
2. Ripening and fermentation
3. Drying in sun
4. Selection and blending
5. Roasting and crushing the beans
6. Grinding
7. Conching
8. Tempering

Let us now study each of these steps in detail.

Harvesting

The cocoa pods on the trees resemble a green elongated oval shaped melon and when they ripen they change their colour from green to maroon to orange to yellow, which indicates that the plant is ready for harvesting. The pods are harvested very carefully so that the branches do not get damaged.

Ripening and Fermentation

After the beans are harvested, they are left to further ripen for a few days. The beans are split open and the seeds which are sticky and pulpous at this stage are collected in large containers or pits and left to ferment for a period of at least five to six days covered with banana leaves; this helps the flavour to develop as the bitterness subsides and the yellow creamy beans transform into light brown coloured beans. These beans are now called *cocoa seeds*.

Drying in Sun

After the seeds are obtained they are further dried in the sun for a period of six days. At this point they are frequently turned around so that they retain only a fraction of their moisture. The cocoa seeds after drying are known as *raw cocoa*.

Selection and Blending

At the chocolate factory, the cocoa seeds are inspected as per the quality checking points laid down by each factory and only the best seeds are selected to be transformed into chocolates. After the careful selection of the right seeds, they are cleaned of any stones, wooden barks, and other impurities. Careful blending of beans is done to produce the chocolates famous around the world. The blending helps to create just the right flavour, which is much desired for that particular kind of chocolate.

Roasting and Crushing the Beans

At this stage the seeds are roasted very carefully and for a brief time. The roasting of the seeds helps in many ways. It helps to reduce the moisture content in the seeds, so that it would be easier to crush them. The roasting would also aid in the removal of the shell around the kernel of the seeds. It also helps the beans to acquire a dark brown colour that is much desired to produce a dark coloured chocolate with the necessary aroma. The roasted seeds are then cooled and passed through a crushing machine, where the machine splits up the seeds and separates the exterior shell from the remaining cocoa bits that are now called *cocoa nibs*, which are ready to be processed further.

Grinding

The nibs are now transferred to grinding mills, where they are grounded into super fine texture. The grinding helps to generate heat due to the friction and the pressure created during the grinding process, the heat slowly melts the cocoa butter present in the mass, which results in a thick liquid mass also known as *cocoa liquor*. Cocoa liquor can be used for making chocolate and its by-products. The mass obtained after grinding is primarily made up of two components—cocoa powder and cocoa butter. To separate both of these, cocoa liquor is passed though hydraulic machines, where a certain amount of pressure is applied to extract the cocoa powder in the form of dry cakes and cocoa butter in melted form. The dry cakes can be crushed to obtain the cocoa powder that finds its application in production of many products in the pastry kitchen. The cocoa butter on the other hand is used for making chocolates and sometimes sold as it is for various uses in the pastry kitchen.

Conching

The next step to produce good quality chocolate is called conching. It is a process that is used for development of flavours in a chocolate. The cocoa liquor is put in large machines, which have powerful stirring mechanism that almost performs a kneading motion and paddles or rolls the chocolate mass. The movement of chocolate mass causes many physical and chemical reactions to take place that are much desirable for a good quality chocolate. The process of conching can last from a few hours to up to a few days depending on the type of chocolate. During this process, chocolate obtains a smooth and velvety texture. At the end of the process, cocoa butter and soy lecithin are added to the chocolate liquor.

Tempering

In this step, the conched chocolate is carefully brought to low temperatures by being stirred constantly. We would discuss the process of tempering in detail in the later part of this chapter. It is only after the tempering process, that the chocolate can be moulded into various shapes and blocks. Melted and tempered chocolate is shaped into drops often called as *callets*, small chips, or in sheets or blocks and then passed through the cooling tunnels before it can be packed for selling in the market and distributed to hotels and its users.

Types of Chocolate and its Uses

Chocolate is classified on various parameters. The most common ones being its colour, taste, and texture. The chocolate is also classified sometimes on the basis of the place of its origin. Two kinds of chocolates are commonly used in the pastry kitchen—Couverture and Compound.

Couverture

Couverture is the French term for covering chocolate. It is a high quality chocolate preferred by pastry chefs around the world for making chocolate confections. A chocolate should have minimum 32% of cocoa butter and at least 22% of cocoa solids or mass, to be labelled as couverture. Couverture is available in milk, dark, and white colour and can be used for dipping, moulding, coating, and making garnishes. It is always necessary to temper the couvertures before using them for any of the uses mentioned.

Compound

This is less expensive than couverture as it is a combination of various other ingredients apart from cocoa liquor and it uses hard tropical vegetable fats and oils such as palm kernel oil. Compound chocolate does not require tempering as it contains very little or no cocoa butter at all. It is used for enrobing chocolates and preparing garnishes as few people prefer it because of its easy to use approach. Unlike couvertures, the compound chocolate can just be melted and used for the same uses as the couverture would be used.

All the chocolates must be melted for most of the uses in pastry kitchen and it is very important to learn the art of melting a chocolate. Whilst melting the chocolate, one must keep the following points in mind.

- Ensure that the chocolate never comes in direct contact with the heat source. Always melt the chocolate on a double boiler.

- Whilst melting the chocolate on double boiler, ensure that the bowl which holds the chocolate is bigger than the pot containing water. This will ensure that the steam rising from the pot does not come in contact with the chocolate. Moisture is an enemy of the chocolate and even the tiniest amount of water will result in thickening of the chocolate.

- Make certain that the pot containing the chocolate does not directly touch the hot water in the pot below. This will result in spot heating of the chocolate and will impact the final product.

- Break the chocolate into small pieces for even melting and stir from time to time to ensure that the chocolate has melted evenly.

- Whilst melting in microwave, do not cook the chocolate; instead melt it by *spurt method*. Heat the chocolate only for 20 seconds. Stir and again heat it for 20 seconds. Repeat this process until the chocolate is completely melted. Though this method is not very conducive for melting chocolates, chefs use it to save time. It is difficult to regulate the temperature of the chocolate in microwave oven and sometimes because of overheating one can easily scorch the chocolate.

- Do not let the chocolate become contaminated by moisture as it will have a harmful effect on the chocolate by changing its consistency and gloss. Excess heat will make the chocolate separate, loss its gloss and become granular in texture.

Now that we have learnt to melt the chocolate, we will move onto the most important aspect of a chocolate known as *Tempering* or *Pre crystallization.* The untempered chocolate will not have the desired sheen and the snap that is required for relishing a chocolate. If the melted chocolate is moulded and allowed to set, it will become hard, but it will have a greyish mat finish colour, that is often referred to as *Bloom*. There can be two kinds of blooms which are:

Fat bloom The fat bloom occurs when the chocolate is heated so much that the butter separates out from the mixture and then when the chocolate sets it shows streaks that are discoloured and hazy.

Sugar bloom The sugar bloom occurs when the chocolate is allowed to cool too quickly or rapidly. The condensation on top of the chocolate dissolves the sugar present in the chocolate and when the moisture evaporates, it recrystallizes the sugar on the surface thereby giving a hazy and dull appearance to the finished chocolate product.

> **CHEF'S TIP**
> To melt chocolate, chop it into small pieces and place in a double jacketed container or bain-marie with water not exceeding 49°C and chocolate temperature not exceeding 40°C.

Because couverture contains cocoa butter it needs to be tempered prior to using. Tempering is a process where the couverture chocolate is melted to specific temperatures and then cooled to enable the cocoa butter fat crystals to bind together. As this process requires considerable skill, time, and effort, most establishments do not bother with it, preferring to use compound chocolate that only requires melting to be ready for use.

The temperatures in tempering process are very important. Tempering can thus also be defined as the process in which the chocolate is melted to 40°C and then cooled to 27°C and then the temperature is slowly brought back to working temperature. These temperatures vary for dark, milk, and white chocolates due to their composition—*dark chocolate* ±31 to 32°C; *milk chocolate* ±30 to 31°C; *white chocolate* ±28 to 29°C.

There are several ways of tempering or pre crystallising the chocolate. The choice of the method solely depends upon the user as all the methods give the same results. There are many methods of tempering a chocolate. Let us discuss them.

Tabling method In this method of tempering, chocolate is melted to 40°C until smooth. Then two thirds of the chocolate is poured on to the marble slab and with a spatula, it is scraped and moved constantly. One would notice that the chocolate starts to thicken and this means that the stable crystals are forming. The temperature of the chocolate at this stage would be roughly 27°C.

The third step is to mix this chocolate with the remaining one third chocolate at 40°C. The chocolate is now brought to the working temperature. Also whilst mixing the chocolate, never use a wire whisk as we do not want to incorporate any air bubbles in the chocolate. Whilst moulding the chocolate, these bubbles will burst and would leave a hole in the figures.

Injection method This method is also known as seeding method or grafting method. In this method, 75% of the chocolate is melted to 40°C and brought down to 2°C more than the working temperature. For example, if the working temperature for dark chocolate is 32°C, then it is cooled to 34°C and 25%

of the grated chocolate is added to the mixture and stirred until the temperature comes down to the working temperature.

Microwave method Though not a preferred method by professional chefs, it comes in handy whilst tempering small quantities of chocolate instantly. In this method, the chocolate is heated in the microwave in spurts. After every 15-20 seconds, the chocolate is mixed and heated again to a stage where a small amount of chocolate is still hard and not melted. Then it is taken out from the microwave and continued to be stirred until the chocolate completely melts.

Machine method Tempering machines are available in the market with different capacities. The machine automatically melts the chocolate stirring it constantly so that it melts evenly. The temperature settings in the machine cool the chocolate to the set temperature and heat it again to the working temperature which varies for different kinds of covertures.

> **CHEF'S TIP**
> To check if the chocolate is tempered, dip the point of the knife in the chocolate. If the chocolate sets with a shine within three to four minutes, then it is an indication that it is tempered.

Uses of Chocolate

Chocolate as we have said before can be used in many ways.

- It can be piped in different designs directly onto sweets, cakes, and petit fours or piped into silicon or greaseproof paper to make decorative chocolate garnishes; some chocolates may need to be thickened for piping purposes. Spirits, liquors, and glycerine are recommended for such uses. Melt the chocolate and add a few drops at a time until it reaches the desired viscosity. Thinly spread chocolate can be cut into a variety of shapes and used for decorative purposes.

- Coating is another commonly used feature whilst working with chocolates. Chocolate can be used to cover a cake, so that the entire sides and top is coated with chocolate. The chocolate needs to be mixed together with dairy cream that has been brought to a boil and allowed to set to firm paste. This product is called truffle. Cakes and pastries are coated with melted chocolate truffle. Truffle can also be used for piping purposes or mixed with whipped cream and used as a filling for cakes, pastries, and a variety of other desserts.

- Moulding is a technique where the chocolate is poured into various kinds of moulds to give it a particular shape and size. Many chocolate showpieces such as Easter eggs and Christmas figures are commonly made by pouring the chocolate into a mould and allowing it to set.

- Enrobing is a kind of process applied to create an array of enrobed chocolates that are sold in high end pastry shops and outlets. The procedure is similar to coating. Here the truffle or flavoured ganache is set, cut into desired shapes and coated with tempered chocolate and garnished as bite size chocolate preparations.

- Chocolate is the most versatile pastry ingredient that is used for preparing garnishes, which add a whole new dimension to the pastry products. Due to its unique properties, the chocolate is the most preferred garnish used by pastry chefs around the world. The ability to colour the white chocolate into interesting shades, makes it worthwhile to use for garnishes and creating chocolate showpieces. Colouring a chocolate is an art. Since water is the biggest enemy of a chocolate, one cannot use liquid colours to colour the chocolate. Powder colours are first dissolved in small amounts of cocoa butter and then added to the melted chocolate. There are also metallic colours available that can be brushed over the chocolate to give it a metallic finish. The metallic colours can be applied in their dry form or they can be mixed with cocoa powder and brushed onto the prepared chocolate garnish.

SUMMARY

It is important to understand the various kinds of commodities used in pastry and bakery and the ways in which they can be used to make a versatile product. In this chapter, we discussed about the structure of wheat grain and saw that the wheat grain is made up of 85% endosperm from where the refined flour is milled. The rest of the grain comprises of 13% of bran and 3% of germ.

The entire wholewheat grain is milled to obtain wholemeal flour, which is healthier as it contains fibres and proteins in the germ. From one wheat grain we can obtain various kinds of flours and by-products.

Apart from the by-products of wheat, we also discussed various types of flours obtained from wheat grain that are used in cooking, especially to produce a variety of breads. Keeping in mind the people who have special dietary requirements such as allergies to gluten or like in India people observe fasts on some religious occasions wherein they do not eat flour that contains gluten, we have also discussed a variety of flours which are gluten free.

We also discussed about a range of fats and oils used in bakery and pastry. Though the usage of oil in pastry kitchen is limited to frying but fats such as butter, coco butter, and margarine are used for a range of applications resulting in different flavours and textures in a product. In this section, we discussed the role of butter and its uses.

Milk, cream, and cheese are one of the most popular dairy products used in preparation of pastry products. Various kinds of creams are used in pastry applications, for cooking or as a base for making pastes and sauces and for whipping that gives volume and texture to a dessert. These days we also have imitation creams that are made from vegetable oils. Cheese also finds a unique place in the pastry kitchen. Though many types of cheeses can be used in bread making, but to create some classical desserts, there are unique cream cheeses.

We also discussed about the types of eggs and their uses in pastry kitchen. Egg is the most widely used ingredient in bakery and we understood its uses in making of meringues.

We also discussed the range of sweeteners used in pastry kitchen and the typical usage of each sweetener in a pastry product. Molasses, treacle, liquid glucose, isomalt, and invert sugars are carefully selected and used in pastry applications for creating a unique experience.

Various types of raising agents that aerate the product chemically and naturally have also been discussed in the chapter. Some of these aerating agents are natural like yeasts and form the basis of many breads and cookies.

One of the most special contributions to the pastry kitchen—the chocolate has also been discussed in detail in the last section of the chapter. The ways to select a chocolate and how to melt and temper it for various pastry applications has been explained in this section.

KEY TERMS

Air cell The air pocket at the large end of the shell

Albumen Protein found in the white of an egg

Atta Indian name for wholemeal flour

Blinis A small thick pancake made from buckwheat flour

Bulgur Cracked wheat used in Middle Eastern countries

Cake flour Weak flour used in cakes

Centrifugal force Spinning of liquids in a machine which allows the two liquids of different densities to separate from one another

Chalazae Fibrous strands that join the yolk and the white together

Charcuterie French for section in kitchen which deals in cold meat preparations such as sausages and salamis. It usually comprises of pork products

Clarifying A procedure usually used for butter, where it is melted to get rid of milk solids, thereby making it stable to cook

Coagulation Firming up of proteins upon application of heat

Cockle cylinder A machine in milling process that separates broken wheat particles from the whole grain

Combinatory A machine in milling process that separates stones from grains

Confit Stewing of duck or goose in pork fat or duck fat to produce soft textured meat

Cooking cream Cream that can be boiled and hence used in cooking

Crackling The crisp piece of meat or skin left behind after the meat has been rendered

Diastatic flour Flour that contains a small amount of natural malt. This process is also known as malting

Emery scorer Machine in the milling process that cleans the surface of the wheat grain

Farina Flour which is ground coarse and is usually of a polished grain

Gluten A protein obtained when the wheat flour is kneaded with water

Hydrogenation Saturating the oils with hydrogen atom

Invert sugar A sugar that has been altered chemically with addition of an acid, this does not let the sugar to crystallize easily

Kuttu ka atta Indian name for buckwheat flour

Leavening agents Products used in aerating a baked good. It can be natural like yeasts or chemicals like baking powder and cooking soda

Lecithin Protein found in the yolk of an egg

Lipid Scientific term for fats and oils

Makki ki roti Popular North Indian bread made from corn meal

Margarine Artificially saturated vegetable oils; sometimes it may also contain animal fats

Meringues Stiffly beaten egg whites with castor sugar to resemble whipped cream. It can be used as a base for desserts or dried in oven and used as garnish

Milling Grinding of a commodity to yield flours of different textures

New York baked cheesecake Baked cheesecake that utilizes Philadelphia cream cheese in the recipe

Pasteurization Heating of milk or dairy products to kill most of the harmful bacteria

Quark cheese Cream cheese from Germany, often used in making baked and chilled cheesecakes

Rendering Separating fats from the muscle or skin by applying low heat

Salts of horn Natural product obtained from the antlers of reindeer

Scones English preparation of self-rising flour and milk. It is served during afternoon tea

Sicilian cassata Italian dessert made with ricotta cheese

Soft flour Another name for weak flour

Strong flour Flour having high amount of gluten

Tiramisu Coffee flavoured Italian dessert made with mascarpone cheese

Trans fats Oils that are saturated artificially

Vitelline A clear seal that holds the egg yolk

WAC Water absorption capacity is the capacity of the flour to absorb water when making dough

Weak flour Flour which is low in gluten content

OBJECTIVE TYPE QUESTIONS

1. List down the most common ingredients used in bakery and confectionary.
2. What are the major components of wheat grain?
3. List down at least five by-products obtained from the wheat grain.
4. What is gluten and how is it formed?
5. How does gluten in the flour help us to bake products?
6. List and describe at least five types of flour obtained from wheat.
7. List down at least five types of flour that can be used for making gluten free breads.
8. What are raising agents and what is their role in cooking?
9. Name at least one natural raising agent and two chemical raising agents.

10. What care should be taken whilst using dry yeast instead of fresh yeast?
11. Define lipids and give one major difference between oils and fats.
12. Name two oils that are solid at room temperature.
13. What is the difference between dehydrated milk and dried milk solids?
14. Name at least three types of creams used in cooking and pastry.
15. Name the various kinds of sweeteners used in confectionary.
16. What is the difference between corn syrup and golden syrup?
17. How would you differentiate between molasses and treacle?
18. What are invert sugars and what are its uses?
19. Name three cheeses that are used for preparing desserts.
20. What is a couverture?

ESSAY TYPE QUESTIONS

1. Draw and label the structure of wheat.
2. What are the various types of dairy products used in the kitchen and what are the specific uses of each?
3. Explain the structure of egg and its uses in kitchen.
4. Write a short note on meringue, its types and uses.
5. What does tempering of chocolate mean and what are the different methods of tempering?

ACTIVITY

1. In groups, make the recipe of bread by just altering the different types of flours such as rye, buckwheat, wholemeal, rice flour, maize flour, and barley flour. Compare the results and write down your findings in the following table.
2. In groups of 3-4, try to melt and temper a dark chocolate with all the methods mentioned in the chapter and compare the results.
3. Make a recipe of pound cake and alter it by adding at least five different types of sweeteners available. Compare the results and understand the effects of various sweeteners on the cake.

Flour	Taste	Texture	Crumbs	Weight	Volume

3 Techniques in Bakery and Pastry

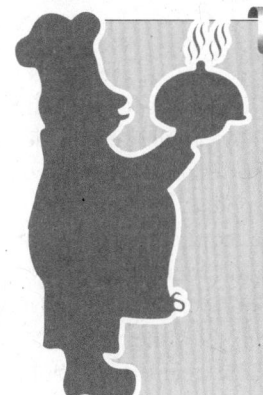

LEARNING OBJECTIVES

After reading this chapter, you should be able to
- understand the pastry and bakery department
- differentiate between the various sections of the pastry kitchen
- remember the terms associated with day to day pastry and bakery operations
- memorise the hierarchy of the department and reporting structure
- know the basic layout of the pastry kitchen and understand its importance
- weigh and scale ingredients as per the required recipe
- identify the large equipment and machinery used in the pastry department

INTRODUCTION

In the last chapter, we learnt about various kinds of commodities used in pastry kitchen and read about many terms such as whisking, lamination, leavening with regards to the processing of ingredients. Unlike Western or Indian cooking, bakery and pastry rely a lot on measurements of recipes as well as the processes used to make a product. It is therefore very important to understand what these processes mean and how should they be carried out most effectively to create a standard product of the highest quality. In the forthcoming chapters, we will learn how to prepare the basic recipes for cakes, creams, and breads, but before we do that it is imperative to understand the various techniques involved in making of pastry and various other products. Most of these techniques are basically done for aeration of the product to make it lighter and softer.

The eating qualities and appearance of baked goods depend very much on the lightness of the products. To achieve aeration, we use leavening agents. They may be physical, chemical or biological and are used individually or in combination to incorporate steam, gas or air cells into the mixtures.

Physical Air and steam are incorporated into mixtures in a specific way, involving physical or mechanical action. Air is introduced into the mixture by a variety of methods, such as *sifting* dry ingredients, *creaming* of fats and sugar, and *whisking* of eggs and sugar.

Steam is a leavening agent found in all baked products. For example, in puff paste, the *laminated* fat incorporated into the paste in layers melts during baking, producing some steam which lifts the layers.

Chemical Baking powder, baking soda, ammonia, etc., are the chemical leavening agents. When moistened and heated, they react to produce carbon dioxide gas. To test whether baking powder is still active, stir some powder in warm water. If it gives off bubbles freely, it is active.

Biological Yeast is a biological leavening agent. Refer to chapter on breads for more information on yeast.

In chapter 2, we discussed about the various types of raising agents which were both biological and chemical. Let us discuss in the following section the various techniques used in preparing bread and then we will discuss the techniques related to pastry making.

TECHNIQUES OF PREPARING BREAD

Several techniques are involved in preparing bread. Let us take a look at some of such techniques in this section.

Sifting

Sifting is associated with flours. The flour is put into the drum sieve and shaken so that it sifts from the small meshes. This is done to incorporate air into the flour and also to get rid of any physical impurities present in it. Sifting also helps to mix certain ingredients in the powder form. For example, mixing of raising agents with flour or sifting cocoa powder and flour for chocolate flavoured sponge. There are drum sieves of various mesh sizes and one must choose the most appropriate one for the required purpose. For example, whilst sifting icing sugar, one would need a drum sieve of finest mesh size to sift off powder from any tiny granular sugar present in the icing sugar, but whilst sifting wholewheat flour, we do not want to use a finer mesh, because we do not wish to separate the goodness of bran present in the same.

In larger kitchen operations, there are mechanical flour sieves that can sift large quantities of flour in very less time.

Autolysis

The word autolysis used in bread making is very different to its biological connotation. In bread making, the word autolysis is derived from the French word *autolyse*, which refers to dough that is allowed to rest in cooler temperatures for a considerable amount of time. This procedure is very important for good bread making as it reduces the kneading time of the dough. When the dough is kneaded for a longer period of time, it undergoes exposure to the atmospheric oxygen which in turn, oxidises or bleaches the enzymes present in flour, thereby discolouring the crumb texture of the bread.

To make an autolyse, combine the flour and water mentioned in the recipe and knead it for 2-3 minutes or until the dough is formed. Now cover the dough and allow it to chill in refrigerator for a minimum of 30 minutes to a maximum of 12 hours. This process makes the dough rest and helps to incorporate other ingredients easily. It also helps the dough to be shaped easily thereby improving the overall structure of the bread.

Kneading

In simple and basic terms, kneading is a mechanical process where dry ingredients such as flour are mixed with water to form dough. Formation of dough through the process of kneading is skilful work and one needs to understand the implications of the same. Improper kneading can result in a poor quality product and therefore, it is important to understand the various kinds of kneading methods. There are usually three most common types of kneading methods.

Short kneading method In this method, the ingredients are mixed for a very short period of time. This is done for a product that needs short texture for example, cookies and tarts.

Improved kneading method In this method, the dough is kneaded at slow to moderate speed to develop the flavours in it and to develop the gluten slowly, thereby improving the texture of the bread.

Intense kneading method As this method suggests, the dough is mixed for a considerable amount of time. In some cases, the dough is kneaded at high speed to develop elasticity and gluten for enriched dough such as brioche or doughnuts.

When the dough is kneaded for long duration of time, the temperature in the dough increases due to friction and this has to be watched carefully as the temperature of the dough should not go beyond 25°C because the yeast will start its work. In such cases, a baker often uses ice to make the dough. Thus, it keeps the fermentation activity of yeast at an ideal rate for gluten ripening. The quantity used will vary depending upon the time of kneading of the dough or the friction factor, and the dough temperature required. Ice used must be in the form of flaked ice so that it is evenly distributed in the bread dough and causes an even cooling of the dough. It can be safely said that 5 kg of ice will be equivalent to 4 litres of water.

One must be careful whilst kneading the dough. Many dough mixers have two speeds such as slow and high speed to knead the dough. Many bread recipes call for kneading the dough at slow speed for a couple of minutes and then increasing the speed to high. Usually, the dough is kneaded until a film is formed when it is stretched. This is also known as *windscreen test*.

Prooving

Also known as proofing, it is a process whereby the yeast is allowed to react with sugars present in the flour to produce carbon dioxide and alcohol. The CO_2 thus produced, helps the dough to rise in volume until it proves to at least double in size. The gases thus released help to ferment the dough and distribute uniformly. The ideal temperature for proving is 32°C. Proving is done in three stages. One is after kneading called *first proving* and the second is after *knock back* and hence, called *intermediate proving* and the *final proving* is done after shaping the bread. So we can say that fermentation is done for the following reasons.

- It helps in production of carbon dioxide gas which aerates the dough.
- It helps to condition the dough. This is through the enzymatic action due to reduction of natural sugars for assimilation by yeast.
- It helps to reduce the proteins to simpler nitrogenous compounds for growth and development of the yeast.
- The enzymes are active during fermentation. The sugars are broken down to release heat, which causes the temperature of the dough to rise. This rise can be controlled by the speed of fermentation and the storage temperature.

We will learn more about bread production in the next chapter.

Shaping

Divided pieces of dough are shaped in the form of loaf or rolls. It should be done on a sparingly floured surface, the dough should be handled gently and should be placed for final proving. After a few minutes of resting, the dough soon reaches its optimum ripening. Thus, the dough is scaled and then shaped. As the dough gets deflated during knock back, it has to be carefully manipulated again since it becomes more resilient after knock back. The dough is rested slightly before shaping to allow for shaping without pressure. This final moulding is essential as the shape of the product and the crumb structure are affected. This step is also known as panning—which means to shape the bread and put in a pan.

There are many shapes that a bread can be shaped into, the most common ones are round balls or ovals but there are more unique shapes such as plaits or knots. Some of these are shown in Fig. 3.1.

The plaited breads are known as *Challahs* and there could be a 3 plait challah or even a 6 plait challah. These breads add to the decorative bread displays. Figure 3.2 shows the different shapes of challahs illustrated with step by step approach of making them.

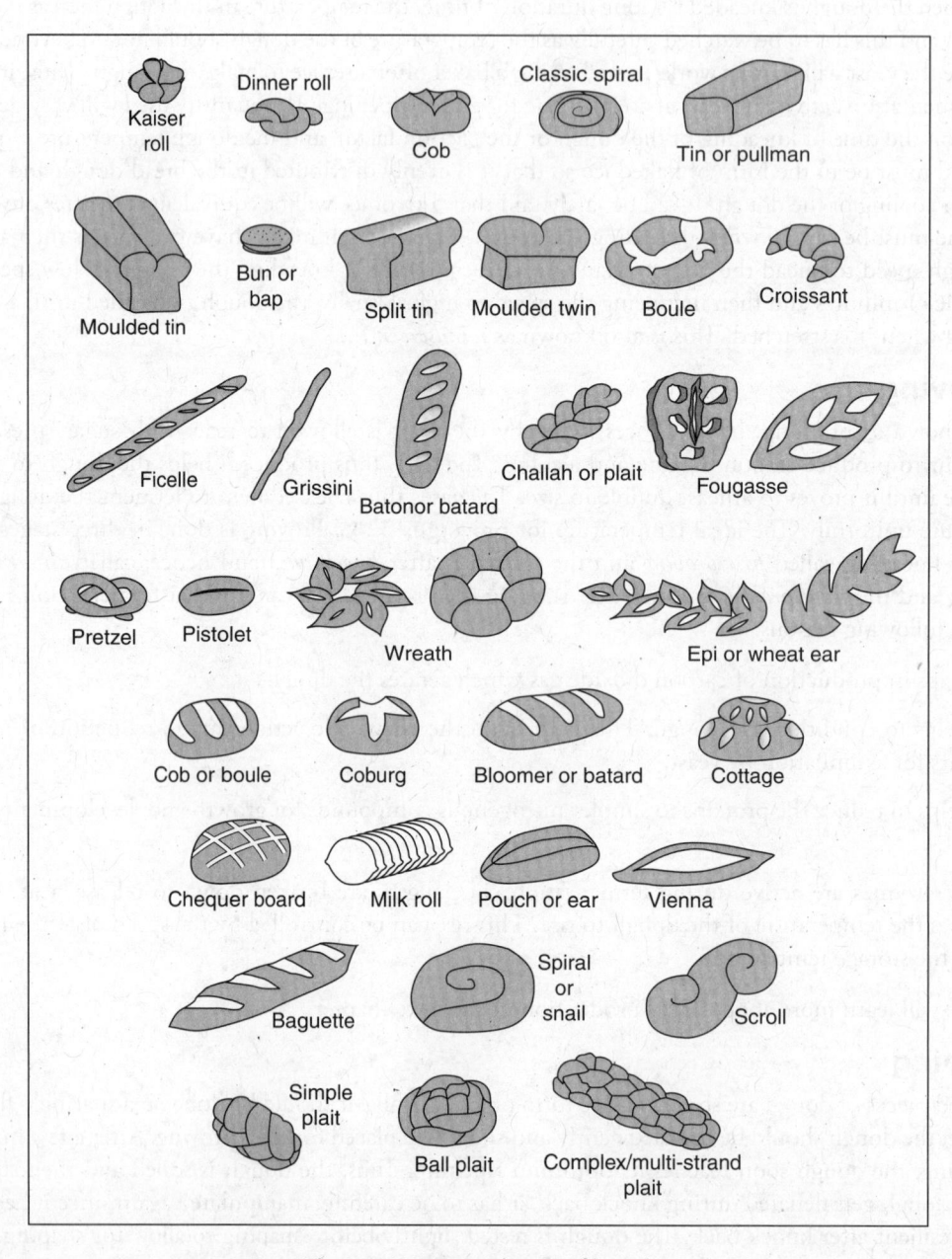

Fig. 3.1 Common shapes of bread

(a) Four-strand challah

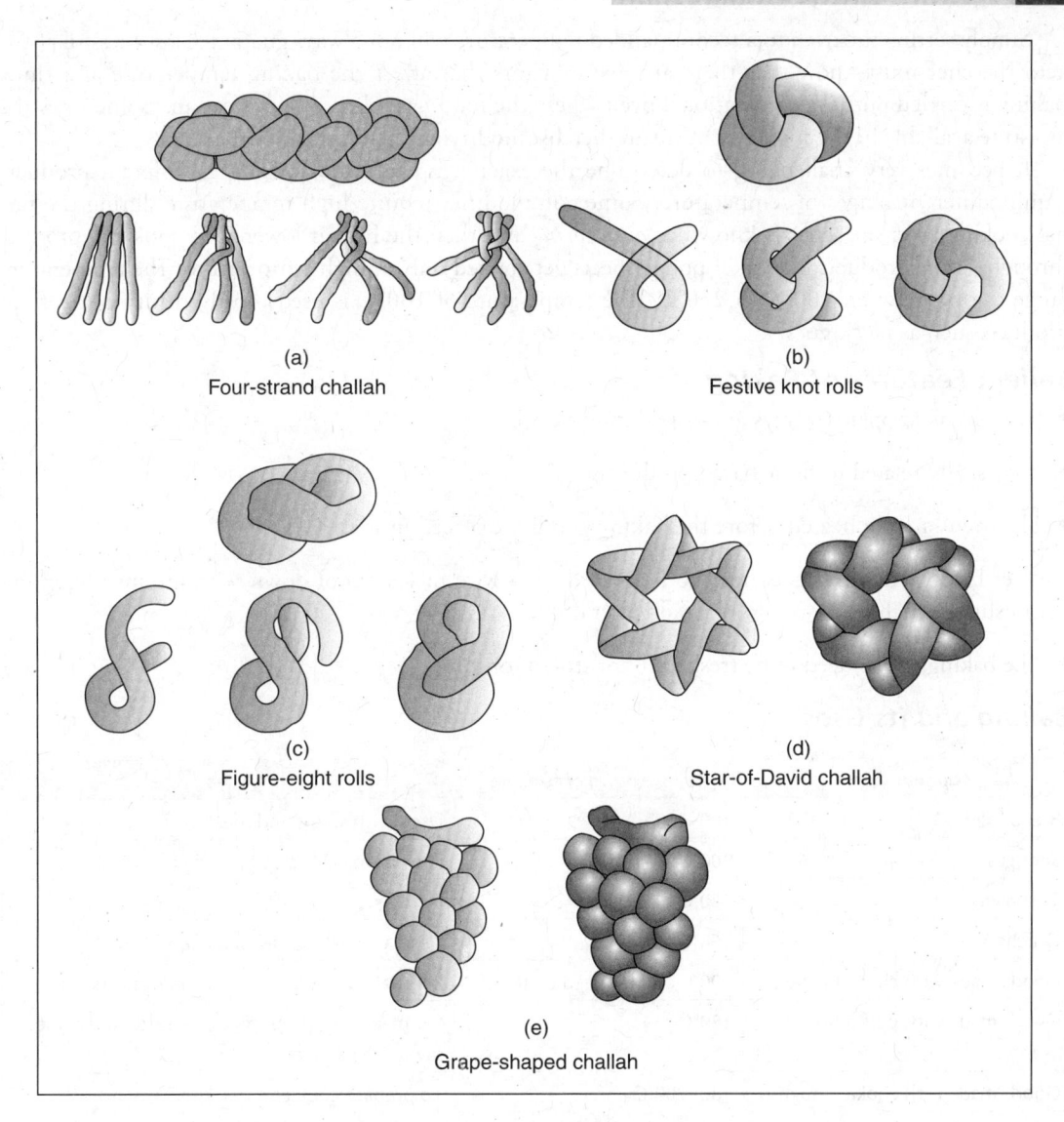

(b) Festive knot rolls

(c) Figure-eight rolls

(d) Star-of-David challah

(e) Grape-shaped challah

Fig. 3.2 Different shapes of challah

Baking

Baking is a cooking principle that is applied only to bakery, confectionary, and patisserie, which are essentially flour-based products. There are few exceptions as some potatoes are baked in their skins and sometimes pastas are also baked. Baking is synonymous to oven and one has to always use the oven to accomplish baking. It is important to have an understanding of the commodities, working terminologies, and types of aeration in a product, but all this knowledge will be futile if we do not understand the nuances of baking. Good and correct baking techniques yield a quality product thereby increasing the productivity of the staff and ensuring good profits for the organisation.

Simply setting the oven to a recommended temperature will not always guarantee a successful product. The chef must know that there are many factors that affect the baking temperature and time. Baking is carried out in a conventional oven where the food is cooked by dry heat and sometimes the moisture available in the food acts as steam thereby, modifying the dry heat of the oven.

It becomes very challenging to determine the exact temperature of baking as different products require different ranges of temperature. Some commodities require high temperature during the initial cooking to create what is known as *oven spring* and then the heat is lowered to cook the product through. Some products like cake sponge sheets get cooked only at high temperature. The temperature range can be between 100°C to 250°C. The temperature of 100°C is used mostly to dry out certain products such as meringues.

Salient Features of Baking

- Food is baked open on trays and is seldom covered.

- It is usually related to flour-based products.

- The ovens are pre heated before the baking goods are placed inside.

- After baking, the products need to be placed on a wire rack to cool down without absorbing any moisture, which could result in mould later on.

- The baking goods need to be fresh and not stored for long.

Baking and its Uses

Commodity	Temperature of cooking	Uses
Bread rolls	180–200°C	Used with soups and meals
Sponges	200°C	For making cakes and pastries
Turnovers	180°C	Used as snacks
Quiches	160°C	Used as snack or main course
Goods made with choux paste	200°C and reduced to 180°C	For making pastries, cakes, and desserts
Goods made with puff pastry	180°C	For making pastries, cakes, desserts, and some savoury products
Goods made with cookie dough	180–200°C	To prepare cookies, tarts, and flans
Fruits	180°C	Baked apples, pears, and quinces are often baked and used as dessert

Scoring

This term usually refers to making a slit in the hand moulded bread loaf with a sharp knife or a blade. The scoring of a bread helps it to expand to a good volume and also helps the bread to expand in the desired direction during the oven spring. Making a slash or slit on bread is an art and one must do it with confidence and ease. Hesitation can hamper a clean slit as it will stop your hand movements resulting in an uneven scoring, which will impact the volume of the bread.

The French bakers use a sharp blade called *lame* for this purpose and it is important to use a very sharp blade to score bread. The bread is usually scored right before baking.

TECHNIQUES RELATED TO PASTRY MAKING

Pastry making is all about right techniques and processes. Let us discuss a few of the most commonly used techniques whilst preparing pastry products or things related to preparation of bakery or pastry goods.

Creaming

Creaming is a method of mixing foods with high fat content in order to incorporate air and make the mixture lighter. Mixing may be either mechanical or manual. There are three attachments of dough mixers—balloon whisk, flat paddle, and dough hook. Creaming is always done using a flat paddle. Creaming refers to beating butter and sugar together to incorporate air and make it light and fluffy. The type of sugar used will depend upon the usage of the final product. For making buttercream that will be eventually used for icing cakes, one would use icing sugar and the one used for sponge will have castor sugar. Following are certain factors that need to be kept in mind whilst creaming.

- Care should be taken whilst choosing the equipment for creaming. One should always use stainless steel as by using aluminium the colour of the butter and sugar deteriorates and becomes grey.
- Take care not to over-cream as the final product might not be able to hold the volume resulting in the collapse of the cake.
- Fats used must be soft and not oily.
- Use a bowl large enough for rapid movement of the paddle as creaming is always done at high speed.

Whisking

Whisking or whipping is a method very similar to creaming. It uses fast movement to incorporate maximum air into liquid ingredients, achieving foam. Like creaming, whisking can also be done mechanically or manually in a suitable bowl. Once the mixture has started to foam, whisking needs to be continuous until the desired stage has been reached. Usually, this stage is referred to as *Ribbon stage* as the emulsion when lifted and dropped falls like ribbons. When whisking egg whites, make sure there is no egg yolk present, since yolks contain fat, and the presence of fat hinders the formation of meringue. The equipment you use must also be fat-free. Egg whites at room temperature will whisk to a foam quicker and produce a greater volume than those straight from the refrigerator, if an acid such as lemon juice is added, it will help stabilise the foam.

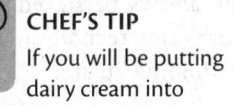

> **CHEF'S TIP**
> If you will be putting dairy cream into a piping bag, do not whip it too much, or the extra manipulation and squeezing in the bag can turn the cream into butter.

Egg white foam starts to break down when it is whisked past the medium-firm peak stage. If it is whisked too much, and then used in cooking, to make poached meringue quenelles for example, the whole structure will collapse because the bubbles have expanded too much.

For the best results when whisking dairy cream, use cream that is old from the refrigerator and a cold bowl. Most of the basic sponges are made by this method.

Rubbing-in

The rubbing-in method is generally used for making short or sweet pastry. The product containing fat and flour is said to be short when it snaps off or crumbles when pressed. First the fat is cut into small pieces. Then, using one's fingertips, the pieces of fat are rubbed into the flour, all the time lifting the ingredients and allowing them to fall back into the bowl. The fat will reduce to small particles the size of breadcrumbs, each with its own coating of flour.

The purpose of rubbing-in is to make a lighter pastry. During baking, the moisture from the fat becomes steam which makes the pastry expand; for best results, all the ingredients should be cold, with liquid ingredients added in all at once to the flour and fat mixture. Do not over-mix as this will toughen the pastry; combine sufficiently to bind all the ingredients. Cover and rest the pastry in the refrigerator before using it.

The other method to make a short pastry is to cut the butter into 1 cm dices and mix with flour. Then roll both the things with a rolling pin until the butter forms flakes. Then combine the dough very lightly and add the required amount of cold water to form into light dough. Over kneading will result in stretchy dough which will hamper the shortening effect of the flour. Rubbing-in is done for the following reasons.

- Fat and flour are rubbed together to create a homogeneous mixture without development of gluten.
- The aim is to reduce the fat to breadcrumb-size particles.
- The fat particles melt during baking, giving off steam which makes the pastry expand and rise.

Folding-in

This is a method of combining other ingredients into the aerated mixture so that there is little reduction in lightness or volume. This is achieved by turning the mixture over gently, using a large spoon or your hand while adding the other ingredients gradually. The mixture must be lifted and folded over gently. Make sure you reach to the bottom of the bowl. Take care not to over mix the mixture. This is also known as *cutting and folding method*. When folding in mixtures with different consistencies (for example, adding whisked egg white to cake batter), soften the heavier mixture first by adding a portion of the softer mixture. Then fold in the rest of the soft mixture. Dry ingredients should always be sieved and added gradually, ensuring they are dispersed evenly throughout the mixture. This technique is very crucial for basic fatless sponge. Certain factors to be kept in mind whilst folding-in are:

- Dry ingredients are added to a creamed or whisked mixture.
- Add gradually and turn gently with open hands and fingers so as to disturb the air bubbles as little as possible.
- One can always fold whilst another person can help him to add the sifted dry ingredients in a continuous flow.
- Proficient chefs can also mix in the dough mixer itself, but just keep in mind that the machine is on the lowest speed possible and the batter should not over mix.

Docking

This means making small holes in pastry goods to allow steam to escape during the baking process. Docking prevents the pastry to puff up which results in poor shape. Docking is also used to avoid shrinkage of the pastry whilst baking.

One can use a docker—which is a tool with spikes all over and used specifically for the purpose of docking or a fork.

Blind Baking

This is the process of baking empty pastry shells that would eventually be used for any filling to make pies or tarts. Pastry moulds are lined with a short crust pastry or sweet paste and a greaseproof paper is placed on top of the pastry and filled with dried beans or rice. This is done to prevent the pastry from either rising, developing bubbles or shrinking during baking. The pastry may be baked half done or completely done according to the recipe requirements. If you want to bake the pastry completely through, remove the paper and beans when the pastry edges are set and lightly browned so that the base can also colour.

> **CHEF'S TIP**
> Whilst putting the rolled pastry on the pastry mould, do not stretch the pastry; let it fall down on its own as the stretched gluten in the pastry will try to come back thereby, creating shrinkage in the pastry.

Pinning or Rolling

Rolling dough or pastry to the thickness and size required is a very important process. You can use a rolling pin or a pastry brake—a roller-type machine turned either by hand or electric motor. It is commonly known as dough sheeter. Best results are achieved when pastry is rolled out on a smooth, cool surface. Avoid over handling the pastry by:

- Preparing the pastry into the shape you want before rolling,
- Rolling out only the amount of pastry you want for immediate use.

To roll out dough or pastry, start from the centre. First roll upwards, then downwards, through the centre to the bottom. Rotate the dough a quarter turn and roll again. Repeat the process, rolling and turning until you reach the required thickness, you should occasionally lightly dust with flour or cornflour to prevent the dough or pastry from sticking. What you use for dusting will depend on the type of dough or pastry you are rolling, and what it will be used for. During rolling, take care to maintain an even thickness. Maintain an even pressure on the pin. Adjust your pressure to suit the type of dough or pastry being rolled.

Never stretch the pastry, as this will cause it to shrink and lose its shape during cooking.

Piping

This is the process of forcing and piping various mixtures through a piping bag. The bag may be fitted with a piping nozzle to achieve certain decorative effects. Before you fill a bag, fit a nozzle if you want one. If the mixture you will be using has runny consistency, twist the bottom of the bag just above the nozzle, and push it firmly into the nozzle. This will prevent the mixture from running out while you are filling the bag. Also whilst filling the bag, fold the top of the bag inside out to form a cuff, which will prevent the mixture from spilling onto the outside of the bag. With one hand inside the cuff, fill the bag using an appropriate spoon or scraper. Avoid trapping air in the mixture. Do not overfill the bag, or you will be in trouble when you start squeezing to do the piping. Twist the top of the bag to close it, making sure it is tightly filled with the mixture.

Hold the bag so that it lies in the palm of your hand, holding it closed with your index finger and thumb. Apply an even

> **CHEF'S TIP**
> Remember that if you are piping with cream, it is best not to use large quantities, because the manipulation and forcing through a nozzle can turn it into butter.
> For writing with a piping bag, make a small piping bag with butter paper and make sure the piping mixture is free of any lumps.

pressure with your remaining fingers, to force the mixture from the bag. Use your other hand only as a guide and allow the mixture to drop onto the surface you are decorating.

Laminating

Laminating is the word used to describe the incorporation of fat between the layers of dough and this is the base of preparing croissants and puff pastry. The chilled fat block is placed between the rolled dough and is encased within the dough. It is then rolled out into a long rectangular shape and folded like a handkerchief. It is chilled and rolled out again. We shall discuss these methods in detail, when we discuss about laminated pastries in later chapters.

Some of the common products that are made in pastry kitchen using laminated dough are croissant, Danish pastry, turnovers, etc.

Icing

Icing is the term used for cakes and pastries only. The basic sponge is sliced horizontally and then layered with flavoured sugar syrup and desired filling. The cake is then covered with the same filling or whipped cream and decorated and garnished with fruits, etc. This whole process is known as *Icing* and we would discuss the various types of fillings that can be used for icing the cakes in forthcoming chapters. Cakes are iced on a cake turn table also known as *Lazy Suzanne* and a flat palette knife is used for spreading the icing on the cake.

SUMMARY

This chapter discusses a range of techniques used in bakery and pastry. These terminologies are often used in the methods of preparation of the products made in bakery and it is important for the students to be aware of these. We understood that whilst baking a product rises in volume due to aeration, which can be incorporated by mechanical means, that is, by whisking or beating thereby making the product light and airy. The aeration can also be caused by chemical means such as by using leavening agents or simply through biological process by adding yeast.

We talked about terms such as autolysis which is absorption of water by the flour, kneading and its types and what are the factors to be kept in mind whilst kneading the dough. We also learnt the art of proving, shaping, scoring, and baking the bread.

In later part of the chapter, we discussed techniques related to pastry making such as whipping, creaming, rubbing-in, folding-in, docking, blind baking, pinning, piping, laminating, and icing. Though some techniques like laminating and icing will be discussed in the chapters to come, the author hopes that you will not only learn these techniques theoretically, but also practice them in kitchen and record your observations.

KEY TERMS

Autolysis Allowing the dough to rest in cool temperature for at least half an hour

Blind baking Baking a short crust or a sweet paste tart shell without any filling

Challah Plaited bread with three or more plaits

Creaming Mechanical aeration by mixing fat and/or sugar to a fluffy mass

Docking Making small holes in pastry goods to allow the steam to escape during the baking process

Folding-in Method of combining other ingredients into the aerated mixture so that there is little reduction in lightness or volume

Improved kneading Mixing flour and water at slow speed for a longer time

Knock back Degassing the dough after it has proved for the first time

Lame A thin and sharp blade used for scoring bread

Lazy Suzanne Another name for cake turn table

Oven spring The initial rise in volume of the product when put in oven at a high temperature

Panning Shaping the bread and putting in a mould

Pinning Another term for rolling with a rolling pin

Rubbing-in Mixing fat with dry ingredients with fingertips to resemble a bread crumb texture

Scoring Making a slit on the surface of the bread with a sharp blade

Sheeting Rolling the dough to desired thickness using a dough sheeter

Short kneading Mixing flour and water for a short time

Sifting Sieving a powdered ingredient from a sieve to separate impurities

Turnovers Savoury or sweet products made with puff pastry, where a filling is encased between sheeted puff dough

Whisking Whipping of eggs/cream to incorporate volume

Windscreen test Mixing dough to a consistency such that, when stretched it forms a thin film without cracking

OBJECTIVE TYPE QUESTIONS

1. Define sifting and list two important reasons why sifting is done.
2. What do you understand by creaming and what considerations should be kept in mind whilst creaming?
3. Define whipping and list down the factors to be kept in mind whilst whipping cream.
4. What happens if egg whites are over whipped?
5. Define rubbing-in and how does it create shortness in the product?
6. What factors should be kept in mind while rubbing-in?
7. Define cutting and folding method and what care should be taken whilst folding-in?
8. Why does docking prevent rising of the dough?
9. What is blind baking and what is its importance?
10. What care should be taken whilst pinning the dough?
11. Why is the bread kept for proving? Give at least three reasons.
12. List at least five different shapes of breads.
13. What are the plaited breads commonly known as?
14. At what temperature would you normally bake sponges?
15. What is scoring and what are its uses?
16. What method would you use for mixing butter and sugar for cakes?
17. List two reasons why rubbing-in technique is used in pastry.
18. What is the name of the equipment on which cake is kept for icing?
19. What do you understand by the word icing?
20. Define laminating.

ESSAY TYPE QUESTIONS

1. What are the various ways to aerate a product? Describe each parameter.
2. Explain the process of autolysis and how does it help in preparing quality bread.
3. Describe in detail the most common kneading methods and how do they impact the product.
4. Describe the science of baking and the factors that influence a product with regards to quality.
5. Describe at least three products that can be made by using the technique of laminating.

ACTIVITY

1. In a group of 4 to 5, prepare a bread dough and create at least 3 types of plaited rolls, 2 large breads for cutting on the board live in front of the guests and at least 5 kinds of decorative breads that can be used for creating bread display.
2. Visit at least 3-4 pastry shops and list down the names of products in them. Now in groups identify, which product was made with which technique and then present to the team for critique and evaluation.
3. Make a chart of baking temperatures and the time taken by a product to bake. Record all this information systematically and paste it on an ideal location next to the baking oven for easy reference.

4 Bread Fabrication

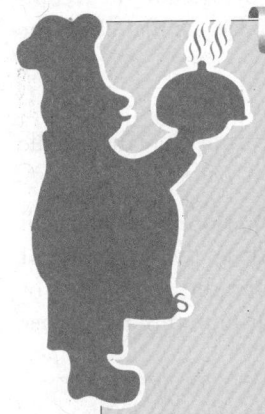

LEARNING OBJECTIVES

After reading this chapter, you should be able to
- understand the different principles of dough and bread making
- know the various steps involved in production of breads with regards to temperature and timings
- prepare various kinds of breads and shapes thereof
- know about various types of international breads
- recognize the importance of ingredients and processes involved in bread making, thereby understanding the basic faults in bread production
- appreciate the storage of various breads, their usage in kitchens, and their serving techniques
- appreciate the difference between lean and enriched dough

INTRODUCTION

Bread making is a combination of art and science. Art because simple bread can be moulded and shaped artistically to make an impact on bread display and science because bread making is more than just a recipe. Apart from the good quality of ingredients, the temperature and the environment have a large role to play in the making of the final product; for the chef to make the standard bread every time requires a great deal of understanding of the science behind bread making. This chapter will give a detailed understanding of the intricacies of bread making. In this chapter, we shall talk about the commodities used in bread making and also see the role of each in the making of the bread.

Once we understand the role played by ingredients, we can then modify our breads to produce a particular product with the desirable structure. This will help us to evaluate breads and if a particular bread does not turn out to be as it was supposed to, then as chefs, we can relate to what went wrong with the recipe. But many times bread is at fault not because of the ingredients alone, but also because of the process involved in making it. For example, we read in chapter on commodities used in bakery, how mechanical kneading of the flour develops gluten. So if a bread does not have a good structure, it will not be good to blame just the flour, as the problem could be in kneading and even in things like baking style, time, and temperature.

This chapter will help us to understand the historical significance of breads and relate it to present technology and methods. It will also give us an insight into the function of various ingredients and how they affect the final product and storage qualities. We will also talk about various bread improvers and how to maximise the effectiveness of each type.

The origins of the first bread are unknown but the wheat has been cultivated since more than 5,000 years ago. The leavening of the bread must have been purely accidental as the previous day's dough would have been left over and the wonderful fermented smell would have enticed the baker to bake it. Till date in many traditional bakeries the concept of *sourdough* or *starter* is still prevalent. Some bakeries have secret guarded recipes for sourdough.

UNDERSTANDING BAKING

It is not enough to have an understanding of commodities, working terminology, and types of aeration to make breads. You also need an understanding of baking to ensure the product would not be sub-standard or spoilt, resulting in a waste of time and materials. Simply setting the oven to the recommended baking temperatures will not always guarantee success. There are many factors that affect the baking temperature and the baking time. They include:

Shape and size of the products being baked Generally speaking, the thicker the product, the longer it takes to bake, the baking temperature must be lower, or else the outside will get burnt before the middle is cooked. Thin products will bake more quickly, and so the oven temperature can be higher.

Oven humidity Oven humidity is critical for some types of baked products. A cake baked by it will need a pan of water in the oven to provide extra humidity. The moisture will delay the formation of crust until full expansion has taken place. The result should be a cake with a flat top and a crust of pleasing colour. On the other hand, an oven full of cakes will provide sufficient humidity for proper crust formation.

Oven overloading Oven loading must be taken into consideration because the temperature of an oven filled with products will fall. The drop in temperature will depend on the type of product being baked and the size and type of the oven being used. To counter this factor, use a higher initial temperature. Whilst placing items to be baked on a tray, place them in an interlocking manner to allow movement of air between the products being baked.

Density of products being baked Products containing a high proportion of sugar, fat, eggs, and fruits will need a lower temperature, and will take longer to bake. You may need to line baking trays with several layers of paper insulation to prevent burning the bottom.

Type of oven Commercial, pastry ovens are thermostatically controlled by three switches. One maintains the pre-set temperature and the other two control the top and bottom heat of the oven. This flexibility allows a chef to bake different items more effectively by having more or less heat in the area required. A convection (fan forced) oven maintains an even temperature throughout the oven. A standard type of oven has varying temperature within the chamber with the top area having a higher temperature. The general rule is that yeast and pastry products are placed towards the top of the oven while cakes are placed towards the centre.

> **CHEF'S TIPS**
> - Get to know your oven as it is an important factor in successful baking.
> - Have the accuracy of your thermostat checked regularly.
> - Do not open the oven door during the early baking stages and avoid opening it too frequently as some products may collapse. If you often open the oven door, the moisture tends to escape from it by dropping the pressure and temperature inside it, resulting in collapse of products.
> - Place items to be baked on a tray in an interlocking manner to allow free passage of air through them so that they bake evenly.
> - Close the oven door slowly.

ROLE OF INGREDIENTS IN BREAD MAKING

Every ingredient used in the making of bread has a particular role to play in achieving the final, desired product. These ingredients however perform only when certain conditions are met and are highly dependent on each other to perform that particular function to the desired level. For example, yeast performs well in the presence of sugar as well as moisture. Thus, it becomes essential to understand the nature of each of these ingredients in detail, how they will affect the final product, and how to manipulate these materials to get the desired products.

Flour The main ingredient used in making breads. We discussed about flours in previous chapters (refer to Tables 2.1 and 2.2) and have understood about various types of flour (wheat, rye, multi grain, etc.). Usually, strong flours are used in bread making. Wholewheat flours have lesser concentration of gluten as the bran content is more and if used for bread making, they lead to a weaker structure in the bread. Also the bran particles being slightly abrasive, cut the gluten fibres resulting in a loaf with a smaller crumb. The presence of the bran particles also allows for higher moisture absorption resulting in short fermentation time. When the germ is present in the flour, there is higher enzyme activity as a result of which the gluten develops faster and the breads are made with a shorter fermentation time.

As explained in Chapter 2, fermentation is a very important aspect of bread making. The yeasts feed on sugar to produce alcohol and carbon dioxide. This process also helps to develop an acidic medium in the dough, thereby enriching the flavour and taste of the bread. The structure and the texture of a bread is carefully controlled by experienced bakers, who allow the dough to undergo shorter or longer fermentations in a controlled temperature and environment.

Water Water is the most commonly used liquid in bread making. It moistens the flour and helps in forming the dough. It also aids in the baking process. The water performs the following three main functions in the bread dough.

- It helps to hydrate and moisten the insoluble proteins.
- It disperses the yeast through the entire dough.
- It binds the flour and other ingredients into a dough.

It is observed that the water content in the dough greatly affects the rate of fermentation. The speed of fermentation is greater in dough with more water content and so, as the fermentation time increases it becomes essential to reduce the water content to effect a higher dough ripening. The amount of water present will also greatly affect the texture of the final product. The amount of water in flour is called hydration and is measured in percentage with regards to flour. The following table lists the hydration levels of various doughs along with their uses.

Table 4.1 Types of textures of dough

Product	Hydration percentage	Uses
Batter	100-130%	Waffles, *jalebi*, pancakes, cake
Exceptionally soft dough	70-90%	Brioche, baba dough/savarin dough
Soft dough	55-70%	Bread rolls
Moderately stiff	50-55%	Crusty bread, malted and rye breads
Very stiff	30-40%	Fancy breads for decoration

Hard water has higher alkalinity and as yeast works best in an acidic medium, fermentation can be slower in the initial stages. However, as the fermentation proceeds the acids produced will neutralise this alkalinity and then the fermentation will proceed at a brisk pace. Also, the alkalinity and the mineral salts will tighten the gluten and thus the dough will be firmer. Very hard water also has magnesium sulphate, which has a retarding action on the yeast. Breads can however be made with both hard as well soft water provided the physical adjustments are made.

When the dough is kneaded for long duration of time, the temperature in the dough increases due to friction and this has to be watched carefully as the temperature of the dough should not go beyond 25°C because the yeast will start its work. In such cases, a baker often uses ice to make the dough. Thus, it keeps the fermentation activity of yeast at an ideal rate for gluten ripening. The quantity used will vary depending upon the time of kneading of the dough or the friction factor, and the dough temperature required. Ice used must be in the form of flaked ice so that it is evenly distributed in the bread dough and causes an even cooling of the dough. It can be safely said that 5 kg of ice will be equivalent to 4 litres of water.

Yeast They are single cell microorganisms, which cause the leavening in the dough. It converts the natural sugar in the flour into tiny bubbles of carbon dioxide that are trapped in the dough and during baking these bubbles expand to give the required texture and lightness to the product.

Yeast is available in three forms—*dry*, *instant*, and *compressed*. The ideal temperature for yeast to act is 25°C. The primary function of yeast is to change sugar into CO_2 so that the dough is aerated.

When dispersed in water with yeast food, the yeast exudes an enzyme that changes sucrose into dextrose, which is then absorbed by the yeast cell. Inside the cell this is broken down into carbon dioxide and other by-products. Yeast also has enzymes which change protein into simpler compounds, which can pass through the yeast cell membrane.

Yeast works best within a temperature range of 25-40°C. Above this temperature range, fermentation becomes rapid but gets weaker successively and is finally killed at 70°C. At this temperature, yeast is completely retarded though it is not damaged. Yeast can never dissolve completely in water, though it is just dispersed well into it. To effectively distribute yeast in water one could use a whisk.

Compressed yeast must be cool to touch and must possess a creamy colour, and should break with a clean fracture. If it is light in colour, and is dry and warm with a pungent odour, it is in poor condition and will not make good quality bread. If it is dark brown in colour with a soft sticky consistency and an unpleasant odour, it is unsuitable for use.

The instant yeast is strongest of all yeasts in comparison to compressed yeast. This means that if converting from compressed yeast in recipes, use half the amount of dry yeast and 1/3 times the amount of instant yeast. For example, if the recipe calls for 30 g of compressed yeast or fresh yeast as it is known, use 15 g of dry yeast and 10 g of instant yeast.

> **CHEF'S TIP**
> When using dry yeast in the recipe, use half the amount of fresh yeast mentioned, as dry yeast is stronger.

The dry yeast needs to be activated with a small amount of water and sugar, whereas fresh yeast and instant yeast can be mixed directly with the ingredients.

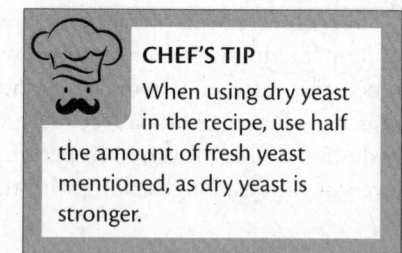

Salt The main function of salt is to control the action of yeast. It slows down the fermentation process and is mixed with flour for best results. It also provides flavour to bread. It also affects the quality of the crumb, crust, and colour of the baked product. Therefore, salt mainly helps in improving the following functions.

- Flavour
- Stability of gluten

- Control on the rate of fermentation affecting the crust, colour, and crumb of the bread
- Retention of moisture

More salt or less salt will adversely affect the final product and we can see that from Table 4.2.

Table 4.2 Impact of salt

Less salt	Excessive salt
Large volume- as there is more breakdown of sugar into carbon dioxide	Tightening of the gluten gives a dense structure
Less crust colour	Dark crust colour as sugars are not broken down
Weak crumb structure	Crumb structure resembles cheese, as not enough gas is produced

Sugar The main function of sugar is to act as food for yeast. It helps in developing flavour and colour. Sugar is the primary food that the yeast feeds on to produce alcohol and CO_2 gas. With the exception of lactose, yeast can breakdown all the other sugars present in the dough, either naturally in the flour or as an addition of sugar, mainly sucrose or sometimes malt. Flour naturally contains about 2.5-3% of sugar in the form of sucrose and maltose. This is enough for the yeast in the initial stage of fermentation. However, in the final proof when maximum of the sugar is required to be broken down for an optimum rise, the natural sugars are exhausted and the addition of sucrose or maltose is required. Like salt, too much sugar or too less sugar will impact the dough texture as described in Table 4.3.

Table 4.3 Impact of sugar

Less sugar	Excessive sugar
Not enough volume	Large volume- as there is more sugar available for breakdown
Less crust colour	More crust colour
Weak crumb structure	Weak structure of bread
Lower yeast activity as yeast works best in 10% sugar solution	Higher yeast activity

Sugar has a solvent effect on gluten and this greatly affects the quality of the crumb in bread loaves. To counteract this, a mineral improver is used and excess salt is used as salt has a stabilising effect on the gluten.

Sugar has many roles to play in dough. Few of these are:

- Being the primary food for the yeast
- Helping to improve the crust colour
- Acting as preservative and anti-staling agent
- Acting as bread improver
- Helping the bread to retain moisture, thereby keeping the bread moist
- Imparting flavours, for example, treacle, honey, and demerara sugar

Milk Provides the moisture, makes the bread whiter and softer and provides a distinct flavour. Milk also has a physical effect on bread in the form of the tightening effect of gluten by the action of Casein or the milk protein. However, boiling or pasteurization neutralises the effect to a great extent. Lactose or the milk sugar is the only sugar which is not fermentable by yeast and hence, it remains in the dough right till the end resulting in a good crust colour. Milk is generally used in powdered and skimmed form and hence, the amount of water taken up in the dough is slightly more though not considerably. If one is concerned about the texture of the dough, then water and milk could be used in a ratio that does not exceed the levels of hydration in the dough.

Egg Eggs are used for richness and to give lightness and colour. Eggs are again rich in protein and hence will tighten the gluten strands, but this effect gets balanced, as the fat in the yolk helps to soften the gluten as well. Eggs will yield softer bread. In many types of bread, such as hard rolls, where a hard structure is required, one does not use eggs in the recipe. Egg is also used at times to give the final brushing on top of the bread before baking. This process gives a dark and shiny surface to the bread, which helps in enhancing the look of the bread.

Oil/fats It is used to provide flavour and softness to the texture. Different kinds of fats are used for different breads like olive oil for *focaccia* (Italian bread). Fats have a physical effect on breads rather than any chemical reaction. Fat being a shortening agent reduces the toughness of the gluten and mellows the final product. Fat also has lubricating effect on the fine gluten strands giving extra volume to the final product. These strands begin to slip over each other and thus, affect the final quality. As the amount of fat increases, the fermentation rate decreases. This is because the fat will form a thin layer on the yeast cell membrane hindering the release and absorption of materials. Thus, yeast quantity is slightly increased.

> **CHEF'S TIP**
> When using high amount of fat in a recipe of bread, always use milk, as the milk protein will have a tightening effect on gluten and thus, it will offset the shortening effect of fat.

Effects of Fat

- Increases the nutritious value of the bread
- Reduces elasticity, softens the crust and the crumb
- Helps to retain moisture in the baked product, thereby keeping it moist
- Increases volume when used in small amounts, if used extensively, volume will be affected
- Gives flavour to the product, for example, butter and lard
- Retards fermentation when used in large amounts

Bread improvers Flour is of variable quality and hence it becomes necessary at times to add something to the dough to bring the final product to a set standard. Bread improvers may be divided into three main categories. These include:

- Those of mineral nature, used by the miller
- Those of organic nature, mainly enriching agents
- Those of both the aforementioned categories which are also yeast foods

Mineral improvers are popular because they increase the yield of the bread by necessitating the use of extra water. Some of the mineral improvers have a slight drying effect on the crumb.

Gluten Gluten is the natural protein available in wheat flour and the flours that are most suitable for bread production are high gluten flours. In some countries including India, we do not have flours sold separately for breads, cakes, and cookies but in Europe and US, the flours are available on the basis of their strength, which is determined by the gluten present in them. So to combat this issue, many bread makers in India add commercially available gluten powder to enhance the structure of their bread.

BREAD MAKING METHODS

There are various stages in bread making and these are very crucial as each of the stage has to be carefully followed to obtain the desired result. Previously in the chapter, we discussed about the role of various ingredients in bread making. Let us now understand how these ingredients are mixed to obtain a wonderful loaf of fresh bread. Refer to Fig. 4.1 for a quick glance of the steps involved in bread making.

Let us now discuss each of these steps in detail.

Collecting the *mise en place* The most important thing required in any pastry operation is to collect the *mise en place*. This will allow you to do things in a planned manner and the product will also come out to be of the desired quality. The *mise en place* for bread making would include:

- Weighing all the ingredients as per the recipe and making sure the ingredients are at the required temperature. If the recipe calls for ice water, then use ice water. Substituting cold water from tap will not give the desired results. Weigh using a digital scale, as accuracy of ingredients is very important in pastry. Sift the flour to remove any impurities.

- Selecting and preparing the bread tins—always use thick and heavy pans for baking bread as they can withstand the high temperatures of the oven, without getting deformed due to the heat. Shapes of bread rely on the mould used. Grease the mould with oil properly to avoid the baked bread from sticking to it.

- Making sure that the temperature of the oven is at the required degree as the temperature of baking is very crucial and would change with different types of breads.

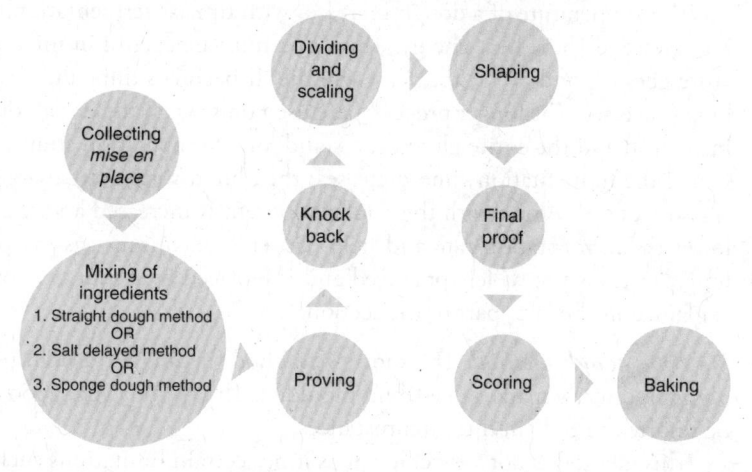

Fig. 4.1 Steps for bread fabrication

Mixing of the ingredients A layman might wonder, what is there in mixing of ingredients, but to professionals like us, it is much more than just mixing everything together to form dough. There are many methods in which bread can be mixed or kneaded and we shall discuss them individually as this forms the basis of bread making. Broadly, these mixing methods are classified as follows:

- Straight dough method
- No time dough method
- Ferment/Sponge method
- Salt delayed method

Let us discuss each of them individually.

Straight dough method This is one of the most popular methods used in production of bread and as the name suggests it is simple and straight forward. The *fermentation* time can vary between 30 minutes to 14 hours. The time of fermentation can also vary with the type of ingredients. Very strong gluten flour will require a long fermentation time to help in the softening and mellowing of the gluten. However, a whole wheat bread or germ bread will require a shorter fermentation time due to the high enzyme activity in the germ of the wheat grain, and the higher water content in the dough.

The most commonly used straight dough processes are those that involve 1-5 hours of fermentation. This is the time from dough making to the scaling of the dough. Most of the doughs are fermented for around 3 to 4 hours in a controlled environment.

The temperature of a dough increases with time as fermentation is an exothermic reaction—involving release of some heat energy. Thus, one must be careful in mixing the ingredients as if the temperature goes beyond 50°C, the yeast will die. It becomes difficult to control the fermentation process in long processes. The longer processes are used only when the dough or the gluten is too harsh to be made into bread and the entire gluten can stand long fermentation strains.

As the fermentation time increases, the gluten softens to a larger extent. Thus, the water content is also reduced. Along with this the salt content is increased and the yeast content is lowered. This will lower the fermentation rate and help conserve maximum gassing power in the final stages. The very long process is not widely practiced and is replaced by a shorter sponge or ferment and dough process explained in the later part of the section.

No time dough method The shortest method, it calls for a high percentage of yeast (2.5%) and the dough is directly made, scaled, and moulded. This is not a very good method of bread making and must be resorted to only in dire circumstances.

This method is not very efficient as it has certain limitations such as:

- There is not enough time for the gluten to ripen or mellow down and the bread contains only CO_2 and in reality there has not been enough fermentation in the dough, so the bread lacks flavour.
- The finished product is generally of poor quality and the bread stales quickly because of insufficient gluten ripening.
- The bread structure also will show uneven expansion as the gas is not evenly distributed in the gluten network.
- The bread will lack the characteristic aroma of a well fermented bread as there is not enough time for the various chemical changes to take place.

Germ breads are made with this method, due to the high enzymic activity that causes the dough to ripen quickly. The dough is made warm preferably to help develop the flavour quickly.

Ferment/Sponge and dough process Breads and buns can be made in two stages to help in fermentation and achieve better dough ripening. These are:

1. Ferment and dough process
2. Sponge and dough process

Ferment is a proportion of water, yeast, yeast food such as sugar, and just enough flour to make a thin batter. The yeast readily disperses in the water and begins assimilating the food dissolved in the water. It begins fermenting immediately and multiplies and is soon active and vigorous. This makes it ready to undertake the harder work of fermenting the dough. Ferment is made and kept until it shows a sign of collapse. This is when it is considered to be at its optimum for bread fermentation. Usually, 30 minutes to 1 hour for fermentation is sufficient for achieving good results.

Ferment is usually used for dough that contains rich ingredients and is high in sugar concentration. Usually, the ideal concentration for yeast to work is 10% sugar. Thus, the ferment made with this concentration will give the bread a boost. A flying ferment is a haphazard guess of water, yeast, sugar, and flour, which is allowed to stand only till the rest of the ingredients are weighed and the dough is prepared, which is approximately 10-20 minutes. This is done to activate the yeast; many books mention it as creating a well in the centre of flour and breaking up yeast with water and sugar and sprinkling little flour on top. When the bubbles start to appear on top, it is an indication that yeast is active.

Sponge can be said to be a stiffer version of the ferment. The rate of fermentation is hence lesser and the sponge is kept for a longer time. It is made by mixing a part of the flour, yeast, sugar, and salt (sometimes not), and some or all the water. The speed of the fermentation is controlled by the amount of yeast added, addition of salt, water content, and the temperature of the sponge as well as the holding temperature. When the sponge rises and collapses, the remaining materials are added to make dough, which is then given bulk fermentation.

The main purpose of the sponge is to help develop a mellow flavour which is the result of the long fermentation. This is done without subjecting all the gluten to the harsh fermentation process and thus, staggering the quantity of gluten present in the final product. This prevents a weak structure or a collapse of the bread. In most bakeries, a portion of the previous day's dough is added to achieve this effect. The dough thus ripens well at a temperature of 5-7°C for a long period of time (16-18 hours minimum) and gives excellent flavour to the bread. The dough is usually placed in a refrigerator overnight. This is also known as sourdough or ferment. In Italian, this ferment is known as *biga* and in French it is called *levain*. In India, it is known as *khameer*.

One must be careful whilst kneading the dough. Many dough mixers have two speeds such as slow and high speed to knead the dough. Many bread recipes call for kneading the dough at slow speed for a couple of minutes and then increasing the speed to high speed. Usually, bread is kneaded until a film is formed when the dough is stretched. This is also known as *windscreen test*.

Salt delayed bread making process An excellent process used initially for harsh gluten flours, but now is widely used for all bread making processes as it drastically reduces the fermentation time without changing quality. This process calls for the omission of salt in the first stages of dough making. As was discussed earlier, salt is helpful in controlling the pace of fermentation by the yeast and hence, when the salt is omitted in the first stages, the action of the yeast increases. The gluten ripens or softens well due to the rapid action of the gases released. The chemical changes that take place in the dough also fasten and the effect of the acids produced is visible in a shorter time.

The salt is added later in three ways, which are:

- By sprinkling the salt over the dough
- By using some water reserved from the original quantity
- By using some fat to incorporate the salt

This process is the best method of conditioning dough without using higher yeast contents or an increase in fermentation temperature or time.

Proving The next step is to let the dough to ferment. Proving means to let the dough rise to at least double its size. This is done to let the yeast break down sugar into alcohol and carbon dioxide. The gases thus released help to ferment the dough. The ideal temperature for proving is 32°C and it is done in three stages. First is after kneading called as *first proving* and second is after *knock back* and hence called as *intermediate proving* and the *final proving* is done after shaping the bread. So we can say that fermentation is done for the following reasons.

- It helps in production of carbon dioxide gas which aerates the dough.
- It helps to condition the dough; this is through the enzymatic action that takes place due to reduction of natural sugars for assimilation by yeast.
- It helps to reduce the proteins to simpler nitrogenous compounds for growth and development of the yeast.
- The enzymes are active during the fermentation period. The sugars are broken down to release heat which causes the temperature of the dough to rise. This rise can be controlled by the speed of fermentation and the storage temperature.

Knock back The fermented dough is punched down to knock off the air bubbles that had developed during the first proving. This is so done to redistribute the yeast and the other ingredients evenly all through the dough. After knocking back, the dough is allowed to rest for a while as the gluten tends to stretch and it will be difficult to mould the bread. This stage is called intermediate proving. It is important not to over knead the dough in the machines as the gluten will lose its resilience. The knock back is also done to equalise the temperature in the dough.

Dividing and scaling This is done to portion the dough into pieces of the required weight. As discussed in the aforementioned paragraph, it is important to rest the dough before dividing and shaping is done. The scaling of the bread that needs to be baked in a mould will depend upon the size of the mould. Though there is no particular formula to calculate the weight, but normally a loaf is calculated by pounds, so one pound loaf of bread will be baked in a one pound mould (the moulds are sold by the volume they can hold). The scaling of rolls will depend upon the final usage of the product. Refer Table 4.4 for weights of certain breads. This should be used only as reference and the weights could change with regards to the usage.

Table 4.4 Sizes of breads

Breads	Size
Breads baked in loaf	Made in moulds of specific weight such as 1 lb, 2 lb
Bread rolls	25-30 g per roll
Burger buns	90-100 g
French baguette	300-350 g per loaf
Bread loaves not made in moulds	450-650 g loaves

Shaping/Panning Divided pieces of dough are shaped in the form of loaf or rolls. It should be done on a sparingly floured surface, the dough should be handled gently and placed for final proving. After a few minutes of resting, the dough soon reaches its optimum ripening. Thus, the dough is scaled and then shaped. As the dough was deflated during knock back, it has to be carefully manipulated again after it becomes more resilient. Machine dividing can be violent and can destroy the structure of the dough. The dough is rested slightly before shaping to allow for shaping without pressure. This final moulding is essential as the shape of the product and the crumb structure is affected. This step is also known as panning, which means to shape the bread and put in a pan.

Final proof As the dough is being shaped, it is temporarily degassed and the gluten tightens. If the dough is mature and the moulding done correctly, the skin surface will be smooth. The objective of the final proof is to allow the loaf to expand completely before baking. The production of the gas and the breakdown of the sugars must be vigorous and the gluten should be in such a condition, that it is strong enough to hold the gasses and expand.

The condition under which the final proof is carried out is important. If there is lack of humidity, the dough surface will dry and there will be a lack of bloom on the crust of the bread. Skinning is the result of draughts of air, and will show as grey patches. Excessive humidity will result in a tough leathery crust, a wrinkled surface, and holes under the top crust of the loaf.

The final proving is usually done in an equipment known as *proving cabinet* or *proving chamber*. Proving chambers have a temperature of 30°C and are maintained at humidity levels of 90%, which is the ideal condition for the yeast to work and ferment the dough. In case one does not have a proving cabinet, it is advisable to place the bread in a warm place sprinkled with water or covered with plastic to avoid the formation of scales on the dough, which will then cause a fault in the bread (refer to Table 4.6).

Scoring It is the process of giving marks on top of the dough with a sharp blade or a knife. It helps the bread to expand during baking without cracking. This step is not mandatory and chefs can choose to do scoring to give a rustic look to the breads. However, certain breads like classical French baguette have scoring marks on them. Some chefs score the breads after the shaping and some choose to do it just before baking. The look of the bread is different in both the cases.

Baking The bread is ready to be baked once it has proved to optimum. Under proving of the dough will yield in cracked loaf and over proving will make the bread collapse in the final baking process. The bread is said to have proved well, if it springs back when depressed slightly. During baking, the dough goes through the following three stages.

- **First stage:** The oven spring occurs and the gas bubbles in the dough expand and it rises rapidly. The yeast activity increases rapidly in the oven and the activity of the yeast stops as it kills the yeasts at 60°C. The gas in the dough expands and so does the steam and alcohol vapour pressure. This causes a sudden burst in the volume of the bread and is called the *oven spring*. Some of the starch is gelatinised to make it more susceptible to the enzymic activity.

- **Second stage**: The dough solidifies because of the coagulation of proteins and transforms into bread. Here the gases escape out of the dough leaving a dispersion of holes, which are responsible for the sponginess of the bread.

- **Third stage:** The dough gets its colour and crust. Enzymes are active till about 80-90°C producing sugars even beyond the yeast activity. This helps in the colouring of the crust. The enzyme activity helps in the crumb, crust colour, and bloom of the bread. As the baking proceeds, weight is lost by the evaporation of the moisture from the crust. As the moisture is driven off, the crust takes on a higher temperature, reaching the temperature of the oven. The sugars caramelize and the breakdown of the soluble protein, blend to form the attractive colour of the crust. The sugars caramelize at 140°C.

The texture of the bread can be altered by regulating the heat at this stage. Crusty bread would require lowering the temperature after the bread is baked 80%. This would help the top crust to get dry thereby giving a crisp crust to the loaf. The crust of the bread can also be altered by giving various types of glazes, which is mostly done in case of bread rolls. Let us look at Table 4.5 for some such glazes and toppings.

Cooling the baked bread When the bread is taken out from the oven, it is essential that it should be demoulded and cooled reasonably quickly, as insufficiently cooled bread when sliced will be subject to mould formation and spoilage. The bread must be cooled on a wire rack because if the bread is placed on a flat surface, the heat from the base will condense and the humidity will let the moulds grow into

Table 4.5 Various glazes and toppings for breads

Glaze/Topping	Description
Egg wash glaze	This gives a darker colour, shine to the roll and also adds a nutritional value. It is advisable to use the egg yolk only; but the whole egg can also be used. The egg is beaten with a little amount of water which is then strained to get a smooth flowing egg liquid. This is then applied with a soft brush or a piece of cloth on the bread.
Salt water glaze	This gives a rustic whitish appearance to the bread. Prior to baking the saline water is brushed on top of the bread. Care should be taken as to how much of glaze is applied, as this could make the bread salty.
Starch glazes	The breads are sometimes glazed with corn starch slurry. This also provides shine to the bread.
Honey glazes	Honey is boiled prior to applying as a glaze, for it is a viscous substance and boiling will allow it to set into a glaze that will stick to the surface of the bread. This glaze is applied after the bread is taken out of the oven. It should be ensured that the bread is still hot, when this glaze is applied. It is mostly done for sweet breads such as *gingerbreads* and *zofp*.
Seeds as toppings	Various seeds such as cumin, fennel, poppy, sesame, and nigella, are sprinkled on top of the bread to improve the look of the bread and add nutritive value and assortment to the rolls on the buffet or in a bread basket. Care should be taken to sprinkle the seeds only after some wash or glaze has been applied to ensure that the seeds stick. The amount of seed to be used will depend upon the intensity of the flavour of the spice or the seed.
Nuts as toppings	Various nuts can be sprinkled on breads prior to baking. Following the same principles as listed in case of seeds, we must also ensure that the nuts are chopped evenly to be able to be used as toppings.
Herbs as toppings	Various chopped herbs can be used as toppings. It is advisable to use dry herbs as fresh herbs will anyways lose their colour when baked in oven. One can create different types of crusts by combining herbs, seeds, and nuts to create unique toppings.
Vegetables as toppings	This is done in specific breads such as Italian *focaccia*—the bread is sprinkled with an assortment of grilled or sautéed vegetables such as onions, bell peppers, olives, which are then spread along with olive oil and rock salt on top before baking. This should not be confused with flavoured breads, as in case of flavoured breads the ingredients are mixed along with the dough and not used as toppings.
Flour as topping	Many types of bread are dusted with large amounts of flour prior to baking. It is important to first glaze the bread with plain water as this will allow the flour to stick to the bread. In case the bread has to be scored, it is always done after the dusting of the flour has been done.
Cereals as toppings	Many cereals such as oats, bran, germ, bulgur, are also used as toppings after applying the water wash on the bread. In these cases, the top surface of the bread is rolled onto the topping so that the entire surface gets coated. This is done right after shaping and the bread is allowed to prove with the topping, which disperses evenly when the bread is proved and is ready for baking.

the bread. Also proper cooling allows for evaporation from the surface of the loaf which would otherwise condense on the crust, and would be known as *sweating*. This will show as moist patches on the crust.

BASIC FAULTS IN BREAD MAKING

Before discussing the various faults in breads, it is vital to look at the various points on which a bread can be judged. They may not necessarily be in the order of importance as each one has a vital role to play in guest satisfaction and each person's preference is different.

- **Volume:** The volume here refers to a large bread that is light for its weight. But there are many breads that are very heavy for their weight, and they are traditionally made in this way, because the recipe calls for it.

- **Bloom of crust:** This refers to the colour and texture of the crust of the bread. However, we can alter the texture of the crust by putting various types of glazes (refer to Table 4.5) on the bread prior to baking.

- **General shape:** This refers to the hand rolled bread which is shaped round, oval or any other shape as required by the bread.

- **Colour of the crumb:** The colour of the crumb will depend upon lots of factors such as type of flour used in dough, oven temperatures, and the ingredients in dough. Bread high in sugar will have a darker colour as compared to the one with less or no sugar at all.

- **Evenness of texture:** The texture here refers to the equal distribution of the holes in the bread loaf.

- **Sheen of the crumb:** The sheen refers to the shine in the dough and this is achieved by kneading the dough to optimum.

- **Moistness:** The amount of moisture in the bread will determine its texture and keep quality. Some breads turn out to be dry when over baked or when less water is used in dough making.

- **Flavour:** Many ingredients such as salt, sugar, and yeast affect the flavour of the bread.

Let us now see the faults of the breads in Table 4.6.

> **CHEF'S TIPS**
> Some breads involve application of steam to make them crisp. A layer of moisture on the bread when subjected to heat will turn into steam and evaporate. When it evaporates, it will take large amounts of moisture away from the surface of the bread thereby, resulting in a crusty roll.
> The standard test for yeast bread is to take the loaf from the baking tin and tap/knock the base of the baked bread. If it sounds hollow, it indicates that the bread is done. The colour should be an even brown from all sides.

Table 4.6 Common faults in bread making

Fault	Reasons
Flaked crust also known as flying tops	-If fermented dough is left uncovered in an atmosphere which is not saturated with moisture (80-85%), water evaporates from the surface of the dough leaving the skin dry. This skin, once formed, is difficult to eliminate and when a skinny dough is knocked back, scaled and moulded, the dry skin breaks off and some which remains on the exterior will get folded into the dough and show as whitish coloured patches which are hard and knotty
	-When moulded dough pieces become skinned, it will give an unsatisfactory bloom of the crust. Also there will be a number of bursts or 'flying tops'

(Contd)

Table 4.6 (Contd)

Fault	Reasons
Lack of volume	-Bread not fermented enough, most of these faults can be said to be a direct effect of insufficient gluten ripening. It has already been discussed in detail how fermentation affects the gluten structure and the final flavour of the bread
	-Over fermentation may also be a reason for lack of volume in bread. Longer fermentation time increases the acid production giving a very sour taste. This activity will weaken the gluten for lack of volume and large holes. It will also give a bad structure to the baked bread which will begin to crumble easily
	-Breads not proved for required length of time
	-Lack of volume may also occur due to improper mixing of the dough, due to which the gluten does not develop, which is directly responsible for the volume of the bread
	-Too much salt in dough
	-Less yeast in dough
	-Oven temperatures too high
Uneven texture, showing large irregular holes	-Breads not fermented enough. When the dough is not fermented long enough, the gluten will not reach its maximum extensibility. As the gluten is not fully extended, the loaf will be smaller in volume. Also, some of the smaller gluten strands will break down under the expansion pressure of the gas, creating irregular large sized holes in the baked product
	-Over fermented dough
	-Under proved bread may show a crack on the base, thereby giving an irregular shape to the bread
Lack of shine on the crust	-Under fermented bread. The sheen of the crumb depends upon the structure of the gluten formation, as kneading increases the number of fine glossy cell surfaces to reflect the light. Greater the web like structure of the gluten, greater will be the reflection of the light
	-Over fermented dough
Lack of flavour and aroma	-Under fermented bread
	-Over fermented dough also gives a slightly acidic flavour to the bread
Rapidly stales	-Bread not fermented for required time
	-Not enough salt in dough
	-Over proofed bread
Crumbly bread	-Over fermented dough
	-Over proofed dough
	-Not enough fat in dough
Lack of colour on crust	-Over fermented dough
	-Insufficient sugar in the dough
Raw inside	-Under baking
	-Baking done in high temperature whereby the crust has got a colour but is doughy in centre

COMMON BREAD DISEASES

The term bread disease is not to be confused with the harmful effects of eating bread or the diseases caused by consuming bread. In this section, we will discuss the diseases that a bread can acquire due to unfavourable environmental conditions. Let us discuss some of these diseases in Table 4.7.

Table 4.7 Diseases caused in breads

Disease	Description
Rope	Rope is one of the main diseases that affect breads. The spores of *Bacillus Mesentericus Vulgatus*, the microorganisms, are responsible for the development of rope. It is usually present in the flour itself. This is not apparent until the bread is some hours old. This develops in the form of patchiness and the crumb becomes sticky. At the same time a peculiar odour similar to that of pineapples develops. This will occur only when the spore is given suitable conditions to develop, increase, grow, and so produce an attack of the disease. These conditions include warmth, moistness, and a deficiency of acid in the medium. Spores cannot develop in an acidic medium. Also as the spores require warm weather rather than cold, it becomes even more important to cool the bread quickly and completely.
	This can be prevented by using sourdough in the making of the bread, as sourdough will have sufficient acid content to prevent the formation of rope. This is also called the *Mature parent dough* method.
Moulds	Moulds is another common disease that a bread can acquire if stored in a humid and warm environment. In such conditions, a green to black hairy growth can be seen on the bread. The moulds are a type of fungus and it can cause foul smell and make the bread unfit for human consumption.
	To prevent mould formation on bread, the bread must be stored in a cool and dry environment and if the bread is to be stored for a longer duration, then it can be wrapped in a plastic film and kept frozen until usage.

EQUIPMENT USED IN BREAD MAKING

Many large and small types of equipment are used in production of bread. It starts from sieving the flour to mixing in dough machines and proving and baking. Let us see the most common equipment used in production of bread in Table 4.8.

Table 4.8 Equipment used in bread making

Equipment	Usage
Sieve	Drum sieve is mostly used to sieve the flours and the size of the mesh through which it will be sieved will depend upon the type of flour being used. The wholemeal flour will be sieved through a coarse mesh as we do not want to sieve away the bran and other nutritious things from it.
	Industrial flour sifters are also used in many hotels which produce breads on large scale.
Weighing scale	Preferably a digital weighing scale should be used, as the accuracy of the ingredients is very important.
Baking trays	Often known as sheet pans, can be of iron, or Teflon coated for non-stick.
Bread moulds	Containers of various shapes and sizes. These are often sold by the volume they are intended for. So one can easily procure moulds of 1 lb, 2 lb, etc.
Proving cabinets	Electric, gas, and pressure steam models are available. It is a cabinet in which water is heated with an element. It maintains the temperature of 25°C and humidity of 90%.

(Contd)

Table 4.8 (Contd)

Equipment	Usage
Retarder prover	A retarder prover is a piece of equipment that controls the rate of proving for the bread to be made. The baker can shape the bread in the evening, while the baking can be done at a later stage, that is, as and when required.
	A retarder prover can be automatically adjusted so that the breads are ready to be baked at programmed timings. This equipment can freeze the shaped bread to stop the functions of yeast and then bring up the temperature whereby the dough comes back to a temperature at which it is cold but not frozen. The machine then brings up the temperature to the required degree and humidity so that the bread can be proved.
Dough mixers	Various kinds of dough mixers are used to knead the dough.
	Spiral dough mixers are used in which the dough hook and the bowl both move in opposite directions, so that the dough is automatically scraped whilst being made. They are also tuned to two speeds—slow and high—as most of the bread recipes call for mixing dough at particular speeds for optimum development of gluten.
Dough dividers	Equipment used for dividing the dough into equal sizes and portions and is also used for shaping it into round balls. It is mostly used in large establishments.
Deck ovens	These ovens can be electrical or gas operated and are usually available as single deck or multiple decks for baking. Few of the baking ovens are available with steam attachment for better baking.
Ovens **Other names:** Batch ovens, rotator ovens	Ovens are traditionally used for baking purposes and they come in various shapes and sizes. The type of the oven largely depends upon the kind of operations. In large operations, where the baked products are required to be made in bulk, large rotary ovens are a good choice. There are also large ovens with automatic feeding belts, where the entire products are loaded and removed from the oven with the help of an automatic feeder. Such an oven is known as batch oven as big batches of products are baked in it.
Convection ovens **Other names:** Combi ovens	These ovens come in various sizes and work on the principle of circulation of hot air. Some models are also available with roll-in trolleys that can be loaded and rolled inside the cabinet. This equipment comes very handy in cooking as well as reheating of food. They are called combi ovens as they have the facilities of both moist as well as dry heat.
Dough scorers	A piece of equipment having a sharp surgical blade in the end, to score the breads at an angle before baking. In French, it is called *lame*.
Dough scrapers	Available in plastic or steel, they are used to scrape the dough and also to cut the dough for scaling.
Wooden table top	Traditionally maple wood is used, as it is non-porous and very hygienic.
	The wooden table tops allow the bread dough to be at the required temperature as wood is a bad conductor of heat and hence, does not take or give heat to the dough. Also the dough rarely sticks to wooden surfaces. However, because of its non-availability and expensiveness, people also use granite or marble table tops. Metal is not preferred as it can react with the dough and discolour it.
Bench brush	A large hard bristle brush to clean the table top and to brush away excess flour.
Spray bottle	Used for spraying water onto the breads, if the ovens are not equipped with steam injections.

Bread Fabrication 77

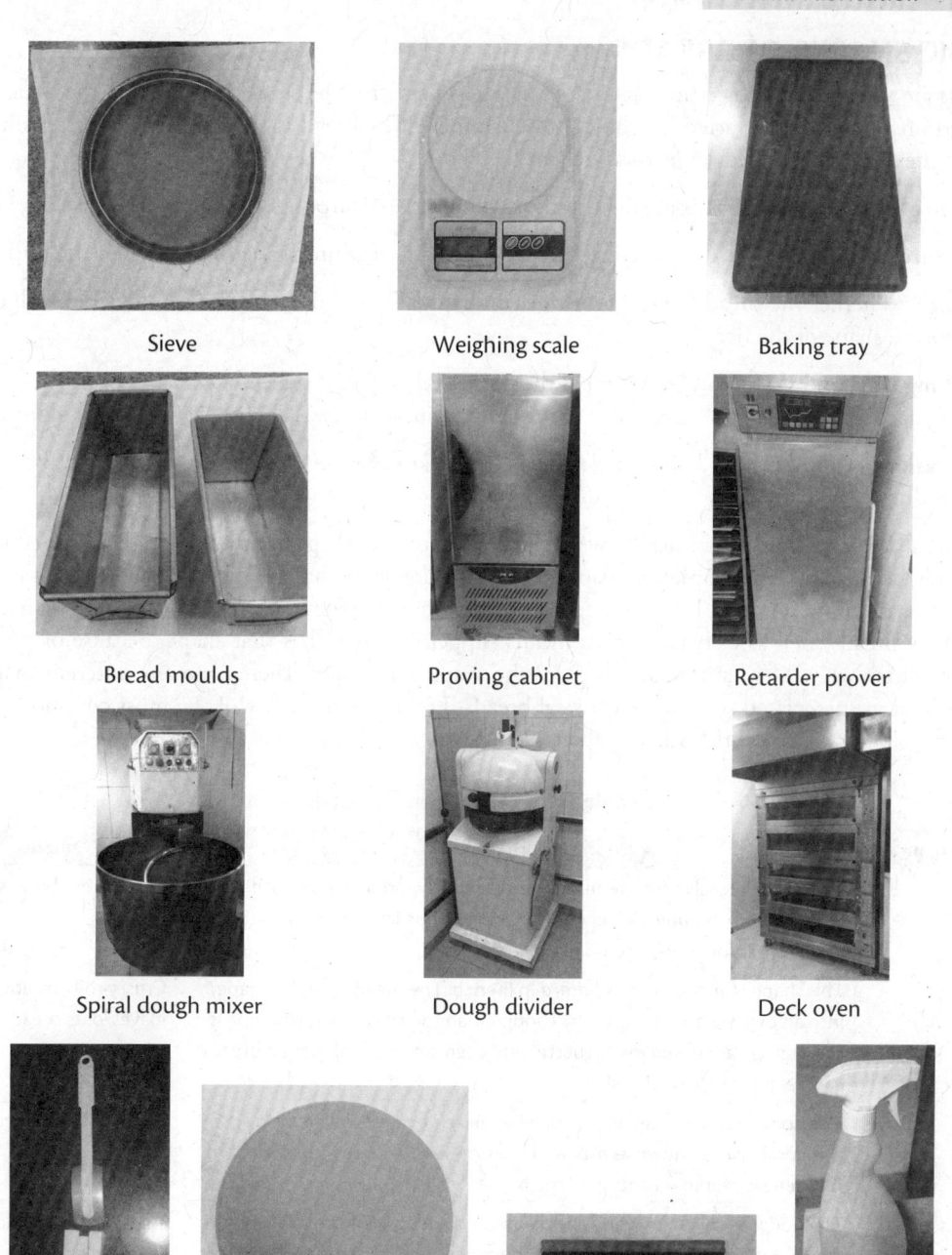

Sieve	Weighing scale	Baking tray
Bread moulds	Proving cabinet	Retarder prover
Spiral dough mixer	Dough divider	Deck oven
Dough scorer	Dough scraper	Bench brush	Spray bottle

Fig. 4.2 Equipment used in bread making

BASIC SHAPES OF BREADS

Breads are versatile and since time immemorial, chefs have tried to create variations in the dough and shaped breads to offer a variety of choices to customers. The bread is shaped for various reasons and earlier the shapes depended on factors such as:

- **Type of bread**: Whether it is a table bread or will it serve a purpose of decoration or display.
- **Texture of dough**: If the dough is firm or slack, will also determine the final shape of the bread.
- **Usage**: Whether the bread will be consumed individually or will be used in sandwiches, will determine the shape of the bread.
- **Baking time and temperature**: Whether the bread will be first poached like a bagel or fried in oil like doughnuts or will it be cooked till crisp in very low temperature, will also impact the shape of the bread.
- **Occasion**: If the bread is being made for a particular occasion or festivity, then it will be shaped accordingly.

The aforementioned points are a few parameters that bakers kept in mind when they shaped breads and now because of some common shapes, the particular shape has been associated with a particular bread. For example, a burger bun is made round and a hot dog bun is made into a small long baton.

Many breads such as ciabatta, which means slipper in Italian has that shape, because of the slack dough, which when lifted automatically gains the shape of a slipper. There are many different shapes of breads that are associated with some classical breads. Let us discuss a few of the most common shapes that are used by bakers worldwide in Table 4.9.

Table 4.9 Common bread shapes

Shape	Description	Examples
Round	The dough is scaled into required weight and then rolled into a ball. It is also known as *boule* in French. The *boule* can be large or made into smaller rolls for consumption in bread basket.	Cob, burger buns, soft rolls
Oval	This shape is also known as *batard* in French. The bread dough is shaped into an oval with tapering ends. Though many a times, a *batard* shape is the preliminary shape for baguettes and even smaller oval shaped breads can be made for bread basket.	Crusty rolls, multigrain loaves, oats bread
Logs	The dough can be rolled into a long baguette or can be rolled even thinner which is known as *fiscelle*. Sometimes a log is cut with scissors to resemble wheat grain and then the bread is called epi.	Hot dog buns, baguette, fiscelle
Sticks	The dough is rolled long and the diameter could range from a few mm to 1 cm. These types of breadsticks are often eaten with soups and used on bread displays.	Grissini, breadsticks
Plaits	The dough could be plaited and the plaits can range from 2 to 9 in number. These breads are used in festive seasons and they also adorn the bread displays due to their unique shapes.	Zofp, challah
Miscellaneous	These shapes can be used to create a variety of bread rolls. The dough is shaped into small ropes which can then be tied to form a knot, or the two ends can be rolled in opposite direction to form an 'S' or any other decorative shape can be given. These shapes are usually given for soft rolls.	Onion knots, cheese roll

Table 4.9 (Contd)

Shape	Description	Examples
Moulded	The breads can be formed into sandwich loaves in a rectangular bread tin or in a circular tube to give the shape of a tube to the bread. The breads can also be moulded into any other decorative mould such as Xmas tree or wheat grain mould.	Pullman loaf, toast bread

INTERNATIONAL BREADS

The human civilisation, since the time it has set its foot in the world has always been evolving. The process of evolution is an on-going process which never ceases to amuse a person who takes a look at history. There have been many noteworthy civilisations which have left their mark on world history. When these civilisations were researched, the nature and character of the people who comprised the civilisation has been very evidently found. We came to know about their food habits, their rituals, as well as the characteristic way of their living and earning livelihood.

Food has always been a very important part of these researches, as it was the sole most significant objective every single individual wanted to strive for, and this has always and will always remain the universal truth. However, the invention of food started with the discovery of grains, specifically cereals, which opened a different world of food products. Before that, people led a nomadic life and survived on natural food which was available in the form of fruits; they also used to hunt down animals to meet their hunger.

Cereals have always been an integral part of human diet, specifically bread, which has become fundamental to human diet in different parts of the world. Let us talk about some common breads from different parts of the world and the way they should be served.

France

In France, bread is eaten with almost every meal and forms a major source of carbohydrate in food. The most famous bread from France is baguette and it has become so popular that it is often known as French bread. So many times when a person refers to French bread, he/she is actually referring to baguette. Let us read about a few of the most common breads of France in Table 4.10.

Table 4.10 Breads of France

Name	Description	Serving techniques
Baguette also known as French bread	This was invented around 1930 and it slowly but surely gained popularity. It has a sharp contrast of a crisp crust with a wonderfully soft interior. It is highly influenced by the soft French flour, and the long kneading and rising which is given to the bread by the skilful baker. Baguettes are always around two feet in length and will always have six scorings on the top.	This bread has a variety of uses in the current culinary world. It can be used as loaf bread, can be sliced to make a crostini, and can be used for making garlic bread as well as bruschetta. Moreover, it can be used as a base bread for open sandwiches and canapés.
Pain de campagne	It literally translates to country bread. These breads can be round or oval loaves and are usually made by using sourdough starters. Pain de campagne is a rustic bread that can contain a small percentage of wholewheat as well.	Mostly used as a loaf bread in a buffet or can also be sliced and made into toasts, or can also be used to make sandwiches and canapés.

(Contd)

Table 4.10 (Contd)

Name	Description	Serving techniques
Epi	It translates as 'wheat ear' and is traditional harvest bread. Its main feature is its unusual shape. Primarily, it is rolled like a baguette and then with scissors, insertions are given at regular intervals and the dough is pointed to alternate directions from the insertions.	Used as a very popular option in the lunch or dinner bread basket to have a good contrast of the shape and the texture. Also can be used to the same effect in case of a buffet.
Cereale	A torpedo shaped loaf which is dusted with flour. This is made with eight different cereals which include wheat, corn, rye, millet, oats, and malted wheat, as well as sunflower and sesame seeds.	Mostly used as a loaf bread in a buffet or can also be sliced and made into toasts, or can also be used to make sandwiches, canapés, and crostini.
Fougasse	Fougasse is also known as 'hearth bread' as it was baked on the hearth of the oven; after most of the bread was baked and the wood charcoal was burnt out, this bread was then baked on the hot ashes, which had a few pieces of smouldering charcoal. The bread is flat in shape and has slashes that resemble the branches of a tree.	Fougasse is traditionally used in bread displays as the unique flat shape with slashes makes it look very appealing.

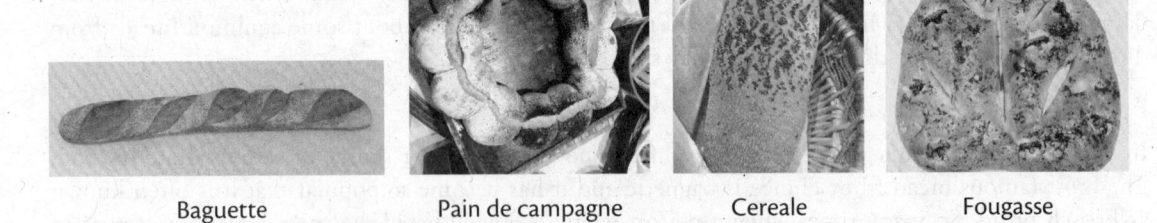

Baguette   Pain de campagne   Cereale   Fougasse

Fig. 4.3 Breads of France

Italy

Bread is commonly known as pane in Italian and like France, bread forms a staple carbohydrate with meals in Italy. Even dishes such as pastas are accompanied with bread and the most common—Italian pizza is also prepared on the base of a bread. In antipasti, bread can be used in various forms. It can be used for preparing open faced sandwiches known as bruschetta or even used for serving with Parma ham as grissini sticks. Left over bread in Italy is commonly combined with salad such as panzanella.

Let us discuss a few famous breads of Italy in Table 4.11.

Table 4.11 Breads of Italy

Name	Description	Serving techniques
Ciabatta	The name means 'slipper' which is justified by the shape of the bread. The dough of the bread is very soft and becomes difficult to handle and hence, lots of flour is used in the dough to give it a shape. This bread is traditionally topped with lots of flour before baking.	Mini ciabatta can be served in the bread basket. It can be used for making sandwiches. It can be sliced to particular thickness and used for open faced sandwiches and bruschetta.

Table 4.11 (Contd)

Name	Description	Serving techniques
Focaccia	The bread has a lot of olive oil, thus it requires to be kneaded for a longer time, which enhances the taste as well as the texture of the bread. The texture is contrasting with a hard and sharp crumb and a soft interior. There are many different flavourings which can be added in the bread such as tomatoes, olives, cheese, and nuts. Prior to baking, lots of olive oil is spread on the surface and one digs one's fingers into the dough to create lots of indentations. This helps the oil to seep in and give more flavour to the bread.	Frequently used as a component of the bread basket, as well as used to give a contrast and variety of shapes in any bread display. Also used for making crostini, bruschetta, and sandwiches.
Panettone	Panettone is usually made in tall cylindrical earthenware pots and is often sold in them. This bread is enriched with eggs, milk, butter, and raisins.	It is a very festive bread and is made during Christmas.
Grissini	These are thicker versions of a breadstick, which are made by incorporating olive oil in the dough. These sticks are shaped and then baked in a moderately hot oven and dried till they get hard. It results in a very crunchy breadstick.	Mostly served along with soups, can also be rolled in poppy seeds or sesame seeds or coarsely grounded sea salt and then baked. They could be rolled with *parma ham* and served as *antipasti*.
Pagnotta	The loaves can be of different shapes and sizes. But mostly pagnotta means a standard wheat loaf, which may be made using wholemeal flour. It is a very country style bread.	Generally used as a family bread which is made in bulk, and is cut and shared.
Pugliese	This bread comes from the region Puglia, which is very famous for its excellent olive oil and wheat. The bread is white, with a floury surface and a dense interior texture with soft crumb.	Used as a bread loaf, and can also be sliced and used individually.

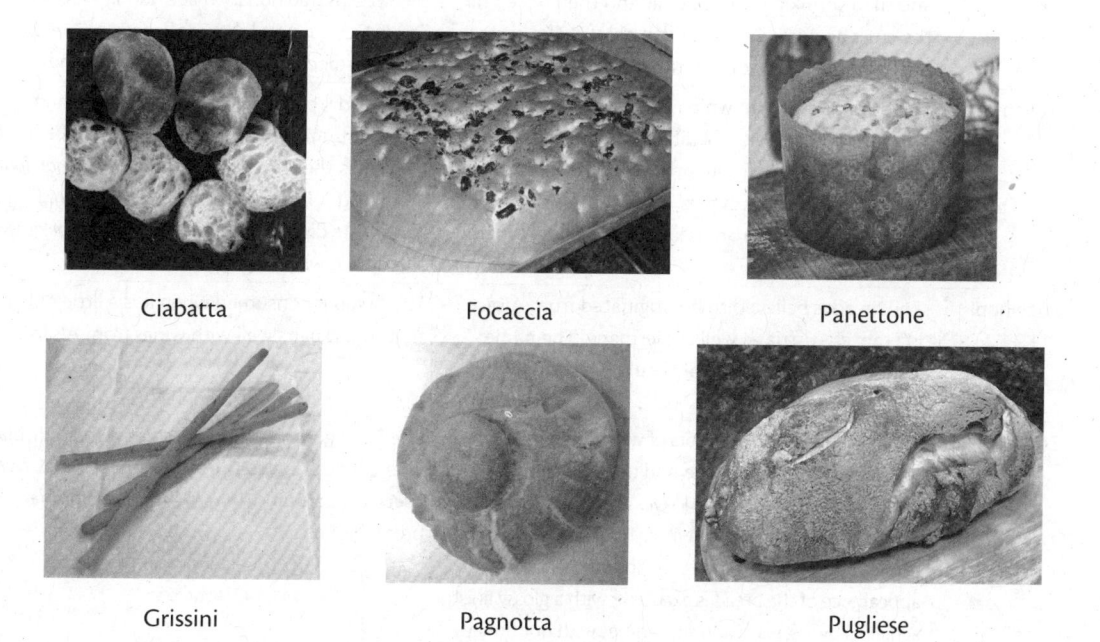

Ciabatta　　　　　Focaccia　　　　　Panettone

Grissini　　　　　Pagnotta　　　　　Pugliese

Fig. 4.4 Breads of Italy

Germany

Germany boasts of the largest collection of hearty breads that are popular in most parts of the world. The German breads are considered to be healthier as they contain wholemeal, rye, and an assortment of grains. German breads are also dense and more flavourful and often eaten with soups and cold meats. Many German types of bread also use spices such as caraway, dill, marjoram, and pepper.

Let us discuss a few of the most common German breads in Table 4.12.

Table 4.12 Breads of Germany

Name	Description	Serving techniques
Kastenbrots	The name means 'box bread' which is derived from the way the bread is enclosed in a tin and is steamed. The bread is made with rye flour or wholemeal flour and is leavened by a natural sourdough.	It is best complimented with a German beer. It can be served thinly sliced with butter or a soft cheese can be used as a spread. It can also be served along with smoked salmon, herring, sausage, etc.
Pumpernickel	It is normally made with rye flour but small amounts of wheat flour is seldom added to the dough to lighten the texture. The bread has a dark colour, dense texture, and a sour and earthy flavour.	It is generally consumed with smoked sausages, marinated fish, and cheese.
Landbrot	It is made in different shapes and sizes, but all are generally made with rye flour and buttermilk, which gives a sweet and sour taste to the bread. The crust is sometimes coated with flour before baking and sometimes not. The bread is chewy and not dense in texture.	Due to its chewy texture and the sour after taste, the bread is particularly good when served along with soups or stews.
Pretzels	They are always made from wheat flour, milk, and yeast. After proving, they are dipped in a lye solution and then sprinkled with sea salt and then baked till the crust acquires a dark golden colour. The crust is salty and the interior is contrastingly sweet.	The lye solution creates a drying effect in the throat and the person would drink more beer, so this bread is traditionally made during October Beer Fest in Germany and they are hanged on pretty wooden stands often known as pretzel stands.
Stollen	It is a very rich bread which has raisins, sultanas, mixed candied peels of fruits, eggs, butter, and milk. Nuts are also frequently added. The bread is heavy with a dense texture, a moist interior, and a brownish crust with an oblong shape and a tapered end.	This bread is particularly associated with Christmas, and is consumed all over during the festival. During Christmas, the bread is often stuffed with *marzipan* and baked. It is then called as *dresden stollen*. The stollens are dipped in clarified butter after baking and dusted with icing sugar.
Kugelhopf	The bread is believed to be originated from Alsace in France, Austria as well as Germany. The name is derived from the type of mould used for baking called *kugel*, which means 'ball'.	The bread is consumed when it is a little old and stale and it pairs well with wines from Alsace.
Zopf	This is a plaited loaf, the roots of which go long back to the Jews, who started the tradition of plaiting bread loaves. These plaited loaves are almost always enriched with yeast, made with white flour and plaited using three or more doughs. In most of the cases, the appearance of the bread is excellent, with a glossy finish achieved by egg wash and sometimes with hot honey.	Used as a good component in any bread display, where it adds on to the appearance. It is also used to a certain extent in lunch and dinner bread baskets.

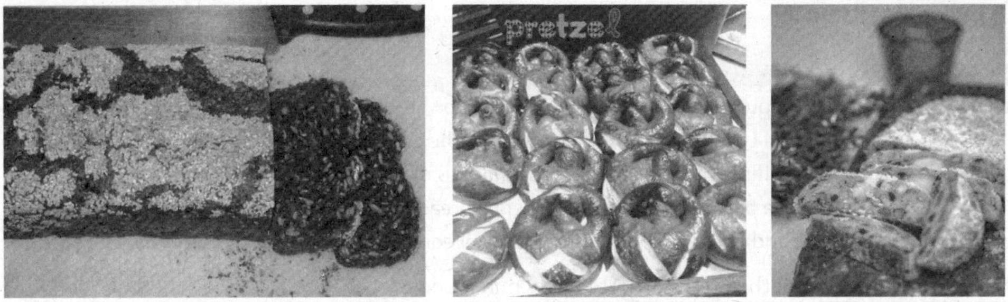

Pumpernickel	Pretzels	Stollen

Fig. 4.5 Breads of Germany

Great Britain

English like other European communities use bread as their staple. Most of the breads in England are however, consumed for sandwiches and a few breads such as English muffins are used for breakfast and others such as hot cross buns are commonly eaten during Easter.

Let us discuss a few of the most popular breads from Great Britain in Table 4.13.

Table 4.13 Breads of Great Britain

Name	Description	Serving techniques
Cob	The name means the head, as the appearance resembles one. Made with wholemeal flour and baked as a plain loaf, it can also be made with white flour or granary.	Basic loaf for family consumption, used as a loaf bread in the buffet.
Bloomer	It has a crusty exterior, complemented with soft interior. It has characteristic five or six scores on the crust and can be made from refined rye or multigrain flour.	Mostly used as a loaf, but can also be sliced and eaten.
Danish	It has firm crust and fine interior. The loaf is cylindrical in shape and dense in volume.	Used as a regular loaf.
Hovis	People began striving for more nutritious food and from this idea evolved the Hovis, which is actually the flour made with the inclusion of the wheat germ that is separated from the bread during milling. Now, it is a proprietary product, and has the name Hovis imprinted on the side of the loaf.	Used as a regular loaf.
Hot cross buns	The bread has a traditional cross mark, which is said to have evolved as a belief that it would ward off evil. This bread is flavoured with raisins, currents, nutmeg, cinnamon, and is enriched with yeast and eggs.	It is a popular celebration bread, eaten especially during Easter.
English muffins	Traditional flat discs of breads which are enjoyed in the winters. It is a very light bread and develops a thin skin like crust when cooked. It is not baked in oven but instead is cooked on hot plates.	It can be slit, toasted, buttered and is mostly preferred to be served along with eggs in a classical dish called Eggs Benedict.

(Contd)

Table 4.13 (Contd)

Name	Description	Serving techniques
Pikelets	Originated in counties such as Leicestershire, Yorkshire, Derbyshire, and Lancashire, they are cooked on the grill like English muffins. The only difference is that it is of the consistency of a batter and thus, the batter is spread on a griddle plate and grilled on both sides until cooked. The surface of the breads is dotted with minute holes.	Used as a base for sandwiches or simply eaten with butter.
Stotie	Rustic bread which comes from the northern part of England. It used to be the last one to be baked at the end of the day and was believed to be ready only when it was dropped on the floor and seen to bounce back.	Used as a loaf.

Bloomer   Danish   Hot cross buns

English muffins

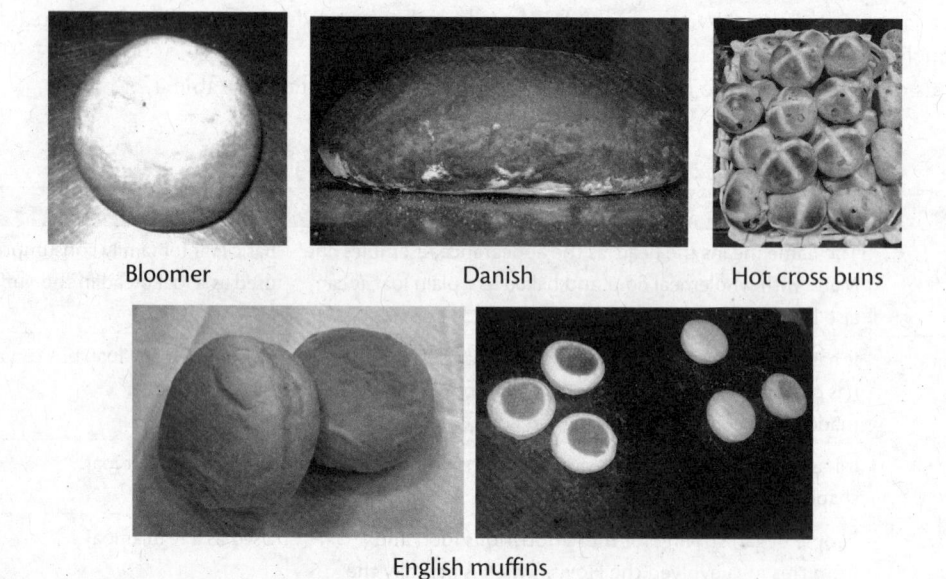

Fig. 4.6 Breads of Great Britain

Jewish Breads

In Judaism, it is customary for the eldest member of the family to break the bread and pass it on to everyone at the table, where a prayer is said expressing that they are grateful to the Lord, who is responsible for giving them the bread. Several varieties of bread are eaten by Jews and some of the most common ones are discussed in Table 4.14.

Middle East

It is believed that the first breads were baked in Egypt and then were spread all across the world by Arabs, who travelled extensively in search of food and fortunes. Today the breads from Middle East are very popular and eaten in all types of meals throughout the day.

Let us discuss some of the most common Middle Eastern breads in Table 4.15.

Table 4.14 Jewish breads

Name	Description	Serving techniques
Bagel	The bread is made with both refined flour, wholemeal and multigrain flour. It can include vegetable oil or margarine or butter along with eggs and yeast. The bread is poached or steamed for a minute or two and a then it is given an egg wash and baked, which helps in the formation of a glossy crust and a dense interior. Bagels are Jewish bread, which resemble a doughnut with a hole in the centre.	Bagels are served commonly in breakfast, but can also be served as sandwiches. Smoked salmon in mini bagels are very famous canapés.
Challah	Made with white flour, it is a leavened bread. It also has eggs, sultanas or raisins, which make it rich. It has a deep brown crust and a sweet white crumb. It can be round or plaited with 3, 6, or 12 strands of dough.	This bread is a festive bread and is consumed on the Sabbath in Jewish families.
Matzo	Also known as poor man's bread, it is a flat bread which is not leavened. History says that when Israelis left Egypt, they could not wait for long hours for the bread to rise and hence, ate these unleavened breads which then became traditional during the week long Passover in which one is not supposed to eat leavened bread.	Matzo bread can be formed into a dumpling and eaten in a broth, or a normal matzo which is a crisp flat bread is broken and eaten as it is.

Table 4.15 Breads of Middle East

Name	Description	Serving techniques
Lavash	It is a flat bread which can be very large. It can be oval, round, or rectangular in shape. It can be made with or without the addition of yeast, but unleavened is more popular. Generally, it is baked in low heat till it becomes very crisp and brittle. In the Middle Eastern countries, the oven in which it is baked is called *furunji*, or it is also baked in a dome covered oven called *saroj*.	This bread gives a good variation of texture when used in bread baskets. It can also be flavoured with ingredients such as poppy seeds, black onion seeds, chilli flakes, oregano, and can be brushed with olive oil and served warm as a snack along with dips.
Khoubiz	It is very similar to pizza base, the only difference is that it is made with wholemeal flour. But it can also be made with refined flour.	Commonly consumed in the Middle Eastern countries as part of their daily diet.
Pita	Pita is very similar to Indian *phulka*; the only difference is that unlike *phulka*, pita is made in oven. The pita is baked on hot stones and is ready to eat as soon as it puffs up.	Pita is served as snack with assorted dips. In Middle East, pita is served with *Falafel* fritters stuffed inside the pita pocket with a salad called *Fattoush*.

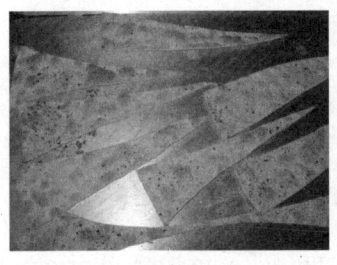

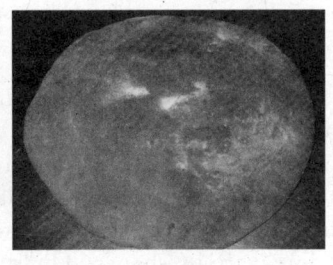

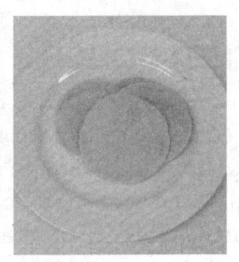

Lavash   Khoubiz   Pita

Fig. 4.7 Breads of Middle East

America

The breads in America are eaten mostly for sandwiches and burgers. Though most of the breads in US are softer as compared to the crusty rolls of Europe. Also a large population of US is gluten intolerant and hence, a range of gluten free breads is very popular in US today.

Let us discuss some of the most common breads of America in Table 4.16.

Table 4.16 Breads of America

Name	Description	Serving techniques
Burger bun	It is made with regular leavened dough, but it is normally kept bland in taste, as it will contain the fillings which will be flavourful. Normally, it is sprinkled with poppy or sesame seeds.	One of the most consumed breads in the world in the form of different burgers. Hot dog buns are made in the same way, the only difference is that they are rod shaped.
Hot dog bun	This is made with soft roll dough and is 6-8 inches elongated roll used for holding a Frankfurter sausage.	Hot dog buns are split open, grilled and served stuffed with grilled chicken and Frankfurter sausages.
Banana bread	The bread is more like a cake. Ripe bananas are used for making it along with baking powder for the required rise. The interior has a very dense texture. It is generally baked in tins.	Very popular tea bread and can also be served in breakfast.

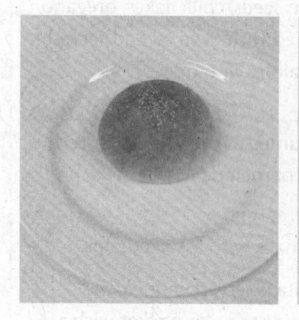

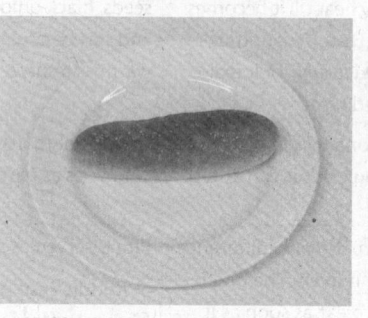

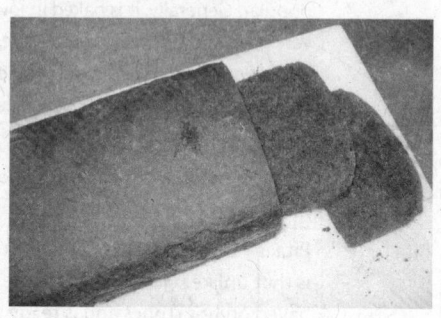

Burger bun   Hot dog bun   Banana bread

Fig. 4.8 Breads of America

ENRICHED DOUGH

As the name suggests, these doughs are enriched with ingredients such as proteins and fats. The protein could be in the form of eggs, milk, sugar and fats in the form of oil, butter, etc. We have already read about the role of ingredients in bread making and that ingredients such as eggs and butter make the dough rich and more flavourful. Such dough is slack and needs to be refrigerated before it can be shaped. The refrigeration allows the butter to firm up, thereby allowing the bread to be moulded into various shapes. The dough without any addition of fat and eggs is referred to as lean dough. The enriched dough can be used for the products mentioned in Table 4.17.

Table 4.17 Products made with enriched dough

Name	Description	Serving techniques
Brioche	There are two concepts, one is that it was made by using *brie*, so the name was given as brioche. Secondly, it has been derived from the word 'brier', which means to pound. Traditionally made as a *brioche à-tête*, or a Parisian brioche in which two balls of dough, a smaller on top of a larger one is placed and baked.	Used as a breakfast pastry, but also can be baked in the form of a loaf and sliced to make toasts or French toasts. Can also be made in a savoury one, generally with the inclusion of cheese.
Doughnut	This dough is allowed to chill for at least 12 hours, and then is rolled and cut with a doughnut cutter. This cutter is special and is a combination of a large and a small circular cutter integrated into each other in such a way, that when the rolled dough is cut, it makes it a circular bread with a hole in the middle.	Doughnuts are deep fried after proving and are popularly served in breakfast. They can be rolled in cinnamon sugar or can be glazed with melted chocolate/fondant.
Berliner	These are made from the doughnut dough and are formed into small balls and allowed to prove. These are then deep fried and filled with raspberry jam and coated with castor sugar.	Popularly served as breakfast rolls.

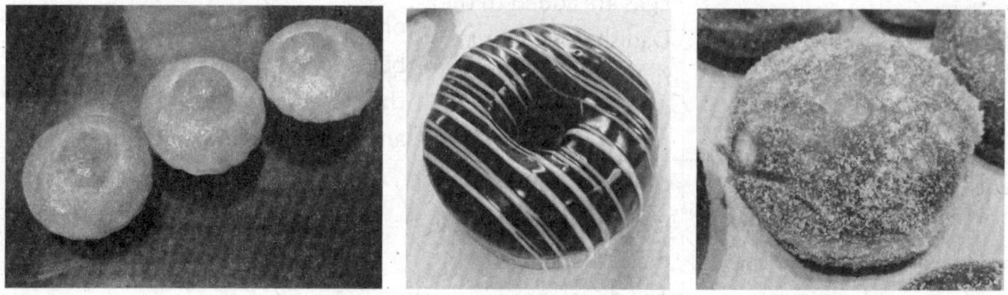

Brioche Doughnut Berliner

Fig. 4.9 Products made with enriched dough

LAMINATED DOUGH

Lamination in cooking terminology means a dough layered with fat in such a manner that layers of dough are separated by fat. This is achieved by encasing the dough with butter and rolling and folding it several times to get the desired effect. Laminated pastries can be made with plain dough to produce puff paste or fermented yeast dough is laminated to produce croissant and Danish pastries, which are the most common breakfast rolls eaten around the world. Sometimes dough is rolled out very thin and then laminated with fat, for example, as in *strudel from Austria*. Very thin sheets of *phyllo pastry* are laminated with fat and used for various purposes.

Whatever may be the name and use, but there are two things that are constant in any laminated pastry and these are—dough and fat. The dough could be of various types such as leavened or plain. Laminated pastries require lots of skill and technical knowledge and are not very easy to make.

Danish and Croissant

Danish and croissants are the two most important breakfast rolls served in the breakfast of any high end hotel. The quality of the croissants is very important. During my initial training at a pastry kitchen, I remember my executive chef telling me, how the impression of the hotel is created or broken by the quality of the croissants served in the breakfast. The Danish and croissant dough are used interchangeably in hotels, but traditionally, the Danish dough is richer than the croissant dough. Danish dough contains eggs and a little more quantity of butter than the croissant dough and that is the reason why sometimes, croissant dough is referred to as lean dough.

The style of laminating the Danish or the croissant dough is same as that of making puff pastry; the only difference is that the Danish and croissant dough are leavened with yeast. The Danish and croissant are flaky to eat, but their texture is soft and not crisp as in case of puff pastry. The other difference is that both the Danish and the croissant are proved like any other bread before being baked in the oven.

Let us discuss the ingredients used in Danish pastry in Table 4.18.

Table 4.18 Ingredients used in Danish and croissant dough

Flour	Fat	Liquid	Leavening	Flavourings
Medium flour is preferred for Danish pastry. The gluten must be well formed and elastic but not over mixed as the pastry will toughen.	The fat used is only butter as it gives a better taste to the product. Unlike puff pastry, the quantity of fat is half in case of Danish and croissant dough.	Cold milk or water or a combination of both should be used as warm water tends to activate the action of the yeast. Eggs are added to the Danish dough for a richer effect.	Yeast is the leavening agent used for Danish and croissant, and the process of making the dough could be same as that of any other bread dough. The only care that has to be taken is to just let the gluten develop and not to over mix.	Salt and sugar are the only flavours added to the Danish and croissant dough. Salt gives a colour and taste to the end product. It also helps in the keeping quality of the product, as it prevents staling.
Eighty percent of the flour is made into a dough with milk, eggs, sugar, yeast, and salt.	Remaining 20% of the flour is creamed with butter and the butter is set into a rectangular shape to make *butter block*. This helps the butter to stretch whilst rolling, thereby ensuring even distribution.	Cold liquid, preferably ice water is used to make the dough. The dough needs to be kneaded until the gluten is formed. The screen test is not required as we will not over mix the dough to get that texture.		

Techniques to Prepare Danish and Croissant

The techniques of laminating the Danish or croissant is similar to that of puff paste with a little bit of difference. Let us discuss this in the following steps.

Danish

Step 1 Combine flour, salt, sugar, milk, and the yeast together in a mixing bowl and knead into a smooth dough. Take care not to over mix the dough, as we want the end product to be soft yet flaky.

Step 2 Cover the dough and keep it for intermediate proving.

Step 3 Do the knock back.

Step 4 Rest the dough and meanwhile prepare the butter block.

Step 5 Roll the dough and laminate the butter in English style. French style can also be used but English is more preferred. Follow the same steps as shown in puff paste; but in case of croissant and Danish, give only three single folds unlike the six given in puff pastry.

- **English style** The dough is sheeted into a rectangle and the butter is placed on two thirds of the dough. The one third part that does not have butter is folded back on to the half of the two third part of the dough which has butter and then the remaining dough is folded over in such a way that a block is made with three layers of dough and two layers of butter.
- **French style** In this style, the dough is rolled out into the shape of a +9(plus) and the block of butter is placed in the centre, then the four ends of the dough are folded on top of the butter to form an envelope. The block is then sheeted for lamination.

Step 6 Cover the rolled pastry with plastic and freeze in the freezer until use. This is so done to avoid the proving of the dough in the refrigerator. Before rolling for final use, one can let the Danish rest at room temperature for sometime, which will bring it back to rolling consistency.

The shaping of croissant is very different from that of Danish pastries. The croissant can be plain or stuffed. The Danish are always garnished with fruits or various other fillings such as pastry cream and crème frangipani, and glazed with boiling apricot jam to give a shiny glaze. It can be drizzled with melted fondant to enhance the looks. The croissant on the other hand is glazed with eggs and baked. It is served plain or dusted with icing sugar if it is filled with sweet filling such as chocolate or almond paste. Let us understand the various types of Danish from Table 4.19.

Table 4.19 Types of Danish

Type of Danish	Method
Custard Danish	Roll out the pastry to 7 mm thickness and cut into 4 inch squares. Fold two opposite corners to meet in the centre and press them with your fingertips. Pipe custard cream in the centre and bake after proving. Glaze with melted hot apricot jam and drizzle with melted fondant. A readymade fondant can be used. To make it, cook sugar with a little amount of water and cream of tartar to 118°C. Spread on a clean marble table and work it with a spatula to make shape 8 on the table. When it cools down, knead it into a smooth white dough. This can be stored until further use at room temperature.
Cinnamon roll	Roll out the pastry into a rectangle of 6 mm thickness. Spread it with custard cream and sprinkle cinnamon powder and some raisins. Roll it like a Swiss roll and chill. Slice it 1 cm thick and prove prior to baking. Glaze with hot apricot jam.
Bear's claw	Roll out the Danish into 6 mm thick and 4 inch square pieces. Place almond paste in the centre and fold over one side to form a small rectangle. You can use egg wash to stick the sides. Now slit the end at small equal intervals, where the joint is and spread into a crescent for it to resemble a bear's claw. Prove, bake, and glaze with jam, and sprinkle roasted almond flakes.
Pin wheels	Roll the Danish into 6 mm thick and 4 inch square pieces. Make a slit from each corner till the centre of the pastry, taking care that the slits do not meet each other. Pipe custard cream in the centre and place a slice of stone fruit such as peach, prune, apricot, or fig, and fold each ear of the slit corner to meet in the centre.
Flower Danish	Roll the Danish into 6 mm thick and 4 inch square pieces. Fold the corners to meet each other in the centre. Pipe custard cream in the centre and place a slice of stone fruit such as peach, prune, or apricot and allow the Danish to prove before it is baked in oven and then glaze with jam.

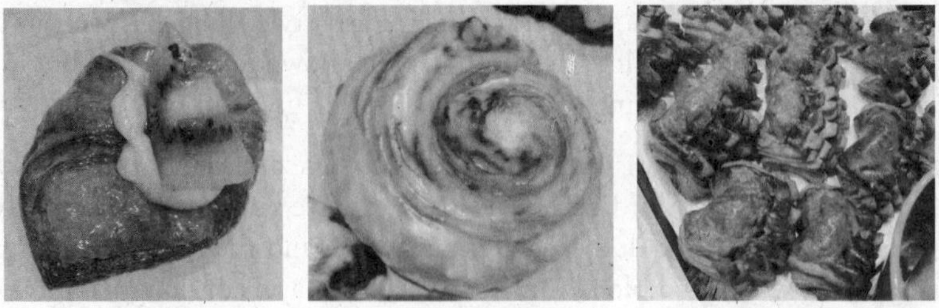

Custard Danish Cinnamon roll Bear's claw

Fig. 4.10 Types of Danish

Croissant

The method of making and rolling the croissant dough is same as that of the Danish dough, but the final shaping of this crab shaped pastry is different from Danish. Let us discuss this in the following steps.

Step 1-6 Similar to Danish.

Step 7 Roll the pastry into about 7 mm thick and around 6-7 inches wide strips.

Step 8 Cut the strips into triangles. Ensure that the base of the triangles is 4 inches.

Step 9 Make a small slit in the base of the triangle and roll the triangle like a cigar, from the base till the tip.

Step 10 Place onto baking sheets and prove until double in size. Glaze with egg wash and bake until golden brown and crisp.

Croissants are usually baked plain, but sometimes they could be stuffed with grated chocolate to make chocolate croissant. They can be glazed with melted chocolate after baking or simply dusted with icing sugar.

STORAGE AND SERVICE OF BREAD

The role of the baker does not end with the production of prime quality bread, in fact that is just the beginning. The chef has to ensure that the good quality product should reach the consumer so that the product is enjoyed and relished by the end user. It is therefore, important to prepare and serve freshly baked breads. In most of the bakeries in hotels and other establishments, the breads are baked close to meal period, so that the consumer gets a fresh product. However, in a few conditions where the bread needs to be stored with a shelf life of a few days, it is important to follow certain storage principles to ensure that it does not suffer in its quality or taste.

Let us discuss a few of these storage procedures.

- When the bread is made in a mould, it should be immediately removed and allowed to cool on a cooling rack. Letting the bread cool in the mould will cause growth of rope disease in bread due to condensation of moisture and thereby, the absorption of the same by the bread.

- Always store bread at a room temperature of 20°C. The place should not be humid as the moisture present in the air can cause moulds in the bread. The bread will keep well for upto two days.

- If the bread needs to be stored for a longer period of time, it must never be stored in refrigerator, as it stales quickly if placed in a refrigerator. Instead wrap the bread in a plastic film and store at a temperature of -18-20°C in a freezer. The frozen bread is allowed to thaw at room temperature and baked in oven again for a couple of minutes. This will refresh the bread and make it fresh again.

The bread is served in various ways and it depends on the timing of the meal, type of the meal, and the kind of establishment where it is being served. Let us discuss some of the common ways in which a bread is served.

- **As an accompaniment**: Individual bread rolls can be served in a bread basket accompanied with butter, olive oil, or vinegar. Certain breads can be made into smaller loaves and served sliced in the bread basket. A bread basket contains an assortment of crusty rolls, soft rolls, breadsticks, and a few pieces of flat bread to provide variety to customers.
- **Buffet display**: The breads can be displayed on buffet counters, where the freshly baked loaves of bread can be sliced by the customers and eaten along with their meal. The bread for breakfast is sliced and kept in buffet. The bread is toasted fresh and served along with breakfast.
- **Pastry shop**: Many hotels have outlets such as pastry shops, where cakes, pastries, breads, chocolates, etc., are sold to customers. In this shop, whole loaves are freshly baked to be sold. It is important for chefs to mention the best by use date on breads, when selling through pastry shops.

SUMMARY

This chapter dealt with basic principles of bread making. Making of bread is a combination of art and science. Care has to be taken whilst producing breads, as badly made bread can spoil the experience of great lavish meals. We spoke in detail regarding the various ingredients that are used in bread making and how each ingredient lends a particular texture and feel to the bread. We understood the effect of heat, mixing techniques and other factors that affect the gluten, which in turn helps in the volume of the bread. We read about flours in chapter 2 and also studied about gluten free breads. In this chapter, we discussed how water is the key element in the consistency of the dough.

More liquid turns the dough into a batter, which is also essential in making certain breads. We studied about dried and fresh yeasts and understood the importance of yeast foods such as sugar. We also learnt how to check the freshness and life of yeasts by doing certain tests. We also studied about temperatures that are suitable for yeasts and learnt that high temperatures such as 50°C can kill the yeast completely. Whilst we discussed ingredients, we also read the comparison of the products having less and excessive quantity of the particular ingredient and how this affects the texture of the final product. We also read about bread improvers, commonly used in bread making in hotels around the world.

After studying about the ingredients and the way they react in different combinations and mixing techniques, we also studied about the principles behind bread making. We discussed the making of breads in 10 crucial steps starting from collecting ingredients and weighing them to cooling of the bread. We learnt about the various ways in which the dough is mixed. The dough can be mixed with hands, but machines provide better results, especially in cases where one would like the gluten to fully develop in the dough. We studied about straight dough, salt delayed, and ferment sponge methods of mixing dough and how each product differs from the other when made with these methods. We studied about proving of breads and understood why it is done in that manner. We discussed the various shapes in which breads could be shaped. We discussed about various kinds of glazes and toppings that are used to create a variety in bread baskets.

We also discussed a very important part on faults in breads and understood how an ingredient or even the process of bread making can result in poor quality bread. We also discussed the range of small and big equipment used in bread making.

We studied about the various breads from around the world and listed a few which are commonly made in our hotels in India. We also came to know a little history regarding some breads and what are the various uses that these breads can be put to. We also discussed some common shapes of breads and understood the difference between enriched dough and lean dough.

In the last section, we discussed an important aspect of dough making known as lamination. Laminated pastries such as Danish and croissant are the soul of every breakfast buffet in a hotel. We also threw light on the storage principles of bread and how they are commonly served.

Theory of Bakery and Patisserie

KEY TERMS

Biga Italian starter used in Italian breads

Compressed yeast Fresh yeast that requires refrigeration

Crust A crisp surface on top of a baked product, usually bread or a cookie

Demerara sugar Kind of sugar that is brown in colour

Fermentation Reaction of yeast and sugar to produce a sour taste and carbon dioxide in dough

Fiscelle Thin baguettes from France

Flying tops Dried patches on top of a bread that look like cracks

Gingerbread Festive bread made with rye flour on occasion of Christmas

Gluten Protein present in the flour

Hearth The floor of the wood fired oven

Hydration The amount of liquid absorbed by the flour, usually measured in percentage

Instant yeast Type of yeast that is available in powdered form and does not require refrigeration

Khameer Indian word for a sourdough starter

Levain French term for a sourdough starter

Maltose Natural sugar present in the flour

Panzanella Italian salad made with vegetables and stale bread

Phyllo pastry Thin sheets of flour based product from Greece

Pullman loaf Another name for a sandwich bread

Rope Disease of a bread that spreads due to improper storage

Sourdough Naturally fermented dough used as a starter for making bread

Zopf Festive bread made in Austria and is glazed with honey

OBJECTIVE TYPE QUESTIONS

1. Apart from the recipe, what are the other factors that influence the making of good bread?
2. Define a sourdough starter and list its uses.
3. What is rope and how does sourdough starter help to prevent the same?
4. Why should the oven be used to its optimum capacity with regards to humidity?
5. What points should be kept in mind with regards to baking of bread in an oven?
6. Why is ice used in certain bread recipes?
7. How many types of yeast are there and how does one test the freshness of yeast?
8. What range of temperature kills the yeast?
9. Write at least five impacts of sugar on the bread dough.
10. What are bread improvers and what is their role?
11. List down the 10 steps of bread making in the correct order.
12. List down the jobs that you would take care of in step 1 of the bread making process.
13. What are the various ways of mixing bread?
14. How does salt delayed process help in improving the flavour of the bread?
15. What is no time dough method and what are its advantages and disadvantages?
16. What is a windscreen test and why is it done?
17. Why is knock back done after the first proving of the bread?
18. Define the process of proving and why it is essential.
19. What is panning?
20. What are the three stages in baking?
21. List down at least five glazes and the effects of the same.
22. List down the reasons of flaked crust in a baked bread.
23. What are the reasons if the baked bread lacks volume?
24. If a baked bread has uneven texture and large holes, what could be the fault?
25. The bread would stale rapidly if.... Complete the statement.
26. Why is a wooden table top preferred to metal ones?

27. List down at least three French breads.
28. Write the names and uses of at least five Italian breads.
29. Which is the dark rye bread from Germany?
30. What is the significance of pretzels during the Beer fest?
31. What is unique about bagels?
32. Name at least three breads from Middle East.

ESSAY TYPE QUESTIONS

1. Bread making is a combination of art and science. Justify the statement.
2. What is the role of water in bread making?
3. What care should be taken whilst making bread with hard water?
4. Analyse the difference between having less salt and excessive salt in bread.
5. Compare the results of having less sugar and excessive sugar in bread dough.
6. What is the effect of fats and oils on the bread dough?
7. Write down the salient features of retarder prover.
8. List down the sizes of bread rolls, burger buns, French baguette, and bread loaves.
9. List down the steps for making laminated dough.
10. Describe at least five types of Danish pastries.

ACTIVITY

1. In groups, make dough using at least five various kinds of flours. Check the windscreen of each dough and wash the dough under running water until it washes no further and the chewy structure is obtained. This is the gluten. Compare the percentage of the gluten in each flour and record your observation. Now make bread using the same flours and compare the results in volume of each bread. Record your observation and now using the same flours make the recipe again, this time put the gluten obtained from the first test in the recipe of the bread. Make sure to add the gluten obtained from the respective flours into the same type of flours. Bake the breads and compare with the ones baked the first time. Compare your results and see how gluten percentage in dough affects the volume of the bread.
2. Divide yourselves into 7 groups. Six of the groups shall make at least one fault in the dough and one of the 7 groups shall make the perfect bread. Compare the results and record observations.
3. Visit various hotels and restaurants in your city and do a study of various kinds of breads and breakfast rolls served in their outlets.
4. Research about various breads made around the world and make those breads for tasting and get them evaluated by experts.

5 Basic Pastes in Bakery and Pastry

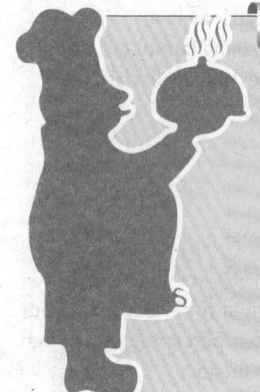

LEARNING OBJECTIVES

After reading this chapter, you should be able to

- know the different types of pastes that can be used as fillings for cakes and pastries to create desserts
- know the various steps involved in production of pastes and the usage and storage of each paste
- prepare various kinds of pastes and understand the various desserts made from them
- know the role played by different ingredients in making pastes
- know about the various types of international desserts made by using these pastes

INTRODUCTION

Pastes form the base of many pastries, while many are used as fillings prior to baking. For example, a classical cake called gateau pithivier is made with puff pastry and filled with frangipani paste or almond paste. The mixture of flour, sugar, butter, and milk or water was initially used in various proportions to create dough or batter. Certain fat rich batters on chilling formed into a dough that could be rolled out and baked. This probably gave rise to pastes in bakery and pastry. Not all pastes are used for making desserts, some of the pastries are savoury in taste and are used to prepare many snacks and products for hi tea.

Even the pastes in bakery and pastry do not just refer to things that are grounded into pastes with addition of liquids; instead many basic pastes such as choux paste are mostly used for making various types of pastries and sweet paste is used for making cookies and tarts. Probably pastry came from the word paste, where the paste of water and flour was used to encase meat while cooking. As the paste baked, it got flavoured with the juices from the meat and was eaten along with the meat. Even today, certain meats are wrapped with doughs or puff pastry and then roasted in ovens. In bakery and confectionery, there are many such pastes that actually resemble dough (sweet paste) but are grouped into this broad group of pastes.

PASTES

In this section, we shall understand the various types of pastes and their uses in the pastry kitchen. It is important for chefs to understand the role played by the ingredients in each paste, as it will help them to critique their product and enable them to provide a different texture by altering the recipe. Many pastes used in confectionery appear to be like dough, but are classified as pastes. The reason is that when they are freshly made they appear like paste, but when refrigerated, the butter sets with flour to give the texture of dough. It must be understood that dough refers to kneading of flour with water to develop the gluten. However, while making certain pastes, such as short crust paste, care is taken so that gluten does not develop in flour otherwise it will lose its 'short' properties. Here short refers to the flakiness of the pastry product. In Hindi, it is called *khasta*.

Short Crust Paste

Short paste or short crust paste is crisp and brittle. It is not elastic and resilient like dough and this shortness in a cookie or many pastry products is much desired to alter the texture and mouth feel of a product. Short crust paste is usually used for making savoury products such as turnovers and pies. Table 5.1 shows the role of ingredients in making short crust paste.

Table 5.1 Ingredients used in short crust paste

Flour	Fat	Liquid
Soft flour is used to avoid elasticity in the product. The product should be resilient and brittle.	The fat used is usually butter; margarines also give a good product, but since margarines are trans fats we should avoid their usage.	Cold water should be used as warm water tends to melt the fat, thereby giving a stretchy texture to the pastry.
Flour is sifted well to provide aeration to the final product.	Fat is cut into smaller pieces and rubbed-in with flour.	Cold liquid, preferably ice water, is sprinkled on the top of rubbed flour and fat is allowed to be absorbed by the paste.

Steps of Making Short Crust Paste

The steps of making short crust paste are given below. Usually, the first two steps are followed for making short crust paste; but if pies or flans are to be made then the latter steps are followed.

Step 1   Mix the butter and flour. This could be done by using the following methods.

- **Rubbing-in method:** The cut pieces of butter are rubbed into the flour to produce coarse breadcrumb size particles. Cold water is sprinkled over and the dough is lightly mixed to form short crust paste. It is chilled in the refrigerator before using.
- **Pinning method:** The butter is cut into small cubes and rolled with the flour until it flakes. The mixture is then collected in a bowl and cold water is sprinkled over it. The paste is collected together to form short crust paste.

Step 2   Chill the paste in the refrigerator. It will be easy to roll later, if the paste is put in a plastic bag and flattened out with the tip of fingers before refrigerating.

Step 3 Pin the dough with a rolling pin (Fig. 5.1). If lining a pie dish, roll into a circle, roll it back on to the rolling pin (Fig. 5.2), and unroll it in the pie dish (Fig. 5.3). Usually 240 g of dough lines a pie dish of 8 inches diameter. There is no need to grease the pie mould as short crust paste contains lots of butter. While making tarts or tartlets in bulk, place the tart moulds close to each other to form a large rectangle. Sheet out the dough and follow the same procedure of rolling it over rolling pin and unrolling it on to the tart moulds. Then press the short crust over the tarts with your palms and then finish each one individually (Figs. 5.4 and 5.5). The trimming left over should not be kneaded together; instead just collect it and roll it again, if needed.

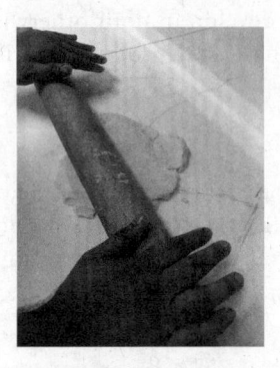

Fig. 5.1 Pinning the dough with rolling pin

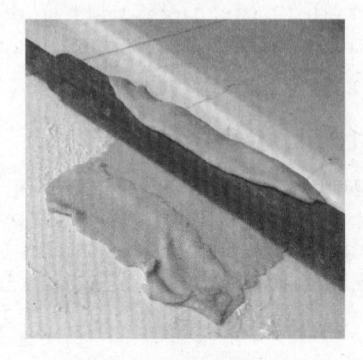

Fig. 5.2 Rolling the dough

(a)

(b)

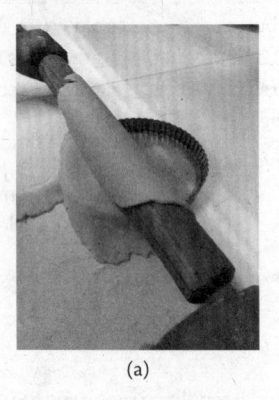

Fig. 5.3 Unrolling the dough

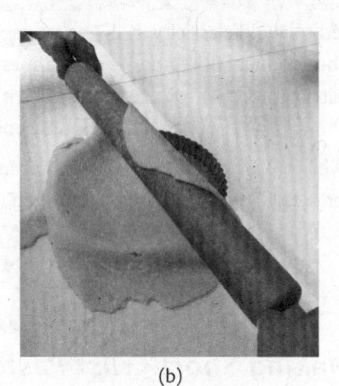

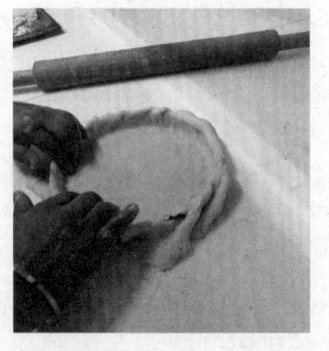

Fig. 5.4 Levelling the tart

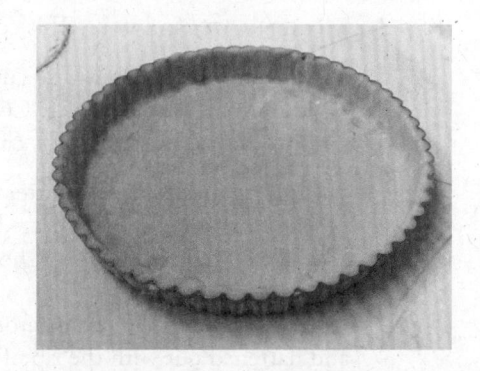

Fig. 5.5 Tart for blind baking

Step 4 Dock the pastry to allow the steam to escape from it while baking.

Step 5 Blind bake the shell. Line with greaseproof paper and fill with beans. The paper does not let the beans stick to the pastry. When half-done, remove the beans and bake the pastry again so that it turns golden brown. At this stage, you can add minced meats and vegetables along with cream and eggs to make a pie called quiche.

Uses of Short Crust Paste

The uses of short crust paste are as follows:

- Short crust can be used for making tarts, pies, and flans. Table 5.2 shows the difference between tarts, pies, and flans.
- Short crust can also be rolled and cut into shapes and used as savoury biscuits.
- It can be crumbled and used as a topping on pies to give a rustic crust.
- Certain meats are encased in short crust prior to baking.

Table 5.2 Difference between tarts, pies, and flans

Tart	Pie	Flan
Tart is a mould which is 3–4 inches in diameter with raised edges. The smaller version of 1 inch diameter is called tartlet.	This is a dish made in a flan mould. Pies are usually sweet or savoury fillings baked in a flan.	Flan is a mould that is 6–8 inches in diameter with raised edges.
Tarts are baked like shells and then cooked fillings and creams are added to them. They are open and never closed.	A pie is usually covered on top with another piece of crust.	Sometimes large tarts which are open are also referred to as flans; we cannot call them pies as pies are always covered.
Tarts are blind baked and cooked fillings are filled in them.	The pie is blind baked till half done and then the filling is put inside and then it is baked again.	Flans are blind baked and cooked fillings are filled inside the shell.
Tarts are usually sweet.	Pies can be sweet or savoury.	Flans are usually sweet.
Examples, fresh fruit tart, lemon curd tart, etc.	Examples, apple pie, Australian leek pie, etc.	Examples, fruit flan, custard flan, etc.

Sweet Paste

Sweet paste is sweet in taste. It is short and brittle like the short crust paste, but its usage is restricted to sweet products. Table 5.3 shows the role of ingredients in making sweet paste.

Table 5.3 Ingredients used in sweet paste

Flour	Fat	Liquid	Sweetener
Soft flour is used to avoid elasticity in the product. The product needs to be resilient and brittle.	The fat used is usually butter. Margarines also give a good product, but as margarines are trans fats the use of these should be avoided.	Eggs are used as liquid in pastes.	Castor sugar or icing sugar is recommended to be used as sweetener. They are more readily soluble, which has a softening effect on the gluten in the flour, in turn influencing the shortening properties of the sweet paste.

Table 5.3 (Contd)

Flour	Fat	Liquid	Sweetener
Flour is sifted well to provide aeration to the final product.	Fat is cut into smaller pieces and either creamed with sugar or rubbed in with flour like short crust paste.	Cold eggs are used as liquid.	Sift the icing sugar to avoid any lumps in the sweet paste. Do not use grain sugar as it will leave brown specks after baking.
If chocolate flavoured sweet paste is desired, then 20 percent of flour is substituted with cocoa powder. Other flavourings, such as lemon zest, can also be added to the flour.		Sometimes milk is added if almond flour is added to the sweet paste.	

Steps of Making Sweet Paste

The steps of making sweet paste are given below. Usually, the first two are followed for making sweet paste; but if pies or flans are to be made then the latter steps are followed.

Step 1   Mix the butter and flour. This could be done by using the following methods.

- **Creaming method:** The butter and sugar should be creamed well. The idea is to make it lighter by incorporation of air. This is the most commonly used method to make sweet paste. The eggs then are added one by one until all the eggs are added. A flat paddle is used to beat the mix. The mixture is then removed from the mixer and carefully folded in the sifted flour to obtain sweet paste. Do not over mix as the sweet paste will lose its shortening effect.
- **Rubbing-in method:** The cut pieces of butter are rubbed into the flour to produce coarse breadcrumb size particles. Beaten eggs are lightly mixed to form sweet paste. The paste is chilled in the refrigerator before using. This method is not very commonly used.

Step 2   Chill the paste in the refrigerator. If the paste is put in a plastic bag and flattened out with the tip of fingers before refrigerating, it will be easy to roll it later.

The other three steps are similar to that of short crust paste.

Uses of Sweet Paste

The uses of sweet paste are as follows:

- Sweet paste is used for making tarts, pies, and flans.
- It is rolled, cut into various shapes, and baked as cookies and biscuits.
- It is used as base for certain cakes and pastries.
- Thin cut out sheets of sweet paste can be used as decorations.

Choux Paste

Choux means cabbage in French. Here baking results in a shape that resembles a cabbage and probably that is the reason why it has been given this name. Choux paste's consistency is between dough and batter and it is used in both savoury items and desserts. This paste may or may not contain sugar, depending upon the usage of the final product. Choux is a versatile, partially pre-cooked paste that can be baked for use in pastries and gateaux, fried for use in potato dishes and fritters, or boiled in gnocchi dishes. Pastry products made from choux paste include éclairs, Paris Brest, gateau St Honore, profiteroles, and many others.

There are many recipes with varying formulae, each giving a product of a different consistency depending on its purpose. When the choux paste is baked, a steam is formed inside which pushes the paste out giving it a hollow texture. This is then baked at low temperature to dry out the pastry to keep it firm and crisp. Otherwise the product will collapse and will be chewy. The tunnel thus created in the pastry is filled with different types of flavoured fillings and decorated. Choux paste is not only baked, but also deep-fried. Table 5.4 shows the role of ingredients in making choux paste.

Table 5.4 Ingredients used in choux paste

Flour	Fat	Liquid
Medium to strong flour should be used, as gluten is required to provide good elasticity and volume to the paste.	The fat used is butter as it gives a better flavour to the product.	Water and eggs are the primary liquids used in choux paste. Water is boiled with butter and flour is cooked until it leaves the sides of the pan. It is then removed from the fire and eggs are incorporated one by one until a paste is obtained.
In India, we would use the normal flour.		The quantity of eggs will depend upon the size of the eggs, degree of cooking of flour, and the amount of flour and fat used.

CHEF'S TIP
While piping éclairs, round tube no. 809 is the perfect choice and if any tip is formed, wet your finger in water and smoothen it out.

Steps of Making Choux Paste

The steps followed in making choux paste are given below.

Step 1 Place the fat and water in a pan and heat until the fat melts and the water boils. The fat and water should boil simultaneously. The fat should be cut into small pieces to help it melt quickly, preventing the loss of water through evaporation. If water loss occurs, the pastry would contain too much fat, making it heavy.

Step 2 Add the sieved flour all at once to the fat and water emulsion and stir continuously with a wooden spoon. This will prevent lumps from forming in the paste. The flour should be added only when the fat and water has come to a boil. This paste, called *panada*, is cooked until it leaves the sides of the pan without sticking.

Step 3 Add the eggs to the *panada* when the mixture has cooled to approximately 60°C. This is done to prevent the eggs from completely cooking in the paste, which would result in a heavy paste. Add the eggs one at a time, working the paste to a smooth consistency before the next egg is added. The final consistency of the paste for pastries should fall off the back of the spoon. Take care when adding the last of the eggs as different flours have different adsorption characteristics. The paste should have a good, smooth sheen. It should be soft and should be able to retain its shape when piped.

Step 4 Pipe the choux paste onto lean baking trays that are lightly greased. They can also be lightly dusted with flour after they have been greased. This paste does not require a resting period. It can be piped immediately and then baked.

Step 5 Bake at a high temperature initially (200 to 220°C, depending on the size). The baking of choux pastry requires a lot of care. While baking, the oven door should not be opened too frequently because the loss of heat may cause the pastry to collapse. Also, if the pastry is not baked thoroughly until it is properly dried, it may collapse. The development of colour is not sufficient indication that the item is cooked properly. If the 'shell' is not firm and crisp, reduce heat and bake further to dry out. The choux paste, after baking, should be light for its weight and when sliced open it should be hollow from inside.

Uses of Choux Paste

Choux paste is a versatile paste and can be used in savoury or desserts. There are many uses of choux paste and some of these are shown in Table 5.5.

Table 5.5 Preparations of choux paste

Item	Description
Chocolate éclairs	Piped in tube shape usually 4 inches long and after baking it is filled with flavoured cream or custard and glazed with melted chocolate or fondant.
Profiteroles	Round-shaped balls of choux paste baked and filled with flavoured creams and glazed with chocolate, caramelized sugar, sifted icing sugar, fondant, etc.
Croquembouche	Profiteroles are filled with custard, flavoured with 'grand mariner' and glazed with caramelized sugar. It is built in a height and is used as a traditional wedding cake in France.
Gateau St Honore	It is a classical gateau from France. It is made by piping a ring of choux paste on a thin disc of puff pastry and baked. The ring of choux paste is then sliced from top and filled with crème chiboust. The ring is decorated with filled profiteroles glazed with caramelized sugar and the centre of the gateau is piped with alternate swirls of crème chiboust and pastry cream.
Paris Brest	A ring-shaped choux paste, baked and piped with whipped cream and decorated with fresh fruits and berries. It is decorated with sifted icing sugar as well.
Swans	Choux paste is piped in the shape of tear drop and baked to make swans. The top is cut and then split in half length-wise to make the wings of swans. The neck is piped in a thin curved shape and baked separately. Swans can be filled with crème Chantilly and assembled to resemble swans.

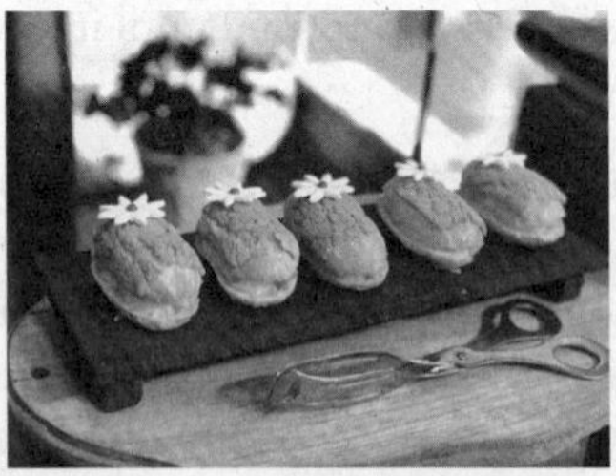

Chocolate éclairs 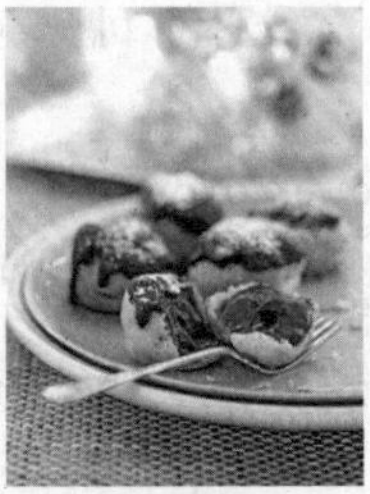 Profiteroles 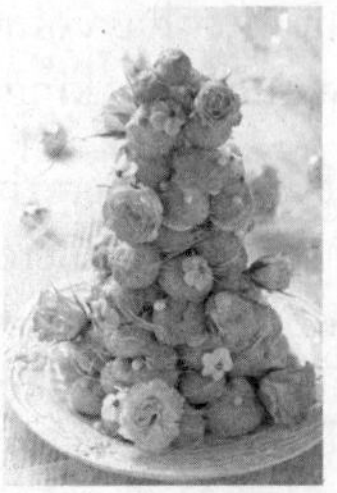 Croquembouche 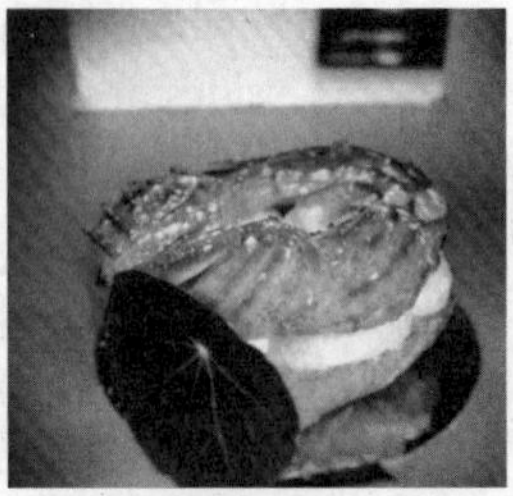 Paris Brest

Fig. 5.6 Preparations of choux paste

Puff Pastry

Puff pastry consists of laminated structure built up with alternate layers of dough and fat. This achieved by rolling out the dough and giving it sufficient turns until there are many layers of dough and fat. When this pastry is baked, the fat melts and releases moisture. As the water vapours turn into steam it helps in separating the layers from each other and gives an illusion of a pastry 'puffing up'. The heat from the oven creates a browning effect, resulting in a delightful, crisp, light, flaky pastry called puff pastry. Though it is a form of dough which is laminated, it is still classified into pastes as it is not baked directly. The puff pastry has been discussed in detail in the previous chapter on breads.

SUMMARY

In this chapter, we discussed various kinds of pastes that can be used as fillings for cakes and for decorating them. After the completion of this section, you would be able to make cakes of international standards. As baking of cakes calls for a lot of skill and patience, it can be perfected by practice.

We discussed various kinds of pastes used in confectionery and read about their versatile uses. We saw how some pastes, such as choux paste and puff pastry, form the base for many desserts, and are used as fillings as well prior to baking. Some pastes are used for making garnishes and decorations.

We discussed short crust paste and sweet paste and understood the uses of the same. We also saw how techniques can affect the final product. If the ingredients in the sweet paste or short paste are kneaded, then they will form into dough; but just by treating the ingredients differently, we get the product that can be used for making cookies and pies. In each category, we also discussed the role played by the ingredients in making of these products and how we can alter them to change the textures. While discussing pastes, we also discussed various other pastry-related things such as differences among tarts, pies, and flans. We focused on the making and usage of choux pastry and various desserts made from the same.

In the next chapter, we will discuss basic creams and sauces used in bakery and pastry, and this will complete our basic and elementary knowledge about bakery and confectionery.

KEY TERMS

Almond paste Almonds grounded into a powder and creamed with butter and sugar. It is used as fillings in cakes and pastries.

Blind baking Baking a pie or tart without any filling.

Castor sugar Another name for breakfast sugar.

Crème Chiboust Pastry cream mixed with a part of meringue, also known as St Honore cream.

Docked Pricking of a pastry with a sharp needle so that it does not rise whilst baking.

Flan Large tarts that are usually sweet.

Ganache One part cream and one and a half parts of chocolate cooked together and whipped to a cream when cold. It is used for fillings.

Gateau pithivier A disc-shaped cake made by sandwiching two discs of puff pastry with almond paste and baked in the oven.

Gluten The protein obtained when the flour is kneaded with water.

Hazelnut A kind of nut enclosed in a shiny light brown shell.

July pan A type of decorating paste.

Khasta Hindi word for short texture.

Lemon zest The outer skin of lemon, without the white pith.

Margarine Vegetable shortening that is hardened by addition of hydrogen.

Panada Starch thickened with liquid to resemble a thick paste or dough.

Pastry cream Milk cooked with eggs, sugar, and starch to produce a creamy product.

Pate à brise Short crust pastry in French.

Pate à sucre French word for sweet paste.

Pie A tart which is covered with pastry dough and baked.

Pinning Rolling of dough with a rolling pin.

Quiche A savoury pie made by combining meat and vegetables with egg based custard and baked.

Short A texture where the product is crisp and snaps in to two pieces when bent.

Streusel A rough crumbly mixture of fat and flour often used as a topping for pies and tarts.

Strong flour Flour that contains high amount of gluten.

Turnovers A sweet or savoury product, where a filling is folded between a geometrical shaped pastry. It can be round, half moon, square, or triangle.

OBJECTIVE TYPE QUESTIONS

1. Define paste in the context of confectionery. How are these different from pastes used in Western cooking?
2. What is the difference between short crust paste and sweet paste?
3. How would you differentiate among a tart, flan, and a pie?
4. What is the role of flour, fat, and liquid in short paste?
5. Short crust paste and sweet paste need to be short. What do you understand by this and how would you ensure that the final product is short?
6. List the steps of making short crust paste.
7. What factors cause shrinkage of short crust paste and sweet paste?
8. Define the role of ingredients in making sweet paste.
9. List five products made by using choux paste.
10. Give names of at least three classical desserts made from choux paste.
11. What is the principle behind rising of the choux paste and the hollow structure?
12. List the steps involved in making choux pastry.

ESSAY TYPE QUESTIONS

1. How is sweet paste prepared? Describe the steps.
2. Explain the role of ingredients used in short crust paste and choux paste.
3. Describe the preparations of choux paste and how one is different from the other.
4. Explain the making of puff pastry.
5. Define the creaming and rubbing-in methods and explain their usage in making pastes.

ACTIVITY

1. In groups, make at least five different paste recipes and compare the pastes and write your observation in the given table.
2. Visit the various pastry shops in your city and write down the types of cakes and pastry products available in these shops. Now make a list of fillings that were used for creating those products.
3. Make pastry cream and add various flavours to the same. Compare the results and add different textured products to the cream such as roasted chopped nuts, chopped chocolate, broken pieces of meringue and taste the products. Make a creative cake with this cream and compare with each other.

Name of paste	Texture	Consistency	Baking effect	Colour

6 Basic Creams and Sauces

LEARNING OBJECTIVES

After reading this chapter, you should be able to

- understand the different types of creams that can be used as fillings for cakes and pastries to create desserts
- know the role played by different ingredients in making creams
- understand the various techniques used in preparing sauces and the faults of sauces
- make different types of sauces with various bases and understand their uses in desserts and pastry making
- make various types of classical and contemporary sauces
- claim an insight into storage and service of creams and sauces

INTRODUCTION

In this chapter, we shall discuss about various kinds of creams and sauces that are used in bakery and pastry. For a layman, a cream is like a whipped dairy cream that is used in cake and pastry making, but for a professional pastry chef, cream in this context has a much broader meaning than just whipped bakery cream. We shall discuss about various types of creams such as *pastry cream*, *crème Chiboust*, and *frangipani*, and how they are used for creating a variety of products. Few kinds of creams are used for icing cakes and pastries, whilst some are used as filling and topping in baked goods.

We shall also discuss about various types of sauces used in pastry kitchens. Many pastry cooks believe that a good sauce is the main feature of good cooking because of the skill needed to prepare and the interest and excitement it gives to food. Sauces are basic but versatile commodities in the pastry kitchen and the professional pastry chef realises the importance of making good sauces. There is no doubt that sauce making requires skill.

Over the years culinary techniques have been developed to produce a consistently good quality product. Various types of hot and cold sauces are used in pastry kitchens. A sauce provides texture, nutrition, and contrasting flavours to desserts and cakes, whilst many are used to give colour on the plated dessert.

In this chapter, we will discuss a variety of hot and cold sauces including liquid fruit purees often known as *coulis*. We will also learn about various components of sauces, their usage and also the usage of the correct thickening agents as well as how to store and reconstitute sauces correctly.

CREAMS

Traditionally, creams are butterfat separated from fresh milk and this can be done physically by allowing the milk to churn in centrifugal machines which helps the cream to rise up. In this chapter when we refer to creams, it is much more than the diary cream. In pastry kitchen, any smooth thick viscous liquid is classified into a broad heading and referred to as cream. For example, buttercream, custard cream, etc. Let us discuss a few creams commonly used in the pastry kitchen.

Marzipan

[handwritten annotation: Ground Almond + Icing sugar + egg/Glucose colour and essence]

Marzipan is a paste made from ground almonds and sugar *[handwritten: castor]* mixed in varying proportions. Better quality marzipan has more almonds and less artificial flavouring. It is more of a commercially made product as it has better taste and texture if made that way. The home-made marzipans are rarely of the consistency and texture as the commercially available ones.

Marzipan is mainly used as coverings for wedding cakes and other rich cakes. It is widely used to make flowers, fruits, and figures as the dough like texture allows the chef to mould it into various forms and figures. Marzipan is also used as filling as in case of *dresden stollen* and in the production of some high quality cake mixtures.

> **CHEF'S TIP**
> Persipan is a mock marzipan made from various kernels of stone fruits such as apricots and peaches. It is less expensive than marzipan.

Let us look at Table 6.1 to understand the role of ingredients in making marzipan.

Table 6.1 Ingredients used in marzipan

Nuts	Sugar	Water	Liquid glucose
Coarsely ground almonds without the skin are used.	Good quality refined sugar is to be used. It is advisable to use high quality castor sugar.	Water is used as a binding agent for almonds and liquid glucose.	It contains dextrin gum that retards the crystallization of sugar.
It is important to check the taste of almonds, as bitter almonds would spoil the taste of marzipan.	Though the sugar will be boiled and one could use grain sugar, but the impurities in the grain sugar will impact the colour of marzipan.	Water is boiled along with liquid glucose and heated up to 121°C.	Liquid glucose keeps the product pliable, and allows you to work with it for a longer time without crystallising the sugar.
Mock almonds, such as kernels of stone fruits are used to make a paste called Persipan.			

Techniques to Prepare Marzipan

Marzipans are better if procured from commercial shops and there are many good reasons to do so—the first being the quality of the product and the second being its consistency. In case of non-availability of commercially made marzipan, one could make one by following the given steps.

Step 1 Blanch the almonds and remove the skin. Dry the almonds well and coarsely grind them, ensuring that the almonds do not become oily.

Step 2   Combine sugar, water, and liquid glucose and boil to 121°C. Make sure that the sugar does not colour and this can be done by ensuring that the sides of the pan are constantly brushed down with a wet brush.

Step 3   Take the liquid off the fire and add coarsely ground almonds to the mixture. Spread the mixture onto a cleaned marble surface and let it cool down.

Step 4   Grind the mixture into a paste. This paste will form into pliable dough when it cools down.

Uses of Marzipan

- It is used for making flowers, decorative figures, and moulds.
- It is used for covering wedding cakes and rich cakes, to make a smooth base for spreading *Royal icing*—Royal icing is a thick paste like icing, made by beating egg whites with icing sugar and a little lemon juice.
- It can be used for modelling purposes and in that case one part of marzipan is mixed with one and half part of icing sugar. The paste thus made will remain more firm and hard when creating modelling structures.
- Marzipan can be used to make high quality cakes. When adding marzipan to a light density mixture, such as egg yolks, it is necessary to first break down the marzipan to avoid lumping. If the preparation uses sugar, blend the sugar with the marzipan first. Sugar is an abrasive which will gradually grind down the marzipan and allow it to disperse when the egg yolks or other liquids are gradually added.

> **CHEF'S TIP**
> Check that the working tables, tools, containers, and storage facilities are spotless prior to commencing work with marzipan. People suffering from excessive sweating of hands should wear gloves otherwise it is unhygienic and there is danger of fermentation.

Almond Paste

Almond paste is commonly known as *frangipani paste* and is composed of ground almonds or marzipan mixed with butter, flour, and eggs. This is used in fillings of many classical cakes such as *gateau pithivier*. This paste unlike marzipan is always baked before eating. It can also be used for making pies and tarts. As it is enriched with marzipan, it produces pies and tarts of rich quality. Let us look at Table 6.2 to understand the role of ingredients in making this paste.

Table 6.2 Ingredients used in frangipani paste

Marzipan	Sugar	Butter	Egg yolks	Flour
Marzipan gives body and texture to the paste.	Castor sugar is better, as it forms an abrasive and helps in creaming the marzipan. Icing sugar can also be used for a finer paste.	Butter helps to cream the almond paste and add flavour and texture to it.	Egg yolks are used for adding a creamy texture and flavour.	Soft flour is carefully folded in and helps to bind the paste together when baked.
It is crumbled into smaller pieces and mixed with eggs and sugar.	Sugar helps in providing the browning effect to the paste when baked or gratinated.	Only butter should be used for making a quality product.	Only egg yolks should be used. If the paste is too thick, then egg whites can be added for thinning down the mix.	The flour should not be over mixed in the paste as the paste will become chewy.

Techniques to Prepare Frangipani

Step 1 Crumble the marzipan and beat it with flat paddle with sugar and butter until a creamy mixture is formed.

Step 2 Add yolks one by one until a creamy mixture is obtained.

Step 3 Add flour and fold with hands and store in refrigerator. This paste can be frozen for later use.

Uses of Frangipani

- It is used for fillings in cakes such as gateau pithivier.
- It is used as filling in breakfast pastries such as Danish pastry and almond croissant.
- It is used as filling for pies and tarts. In a flan or tart, frangipani is added to the tart base and sliced fruit such as pear is arranged on top and baked at 180°C until golden brown. The almond paste rises up encasing the fruit.

Touille Paste

Touille is derived from the French word that means *tiles* and this name is probably given to it because this paste is baked in thin sheets that look like shingles or tiles. Touille is often used for making thin petal like cookies for garnishes and decorations. A design is first drawn onto a cardboard, usually of 2-4 mm thickness, and then cut out. For regular work, it is best to use plastic or heavy aluminium stencils which are available in the market for this purpose. The stencil is laid on lightly greased and floured baking trays and the mixture is spread in the centre of the cut out.

When spread, the stencil is lifted off carefully. The mixture is then baked evenly at approximately 190°C until golden brown. When the paste is just baked, it is soft and can be moulded into various shapes such as curls and twists to give a dimension to the garnish. Many types of touille paste are used for garnishing pastries and each has a different texture and mouth feel, though the purpose of each is the same and that is garnishing and decorating. Touille paste can also be used to make cups and cones for serving desserts or ice creams in them. Let us look at Table 6.3 to understand the different types of touille paste.

Table 6.3 Different types of touille paste

Type	Description	Uses
Basic touille	Made by creaming butter and icing sugar. Eggs are added and folded in flour to form a paste.	Used for making cones, swirls, and various garnishes.
Almond touille	Made as per the recipe of basic touille, but 20% of the weight of flour is replaced with almond powder or marzipan.	Used for garnishes and decorations. It can also be served with ice creams.
July pan	Equal amounts of milk, icing sugar, and flour mixed together to make a paste.	Used as garnishes for eggless desserts. Used for making springs as it takes longer time to set to brittle texture as compared to other touille.
Brandy snaps	This touille is very different from the aforementioned touille pastes, both in terms of making the mix and appearance. This bakes to very thin dark brown sheets with large holes. The butter, sugar, and honey are cooked until the mixture comes to a boil and flour is added to make a paste. It is then cooled and baked on silpats. It is usually spread out on a sheet.	Used for decorations and served as crisps with ice creams.

Pastry Cream

Pastry cream or custard cream or *crème patisserie* as called in French, is one of the most common creams used in cakes and pastry products. This cream can also be baked and hence, is used in both hot and cold desserts. Pastry cream is basically a mixture prepared from vanilla flavoured milk, egg yolks, sugar, and starch. It is boiled until a thick mixture is obtained and butter is added on top to avoid skin formation. This cream has the same value and uses as the white sauce in Western cooking.

Pastry cream however has a variation as well. When a part of whipped meringue is added to the pastry cream it is known as *Chiboust cream* or *St Honore cream*, as it is used as a filling for Gateau St Honore. In this book, when we refer to pastry cream we will be referring to custard cream. It can be enriched with a part of whipped cream folded in to make the mixture more delicate thereby, making it more useful in fillings for cakes and pastries. Adding of cream to the custard cream however, renders it useless for baking purposes.

The pastry cream is used as a filling for choux buns, fruit flans, éclairs, etc., without the whipped cream being mixed, it can also form the base of many hot desserts such as *cobblers* and *pies*. It is also used as filling in breakfast Danish pastries.

Let us look at Table 6.4 to understand the role of ingredients in making pastry cream.

Table 6.4 Ingredients used in pastry cream

Milk	Sugar	Egg yolks	Starch
Usually, whole fresh milk is used for better flavour.	Granular sugar is used as it will be dissolved when cooked with milk.	Egg yolks are beaten with sugar. This is done to break the yolks, so that they cook uniformly.	Common, proprietary custard powder is used, but one can use a mixture of cornflour and custard powder in the ratio of 1:1. Some recipes just use plain flour but in that case one has to cook for long time to get rid of the raw flavour of the flour.
After the pastry cream is made it can be cooled and mixed with a part of whipped cream.		Whole eggs could be used, but it will give a much lighter product.	

Techniques to Prepare Pastry Cream

Step 1 Boil milk and half the sugar with scrapings from vanilla bean. This is done to test the quality of the milk. If the milk is old or sour it will curdle and secondly, hot milk will form the emulsion of eggs fairly quickly and will also help the starch to swell faster.

Step 2 Beat egg yolks and the remaining sugar together along with the starches to form a smooth creamy mixture. If making in large quantities, one can also whip this mix to form a smooth emulsion.

Step 3 Temper the egg and flour emulsion. Tempering means adding little amounts of hot liquid into the egg mix whilst mixing continuously. This helps to bring both the mixes at almost the same temperature and hence when added, the egg and starch mixture will disperse equally and will not form lumps.

Step 4 Boil the pastry cream until it starts to bubble.

Step 5 Remove from fire and add butter and mix well.

Step 6 Use immediately or wrap with plastic and keep refrigerated until further use.

Uses of Pastry Cream

- It is used for fillings in tarts, pies, and flans.
- It is used for filling between sponge cakes to create gateaux and pastries. This is a neutral cream flavoured with vanilla. It can be flavoured with any other desirable flavour as well.
- It is used as a base for hot desserts, as it can be baked also.
- It is used for filling choux pastry items to create desserts.

Chantilly Cream

Crème Chantilly is a basic bakery cream that is whipped with sugar and vanilla flavours to be used in various desserts, cakes, and pastries. This cream finds its use in almost all the cakes and pastries in one way or the other. Chantilly cream is one of the most important ingredients used in a *mousse* and *soufflé*. Let us look at Table 6.5 to understand the role of ingredients in making Chantilly cream.

Table 6.5 Ingredients used in chantilly cream

Cream	Sugar	Flavourings
Bakery cream with at least 40% fat content is best suitable for whipping.	Castor sugar is used as it will dissolve well.	Vanilla pods are scraped and used to flavour the cream.
Cream should be cold and even the bowl and other equipment used in whipping cream should be cold as cream whips faster and to a good volume.	Usually 200 g of sugar is used to sweeten 1 litre cream.	Many other flavourings such as citrus fruit zests and fruit purees are added to flavour. It is always advisable to use natural flavourings as against synthetic ones for better quality.

Techniques to Prepare Chantilly Cream

Step 1 Collect all the ingredients. Make sure that the cream is chilled and that the bowl and whip are also at a cold temperature.

Step 2 Add sugar and scrapings from the vanilla pod and whip the cream at medium speed.

Step 3 Keep the consistency of the cream slightly under whipped, as it will be mixed or folded again into desserts or while making cakes. If it is not whipped to the right degree, then it might split to form butter and water whilst mixing.

If you are using imitation cream, make sure the cream does not have any ice crystals, as this cream always comes frozen. Whip normally to the right degree and ensure that it is not under whipped, as it will give a synthetic taste if not whipped to the right consistency.

> **CHEF'S TIPS**
> - If the cream gets over whipped, do not throw away, and instead whip it further to get butter, which can be used for various other purposes.
> - Mix a part of Chantilly cream with a part of imitation cream to get a well textured and good flavoured dessert.
> - The imitation cream can be refrigerated for upto two days, but freshly whipped Chantilly cream must be used immediately.

Uses of Chantilly Cream

- It is used as filling between sponge cakes to create gateaux and pastries.
- It is used for making various desserts such as mousse and soufflés.
- It is served with coffees and milkshakes.
- It is used as a condiment with fresh fruits such as strawberries and mango.
- It is used for preparing bases for other creams such as Bavarian cream, caprice cream, and fruit creams.

Caprice Cream

Caprice cream is a variation of crème Chantilly. The only difference is that it is whipped without sugar and when the cream is whipped, $1/5^{th}$ part of the whipped cream is replaced with broken pieces of meringue. The cream is refrigerated until further use. It is mostly used in the filling of cakes and pastries.

Buttercream

Equal quantities of unsalted butter and icing sugar are creamed to produce a smooth aerated creamy mixture called as buttercream. It should be stored in a sealed container in a cool place. One has to refrigerate it because of the perishable nature of butter; but it needs to be creamed back to a creamy consistency before being used. Buttercreams are used as fillings and toppings for sponge to make cakes, cupcakes, and pastries. This is one of the oldest creams used in cake fillings and can be flavoured with any kind of flavourings. One can also add colours to the buttercream to make fancy shapes for children's birthday cakes. The ingredients used in buttercream are very simple—only butter and sugar, but the quality of the ingredients is crucial, as this filling is never cooked and is used as it is.

Let us look at Table 6.6 to understand the role of ingredients in making buttercream.

Table 6.6 Ingredients used in buttercream

Butter	Sugar	Flavourings
It is important to use only unsalted butter. Fresh white butters that are home churned, sometimes have an odd flavour and too much of water in the mix. So care must be taken to beat the butter alone to remove any water present.	Only good quality icing sugar is to be used. It is important to sift the sugar so that there are no small granules of sugar in the mix. As this cream can also be used for writing on cakes, it becomes a nuisance when the small sugar crystals get in the way and block the flow of icing.	Buttercreams can be flavoured with melted chocolate, vanilla pods, zest of citrus fruits, or even synthetic flavours, as combining it with fresh fruit purees will not form an emulsion and the cream will split. Liquors and spirits such as rum, whisky can be added to buttercreams. Before adding powdered colours, mix the colour in a few drops of water and then mix it in the buttercream.

Techniques to Prepare Buttercream

Step 1 Collect all the ingredients. Make sure that the butter is at room temperature, as it creams well if it is not very cold. Cut the butter into smaller pieces and beat it on slow speed with a flat paddle for 5 minutes.

Step 2   Sift the icing sugar and mix it into the butter. Make sure that the speed gear of the machine is turned to one as the icing sugar might fly out if the mixer is run on medium or high speed. Let the icing sugar incorporate and then run the machine on high until the cream is light and fluffy.

Step 3   Remove from the mixer and scrape out into a clean plastic bowl and store in a cool place.

There is another variation of buttercream known as *Italian buttercream*. It is made by making Italian meringue. Italian meringue is made by whipping egg whites with a little amount of sugar with the rest of the sugar being cooked to 118°C and slowly added to the egg whites to form Italian meringue. These types of meringues are more stable than the French or *Swiss meringues*.

The French meringues are plain egg whites whipped with sugar to form a thick fluffy mixture whereas Swiss meringues are cooked meringues. The recipe of the Swiss meringue is similar to that of French meringue, the only difference is that Swiss meringue is whipped over a double boiler and hence, the meringue is more stable than the French one. A part of Italian meringue is folded in buttercream to make Italian buttercream, which is lighter as compared to the French buttercream.

Uses of Buttercream

- It is used for filling between sponge cakes to create gateaux and pastries. This is a neutral cream flavoured with vanilla. It can be flavoured with any other desirable flavour as well.
- It is used in piping bags to decorate cakes and pipe wordings on the cakes.
- It is used to pipe swirls on top of cupcakes.

Lemon Curd Cream

Lemon cream is commonly known as lemon curd and is a smooth, creamy paste that has a balanced taste of sweet and sour. It is often known as curd because of the slow poaching of eggs in butter and lemon juice with sugar. The lemon curd was initially invented for usage with scones in England instead of jam, but slowly people started to use it as a topping and filling for cakes, muffins, and tarts as well. When piped into a tart, the mixture is very tarty and sharp, so to cut down on the sharpness, whipped meringue is topped onto the tart and gratinated. This is very commonly eaten as lemon meringue pie in USA and England.

Let us look at Table 6.7 to understand the role of ingredients in making lemon curd.

Table 6.7 Ingredients used in lemon cream

Butter	Lemon Juice	Egg yolks	Sugar
Unsalted butter is used and it helps the curd to set into a creamy texture when it becomes cold. If oil is used instead, the mixture will be runny.	Lemon juice is used traditionally to make lemon cream. Many other fruit juices might become bitter after cooking.	Egg yolks help to form a creamy texture. The proteins present in the egg, coagulate with the application of heat and gel up together with butter and juice to form a cream.	Granular sugar will be a good choice as it will get dissolved in the lemon juice.

Techniques to Prepare Lemon Cream

There are two methods of making lemon curd. One method is to combine the butter, sugar, and reduced lemon juice on low heat until the sugar gets dissolved. The mix is then added into a machine with wire whisk and egg yolk is added one at a time until all the eggs are incorporated and the mixture has become thick. Then the mixture is removed from the bowl and put in a plastic container and chilled until set. Metal containers might react with the acid present in the lemon curd and hence, it is preferable to store it in plastic containers.

The second method is the most commonly followed method in making lemon cream as it is one of the easiest and hassle free methods. Following are the steps of this method.

Step 1   Combine butter, egg yolks, sugar, and lemon juice and mix well to break the egg yolks with sugar.

Step 2   Cover the bowl with aluminium foil and place over a bain marie. Remove at intervals of 15 minutes and mix again to form a homogeneous mix. Place it back on the double boiler and cook for another 1 minute.

Step 3   Remove from the fire and allow it to cool. It will thicken into a thick cream which can be piped into tart shells.

Step 4   Use immediately or wrap with plastic and keep refrigerated until further use.

Uses of Lemon Cream

- It is used as filling in tarts, pies, and flans.
- It is used for filling between sponge cakes to create gateaux and pastries. This is a neutral cream flavoured with vanilla. It can be flavoured with any other desirable flavour as well.
- It is used as a condiment in place of jam with scones and dry cakes.

Ganache

Ganache and truffle are made with chocolate and cream. Both the truffle and the ganache have the same ingredients but they are slightly different to each other in ratios, preparation, and usage. Though many chefs use these words interchangeably, let us understand the basic difference between the two from Table 6.8.

> **CHEF'S TIPS**
> - When filling the tart shells with any cream, brush the inside of the tart shell with melted chocolate. This will form a film and prevent the tart shell from getting soggy from the liquid in the creams.
> - The truffle if mixed with small amounts of sugar syrup, will get a shine. Some chefs add a small amount of gelatine to the truffle and it sets like a thin shiny glaze on top of the cake.

Table 6.8 Difference between ganache and truffle

Ganache	Truffle
Cream is brought to a boil and chopped chocolate is added in the ratio of 1 part cream and 1/2 part chocolate.	Cream is brought to a boil and chopped chocolate is added in the ratio of 1 part cream and 1 and 1/2 part chocolate.
The mixture is cooled down and then whipped to creamy consistency.	Truffle sets into a dark creamy paste.
Ganache is used for fillings in cakes and pastries.	Truffle is warmed slightly till it becomes flowy and is used to glaze the top of chocolate cakes. It can be used as filling to produce dark chocolate truffle cakes, which are very rich.

Let us look at Table 6.9 to understand the role of ingredients in making ganache.

Table 6.9 Ingredients used in ganache

Cream	Chocolate
Bakery cream with high fat content is used as it helps to whip to a thick mousse like texture which is desirable for filling in the cakes.	Dark, milk, or white chocolate can be mixed, depending upon the end usage of the chocolate.
Milk can also be used, but it will not whip properly and will give a very thin and flowy ganache.	Use coverture chocolates only, as compound chocolates do not have good quality taste.

Techniques to Prepare Ganache

Step 1 Boil bakery cream and take it off the fire.

Step 2 Add chopped chocolate and mix with wooden spoon till all the chocolate has melted to a smooth paste.

Step 3 Cool the ganache until chilled and whip it into a creamy mousse texture.

Step 4 Use immediately or wrap with plastic and keep refrigerated until further use.

> **CHEF'S TIP**
> When making ganache or truffle in bulk, chop the chocolate and put into a dough mixer with flat paddle. Boil the cream and pour on top of the chocolate. Let the chocolate soften and then put the mixer on low speed to create a smooth paste.

Uses of Ganache

- It is used for filling between sponge cakes to create gateaux and pastries. It can be flavoured with any other desirable flavour such as whisky and rum.
- It is used for filling choux pastry items to create desserts.

SAUCES

The sauces discussed in this chapter will be only sweets sauces or sauces that can be served with desserts or cakes and pastries. The purpose of serving sauces with desserts is almost same to their purpose in Western cooking. Sauces add colour to desserts and provide the necessary moisture to dry cake or pastry. It also enhances the nutritional value of the particular dessert and more often gives a contrasting taste to a particular dish.

The sauces in pastry are broadly classified as:

- Hot sauces
- Cold sauces

They can also be classified on the basis of their texture such as smooth sauce and chunky sauce. Let us see the classification of sauces in Table 6.10.

Whilst discussing about various sauces, we will come across terminologies such as *crème anglaise*. Though literally it translates to English cream, it is not classified under the creams listed above, instead it is grouped under sauces. However, when *crème anglaise* is mixed with whipped cream and set in moulds with the help of gelatine, the dessert is then known as *crème bavarois* or Bavarian cream. The name of the dessert is coined as per the fruit or ingredient used, for example, Mango Bavarois, Chocolate Bavarois, etc.

Table 6.10 Classification of pastry sauces

Classification	Description	Uses
Puree based	There are various types of fruit purees such as coulis, in which the fruit is stewed with some amount of sugar and cooked till soft. The sauce is either left coarse or passed through a sieve resulting in a coulis.	Berry coulis is served with desserts and ice creams. Coulis folded in with whipped cream results in a dessert called *Fool*. Used as a topping or filling for cakes and pastries.
Custard based	Refer to Table 6.11.	Refer to Table 6.11.
Chocolate based	Chocolate based sauces can be made in various ways such as: ♦ Boiling cream and chocolate yields truffle that can be thinned down with milk, cream or sugar syrup to obtain chocolate sauce. The colour of the chocolate sauce can be regulated by adding milk and cream in the required proportions. ♦ Another kind of chocolate sauce is obtained by adding chopped chocolate to crème anglaise whilst the mixture is still hot and blending it with stick blender. ♦ Chocolate sauce can also be made by combining water, sugar, cocoa powder, and butter and cooking the mixture like a pastry cream. The consistency of the sauce can be adjusted by using sugar syrup or cream. ♦ Another method of making chocolate sauce is to boil water and liquid glucose and then add chopped chocolate to obtain a smooth sauce.	Served with ice creams, desserts, cakes, and pastries.
Cream based	Reduced cream with flavourings is widely used in confectionary. Caramel sauce, butterscotch sauce are a few examples of cream based sauces.	Served with ice creams, desserts, cakes, and pastries.
Miscellaneous	These sauces are basically reductions of liquids such as wines and fruit juices.	Served with ice creams, desserts, cakes, and pastries. Mixed with whipped cream to make fillings for cakes and other desserts.
Syrup based	Sugar can be cooked until thick and then combined with diced fruits and herbs to make clear and syrupy fruit based salsa sauces.	Served along with sour desserts such as lemon tart and used in plated desserts.

These types of sauces which are made by using milk or cream and thickened with eggs come under the category of *custards*. These should not be confused with custard cream or pastry cream as discussed earlier in the chapter. Let us see Table 6.11 to understand the different types of custards and their uses.

Table 6.11 Types of custards

Type	Description	Uses
Basic custard	This is the uncooked mixture of milk or cream with eggs and sugar. Usually 1 litre of cream or milk or both depending upon the usage are combined with 200 g sugar and 10 whole eggs.	It can be poached in moulds lined with caramelized sugar to produce the famous dessert called *crème caramel*. It can be poured onto diced, leftover breakfast rolls and baked to produce a baked dessert called diplomat pudding or bread and butter pudding.
Crème anglaise	Milk or cream is boiled with sugar. Egg yolks are beaten with whisk and then tempered with hot milk or cream. The egg yolk mix is then mixed back into the liquid, being stirred all the time with a wooden spoon, until the custard is thick and coats the back of the spoon. The ratios are same as that of basic custard, only difference is that instead of whole eggs, only yolks are used.	It can be used to make a base for many desserts such as Bavarois. When the Bavarois is filled in a mould lined with slices of Swiss roll it is then called *Charlotte Royal* and when it is lined with sponge fingers, it is called *Charlotte Russe*. It can also be served as a sauce. It can be flavoured with many flavours such as citrus zests, caramelized sugar, and spirits such as brandy, rum, and whisky.
Sabayon	Egg yolks are mixed with sugar and a few tablespoons of liquid such as milk, cream, or liquor and the mixture is then whipped over bain marie until it forms ribbons.	It is used as a base for desserts such as mousses and soufflés. It is served as a dessert all by itself, for example, *zabaglione* from Italy. It is also used as a gratinated topping upon fruits and berries.

Types of Sauces

Sauces used in pastry do not have classifications as in Western sauces, but broadly the sauces are classified on the basis of the major ingredient used to prepare them. Sauces can also be classified based on their textures. Pastry sauces have two basic types of textures—Strained and Chunky.

Strained sauces Certain sauces are made by stewing the soft fruit especially berries. These are then pureed and served strained. These are commonly referred to as *coulis*. Few examples of such coulis are strawberry coulis or raspberry coulis. Most of the sauces can be served hot or cold depending upon their usage.

Chunky sauces As the name suggests, these sauces are not strained and hence, have chunks of ingredients in them that add flavour as well as texture to the sauce. Fruit salsa, nutty chocolate sauce, and passion fruit sauce with its seeds are a few examples of chunky sauces.

Components of Sauce

The function of a sauce in a dessert is to add flavour and colour that complements, supports, or contrasts the main ingredients of the dish. The components of a sauce however remain the same, whether we are talking about the savoury sauces served with meats in Western kitchen or preparing the sauces for desserts. Figure 6.1 represents the components of a sauce.

Let us understand each of these components and the impact that they have on the overall product.

Liquid

Liquid component in a dessert sauce can range from plain water to milk and even liqueurs. Unlike Western hot kitchen sauces where the juices from the roasted piece of meat can form a flavourful base of the sauce, in pastry kitchen the chef has to rely on the addition of external liquid to prepare a sauce.

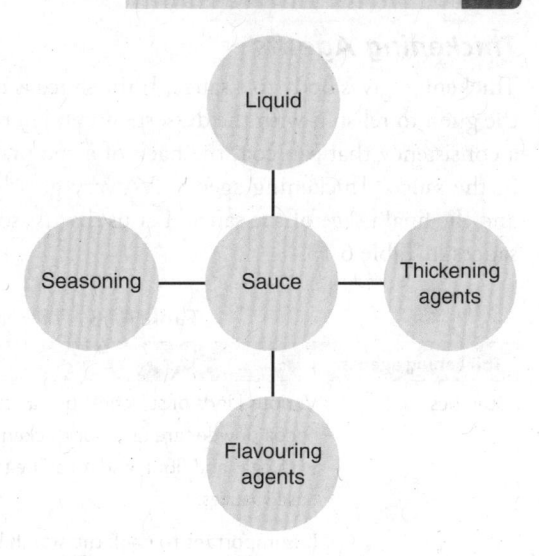

Fig. 6.1 Components of a sauce

Let us discuss some of the commonly used liquids and their effects on the final product in Table 6.12.

Table 6.12 Liquid components of a sauce

Liquids	Description and effects
Water	Water is commonly used in preparing pastry sauces. Since water is neutral in flavour, it is important to flavour the sauce with other flavourings.
	Usage of water results in clear sauces and water can be used in a variety of ways to prepare sauces. For example, water and sugar are combined and heated to yield a clear caramel sauce, and sometimes water and sugar are heated to make thick syrups that can be flavoured with herbs and chopped fruits to make chunky fruit sauces.
Fruit juices	Juices and pulps from fruits are most commonly used in pastry kitchen to make sauces. The selection of the fruit for a sauce would depend upon the particular dessert. Juices from citric fruits such as, lemon and orange are commonly combined with chocolate based desserts. Pulps from fruits such as passion fruit and mango are also combined with thick sugar syrup to make sauces that can be served as toppings for various ice creams, sundaes, and other desserts.
Milk	Dairy products such as milk and cream are synonymous to pastry kitchen as their usage is very varied and unique. Milk can be used for making cakes, breads, sauces, and many more products. Milk is combined with sugar and thickened with eggs, starch, etc., to yield an assortment of sauces.
Cream	The art of skilfully blending cream with other ingredients yields some of the most famous sauces that are used along with desserts and for other purposes in the pastry kitchen. Cream can be boiled along with chocolate to yield ganache and truffle that are used as sauces as well. Whipped cream's consistency is adjusted to be used as a sauce.
Spirits and alcohol	Spirits and alcohols such as rum, whisky, brandy, and a range of liquors are used for preparing sauces. Wines also are commonly used for making sauces and they are boiled off to get rid of the alcohol content. These are then thickened with eggs or other thickening agents that we shall discuss in Table 6.13.

Thickening Agents

Thickening gives body to a sauce. If the sauce is not thick it will run on the plate, making it difficult for the guest to relish it with the dessert. When referring to thickness in the dessert sauce, it is referred to as a consistency that can coat the back of a spoon. Too much thickness in sauces would spoil the texture of the sauce. Thickening agents also vary greatly, depending on the nature and flavour of the source and the final usage of the sauce. Let us discuss some of the commonly used thickening agents in pastry sauces in Table 6.13.

Table 6.13 Thickening agents used in sauces

Thickening agents	Description and effects
Starches	Various kinds of starches such as custard powder, cornstarch, flour, tapioca, potato starch, and cocoa powder are used for thickening sauces. Pastry cream is made by boiling milk and sugar with eggs and flour, and it can be thinned down with milk and sugar syrup to make custard based sauces. It is important to cook the starch based sauces for a longer time to get rid of the starchy flavour.
Eggs	Whole eggs or the yolks are the most commonly used ingredient to thicken sauces. Since eggs give a wonderful colour and texture, they are widely preferred over other ingredients. Eggs yolks whisked with sugar and spirits over a bain marie result in very flavourful sauces that are used with many popular desserts. Care should be taken to cook such sauces on slow heat, such as water bath also known as bain marie, with gentle agitation to prevent overcooking.
Chocolates	Chocolates are also commonly used for providing thickness to the sauce. Care has to be taken as consistency of chocolate based sauce fluctuates with temperature changes. If after chilling the sauce is too thick, then it can be thinned down with either more cream or sugar syrup. Thinning down with cream will give a muddy finish, whereas thinning down with sugar syrup will yield a dark and shiny sauce.
Gelatine	Gelatine is used sometimes to give the necessary thickness to thin sauces. For example, a fruit juice would be thickened with gelatine and then rested in a cool place until set. The set gel is then blended and strained through a sieve to obtain a thick sauce.
Cream	Cream can be reduced for thickening. It can also be whipped to the required consistency and then flavoured to yield a sauce. Whipped cream can also be added to liquids to yield sauces.
Sugar and its products	Sugar heated until it melts is also used as a thickening agent in sauces. The consistency of the sugar syrup depends upon the temperature of the syrup.
Air	Air increases viscosity of purees. Purees agitated in mixer at high speed incorporate many small air bubbles, which gives thickness to the sauce.
Fruits and vegetables	Fruits and vegetables usually pureed are commonly used for thickening sauces. The consistency of the sauce can be adjusted by adding the required amount of puree and then adjusted to a coating consistency. Various fruits and vegetables such as berries, mango, and apricots are commonly used for thickening sauces.

Flavouring Agents

Flavour is the total sensory impression formed when food is eaten. It is a combination of the sensations of taste, smell, and texture. Many of the sweet sauces are based on specific flavouring agents, for example, vanilla, fruit pastes, nuts, spirits, etc. Skilful blending of flavouring agents with a basic sauce is the key to successful sauce making. The result is an almost endless range of sauces that have individual and characteristic flavours. If you have a natural alternative, it is best to avoid artificial flavours which can be overpowering.

Condiments, herbs, spices, and flavourings are used to modify, blend, or strengthen natural flavours. The use of these materials may create the difference between a highly palatable food and a drab, tasteless one. Let us discuss about a few flavourings used in pastry sauces in Table 6.14.

Seasoning

Seasoning in desserts is referred to addition of sugar and sometimes salt to bring out the tastes and to heighten the flavours in a sauce. Let us understand some of the common seasonings used in pastry sauces in Table 6.15.

Table 6.14 Flavourings used in pastry sauces

Flavourings	Description and effects
Salt	Salt is most widely used for seasoning food; but its application in the preparation of sweets is limited. It is used to bring out the natural flavours in the food.
Acids	Acids in the form of vinegar and lemon juice are commonly used to flavour food.
Extracts	These are derived from natural flavouring materials. The flavour is extracted by macerating the natural source, for example, vanilla, ethyl alcohol, etc. These extracts are the best flavouring materials, but also the most expensive.
Herbs and spices	The art of skilfully adding the right amount of spice or herb to a food is a basic for successful pastry cooking. Frequently used spices are cinnamon, nutmeg, cloves, and herbs such as mint.
Essential oils	These contain the principal flavour of all fruits, nuts, and flowers. Lemon and orange oils are most useful in patisserie work, as they are able to withstand high temperatures without deterioration.
Essences	Many flavours can now be made artificially. Used with discretion, they are very useful when the natural substitute is not available.
Blended flavours	These are compounded from both natural and artificial sources. Such essences have the true bouquet of natural flavours, reinforced with the strength of the artificial essence.
Fruit pastes and concentrates	These are products that impart the true flavour of the fruit.
Spirits and liqueurs	Such flavouring agents are expensive and therefore, should be used with discretion. Since they are volatile substances that can evaporate when heated, their use should be confined to creams, icings, and sauces. They should rarely be used as ingredients in goods that are to be baked. Some are available as concentrates and are ideal for cooking purposes.

Table 6.15 Seasonings used in sauces

Seasonings	Description and effects
Salt	Salt is most widely used for the seasoning of food; but its application in the preparation of sweets is limited. It is used to bring out the natural flavours in the food.
Acids	In the form of citric juices such as orange and lemon juice are commonly used for seasoning and flavours.
Sugar	Sugar in many forms is used for adding seasoning to dessert sauces. Honey, corn syrups, treacle, and molasses are also used for both flavouring and seasoning sauces.

Uses of Sauces

Unlike Western kitchen, sauces made in the pastry kitchen have many more uses other than being served along with a dessert. In cakes and pastries, certain chocolate based sauces are also used as icing. So sauces in pastry kitchens have unique and varied uses. Let us discuss some of these uses.

Sauces as accompaniments When the sauce is used as an accompaniment to a dessert, it serves the same purpose as the sauces in Western kitchen. The sauces are primarily served to enhance the flavour of the dish, to add moistness, colour contrast, and nutrition to the main dish. Sometimes the sauce is used to enhance the presentation of the dessert on a plate. Selection of sauces for this purpose is very important as the accompanying sauce should not overpower the main dessert, but should complement it.

Sauces as toppings and fillings Sauces are commonly used as toppings on ice creams, coupes, and sundaes. They can also be mixed with gelatine and used as a topping or icing for cakes and pastries. Sauces can also be used for filling tarts, pies, and even moulded chocolates and truffles. Sauces should be reconstituted to desired consistency for each usage.

Sauces as bases for desserts This is one of the most versatile uses of sauces in pastry kitchen. Crème anglaise is the most commonly used sauce as a base to create many desserts apart from being served as a sauce by itself. Sauces are combined along with whipped creams to create desserts such as mousse, soufflés, and fools. Sauces can be heated and thickened with starch and made into desserts such as *fruit cobbler*. Crème anglaise is also known as Bavarian cream and it is combined with whipped cream, gelatine, and flavours to create desserts called *Bavarois*.

Factors for Choosing an Acompanying Sauce

Choosing the right kind of sauce for the right product is very important and this depends upon various factors such as sweetness of dessert, texture, mouth feel, and even the style of service of the dessert. Let us discuss some of these factors in detail.

Sweetness of dessert The amount of sugar in the dessert would also determine the kind of sauce that would be served with it. Meringue based desserts which are very high on sweet content are served with tarty sauces such as citrus sauces and tropical fruit salsas or coulis. The acid in the sauce would cut down on the sweetness in the dessert and provide a contrasting taste and flavour. Crepe suzette is a classical dessert that is served with caramelized sugar based sauce. Since the crepes have little or no sugar, hence the sweet sauce compliments them.

Texture of dessert The texture of a dessert would also be one of the guiding factors towards the selection of the sauce. A creamy dessert would be served with a chunky sauce or sauce that has crushed nuts or any substance that can break the creamy texture of the dessert. Desserts with crumbly textures would rather be served with smooth sauces. For example, plum pudding is classically paired with brandy sauce.

Service of the sauce The style of service and presentation of sauces at the time of service also determines the kind of sauce to be used or the consistency of the sauce. There are many factors that must be kept in mind whilst deciding what kind of sauce should be served with what dish. The following guidelines will help you to effectively use sauces to enhance the presentation of a dish.

- In silver service, the sauce is always served separately. This allows the customer to decide how much sauce will be served. Too thick sauces would be difficult to serve and too thin would flow on the plate. Medium thick sauces that coat the back of a spoon are the best option in this case.

- For pre-plated desserts, consider whether the sauce will be best on the dessert, under the dessert, or partially coating the dessert as in case of ice cream toppings. The placement of the sauce would determine its consistency.

- Should the sauce be spooned, ladled, poured, or piped? Sometimes sauces are served decorated on the plate and in this case the sauce needs to be piped in designs. All these factors would determine the kind of sauce to be used and its consistency.

- To strain or not? Should you strain a sauce to remove, say raspberry pips or chips of chocolate? This is often simply a matter of taste and style. Think about the effect that you want to create.

Colour combinations The colour of sauces will vary, but it must be appropriate to the sauce being made. Try to avoid artificial colours, though they may be useful on certain special occasions and festive preparations. Using contrasting colour of sauces would also determine the choice of the sauce to be served. Sometimes dark and white coloured sauces such as chocolate sauce and crème anglaise are placed on the plate and given a marbled effect to create designs and enhance the presentation on the plate.

Classical and Contemporary Sauces

A range of classical and contemporary sauces are used in pastry kitchen for varied uses. Though like Western kitchen, the pastry sauces are not classified into various mother sauces, but few of the most common classical and contemporary sauces used in the pastry kitchen are discussed in Table 6.16 along with their uses in cakes, desserts, and pastries.

Table 6.16 Classical and contemporary dessert sauces and their uses

Sauces	Description	Uses
Crème anglaise/ Vanilla custard/Vanilla sauce/Bavarian cream	Sauce anglaise is warm egg custard sauce that apart from being served on its own is used as the basis for other sweets. This sauce contains no starch. Egg yolks, sugar, and warm milk with the addition of a few drops of vanilla essence are mixed together, and over gentle heat on a water bath, stirred with a wooden spoon until it thickens and coats the back of the spoon. The sauce should not be allowed to re-boil as it will curdle. There is the danger of overheating and toughening of proteins. This sauce has to be strained and kept warm in a warm water bath. It is not recommended for reheating. Sauce anglaise based sauces must be held in a warm place at about 37°C. This is critical because if the temperature is too hot, the sauce will separate (split). Egg yolks based sauces such as sauce anglaise need slow heat (water bath) and gentle agitation to prevent overcooking.	These sauces can be used as base for many classical desserts such as cold soufflés, Bavarian creams, and ice creams. Vanilla sauce can also be flavoured with brandy to make brandy sauce that is classically served with Christmas plum pudding.

(Contd)

Table 6.16 (Contd)

Sauces	Description	Uses
Chocolate sauce	Chocolate sauce can be made in a variety of ways. It can be made by boiling cream and blending with chopped chocolate or by boiling milk with cocoa powder and other ingredients. Chocolate sauce tends to thicken when it cools down and hence, must always be reheated before adjusting its consistency. The consistency of chocolate sauce varies with temperature. It tends to thicken when cold and flowy when too hot.	Chocolate sauce is served along with ice creams and hot chocolate brownies and fudge as well.
Melba sauce	Melba sauce is a coulis that is made by stewing fresh or frozen raspberries with sugar and water and then passing it through a wire mesh strainer to obtain a smooth sauce. It can be seasoned with a few drops of lemon juice. Melba sauce is usually served cold.	This is one of the most classical sauces and is utilized commonly as a topping for coupe known as peach melba.
Caramel sauce	Basic caramel sauce is made by heating a mixture of sugar, water, and liquid glucose until the sugar starts to caramelize and attains a dark golden colour. The pan is then removed from the heat and the bottom is immersed in cold water to arrest the cooking. This sauce will set hard after this, therefore, water is added to the mixture and brought to boil again, so that the crystals that were formed after adding water get dissolved and the sauce is syrupy and flowy.	Caramel sauce is a basic sauce and forms the base for many other caramelized sauces such as fudge and butterscotch.
Butterscotch sauce	Butterscotch sauce is made by the same method as caramel sauce. The only difference is that softened butter is incorporated into the caramel sauce after it has cooled down to 30°C. Sometimes cream is also added to give a rich and creamy texture.	This sauce is served with ice creams or used as an accompanying sauce to plated desserts.
Crepe suzette sauce	To make this sauce orange juice, lemon juice, and zest are combined and heated in a pan until warm. The mixture is then left to macerate for a few minutes. Sugar is allowed to caramelize in another pan over low heat until it gets a golden colour. The pan is removed from the heat and chilled butter cubes are added and cooked again until the butter is dissolved in the sauce. Warm juice of citrus fruits is now added. Traditionally, this sauce is flambéed with brandy. Flambéing is a technique used in kitchen, where alcohol is poured over a dish and then lighted with fire so that the alcohol burns off. This creates an unusual impact in the restaurant and also helps to burn the excess alcohol away.	This sauce is classically served with French pancakes also known as crepes and hence, the name. It is one of the most classical desserts that is prepared in front of the guest on a *gueridon trolley*.

Table 6.16 (Contd)

Sauces	Description	Uses
Strawberry coulis	Strawberries are cut into quarters and cooked with sugar and water. When soft, they are removed from the heat and blended until smooth or passed through a wire mesh. The choice of blending or passing through a wire mesh determines the texture and consistency of the coulis.	This sauce is served with ice creams or used as an accompanying sauce to plated desserts. This sauce is also served with waffles and pancakes.
Apricot jam sauce	Commonly made in France, this jam sauce can be made with any jam. The jam is combined with sugar and allowed to boil. The consistency of the sauce is adjusted with cornflour slurry.	This sauce is served with ice creams or used as an accompanying sauce to plated desserts.
Sabayon sauce	This sauce is very unique as it has to be served immediately and cannot be stored for long. Sabayon based sauce is made by combining egg yolks, sugar, and the desired flavour in the form of alcohol. The alcohol base also helps in providing the liquid to the mixture which is now whisked over a water bath so that it becomes thick and frothy. If you are omitting the alcohol, then a few teaspoons of water should be added to the egg yolks.	This sauce is used for classical desserts such as gratinated berries. An assortment of liqueur macerated berries are topped with sabayon and gratinated. Sabayon can also be used as a base for many creams that are used as fillings.
Tropical fruit salsa	This is a contemporary sauce made in a variety of ways. Fruits such as kiwi, pineapple, and strawberry are cut into small dices and combined with thick sugar syrup or thickened fruit juices to make this chunky fruit salsa.	The acidic flavour of tropical fruits makes it an ideal accompaniment for meringue based desserts as it helps to cut down the excess sweetness in these desserts.

Storage and Service of Sauces

The storage and service of a sauce would depend upon its temperature. Whether the sauce has to be served cold or hot, would determine the sauce's consistency and style of service. Ideally, hot sauces should be made immediately before serving. However, very few establishments can afford the time and expense this entails, and many prepare sauces beforehand. But there are disadvantages in keeping a hot sauce in a bain marie. These disadvantages could be:

- The consistency of the sauce may change. Chocolate sauce may become too thin if it becomes very hot.
- The colour and structure of the sauce may change.
- If cream has been added, fat separation may occur.
- If the sauce has cream added to acid, curdling may happen.

The temperature for holding and serving hot sauces should be around 80°C. The temperature for a cold sauce would depend on its application. Warm sauces that are thickened with eggs, such as custard, should not exceed 50°C or else there are chances that they may curdle.

When serving sauces, the general guideline is to serve approximately 50 ml of sauce per person. However, the amount of sauce to be served will be guided by the nature of the dish and the type of establishment. Sauces used as a base on a plate may be considerably less than if served separately in silver service.

Storage of sauces is one of the most crucial aspects of pastry kitchen. Since the pastry sauces are rich in high protein foods such as milk, cream, and eggs, they are more susceptible to bacterial contamination. If a cooked sauce is to be stored for any period of time it is used, it must be cooled as quickly as possible then covered and refrigerated. The best method of cooling a sauce is to place it on a rack to allow air to circulate around. It should be stirred frequently to ensure an even rate of cooling.

Due to evaporation from the surface, a skin will form rapidly on the sauce if it is left to stand. This can be prevented if the sauce is covered with a plastic wrap or a tight-fitting lid.

Sauces may be stored at a temperature of 1-4°C. Depending on its ingredients, they may not hold for any length of time; it is a good practice to make fresh supplies as often as required, if sweetened fruit purees are used as a sauce there is the danger of fermentation and rapid bacteria growth. To extend the keeping time, coulis and purees can be cooked before storage.

It is important that all sauces are labelled and date tagged to follow the first in first out procedure.

Common Faults in Sauce Making

To err is human, and many a times the dish does not turn out to be as good as desired. The reasons could be many, especially in case of bakery and confectionary, where each process is weighed and scaled, the temperatures are to be taken into account and various other factors that influence the outcome of the product. The quality of flour varies in different countries, because of the soil and processing techniques. So chefs have to adjust their recipes in every country. Certain errors that occur could be technique and process related and can be fixed, once we know the source of the problem. The most common faults that could occur during making sauces for pastry are:

Lack of flavour (poor base) Less flavouring used or the quality of flavouring is old and lacks the desired flavour

Too strong a flavour Too much flavouring used

Starchy flavour Insufficient cooking of the sauces, which utilized starch for thickening

Too thin Insufficient thickening added, or the mix was not cooked to the desired consistency

Sauce ferments Too old, incorrect storage

Incorrect colour Too much artificial colour

The storage of sauce is of utmost importance as the ingredients used in pastry kitchen are very prone to bacterial contamination and hence, they must be stored under refrigeration and wherever possible they should be made fresh and served fresh.

Once you follow these educational tips and with regular practice, one fine day you will achieve greater success as a pastry chef. In the next chapter, we will discuss about basic sponges and cakes, and utilizing the knowledge of this chapter you will be able to prepare good quality cakes and serve them with accompanying sauces.

SUMMARY

We discussed about various types of creams apart from whipped cream and understood how the creams can be flavoured to enhance the texture of a cake. The crunchy texture of cream caprice will be so different from crème Chantilly and the usage of each in a cake will provide a different mouth feel or texture to the guest. We also discussed in detail about buttercream that is the most commonly used filling in cakes around the world. Lemon curd and ganache were also discussed and the difference between ganache and truffle completed our understanding of uses of each.

The chapter described sauces in detail, which are one of the most important aspects of a pastry kitchen. The most delectable of dessert would not look as appealing if served without a sauce.

Unlike Western kitchen where sauces are made from the liquid in which the food is cooked, in the pastry kitchen a range of liquids is used to transform them into many different kinds of sauces. In this chapter, we discussed a range of ingredients, in tabular form, used as components in sauces.

Various types of sauces such as fruit based, egg based, chocolate based, and starch based are also discussed in detail along with examples. Though unlike Western kitchen there are no mother sauces in pastry kitchen, however many variations can be made from one type of sauce. For example, chocolate sauce can be made from crème anglaise as a base or it can also be made by starch based method or by boiling water with liquid glucose and adding chocolate to it.

The uses of sauces in pastry kitchen have also been explained in the chapter. Apart from being served along with the main dessert, these sauces can be used as a base for various desserts and puddings ranging from soufflés to mousses to even ice creams. Some sauces are served as toppings on ice creams whilst some are piped on a plate or spooned over desserts. In this chapter, we also discussed various factors that determine the choice of sauce that would accompany a dessert. Various factors such as sweetness of dessert, its texture and style of service decide upon the consistency and type of sauce to be used along with the dessert.

Several classical and contemporary sauces served with desserts have also been described in the chapter along with what makes them unique and special. Sauces such as Melba sauce and crepe suzette sauce are one of the oldest sauces used in confectionary. We also threw light upon the factors to be kept in mind whilst storing and serving sauces and lastly, we talked about the common faults that may occur while making sauces.

KEY TERMS

Bavarois Dessert made by combining crème anglaise with gelatine and whipped cream

Brownies Rich chocolate dessert often served hot with chocolate sauce

Cognac Kind of brandy from France

Corn syrup Chemically refined syrup obtained from corn kernels

Coulis Sauce obtained by stewing and puréeing fruits

Crepe suzette Flat pancakes cooked in citrus flavoured caramel sauce

Flambé Adding alcohol to a dish and flaming it with fire to burn it off

Fruit cobbler Hot dessert made by baking cooked fruit sauce

Gueridon trolley Mobile trolley used in restaurants, often used for cooking live in front of the guest

Liquid glucose Sticky syrup obtained by treating corn syrup with acid. Liquid glucose prevents crystallization of sugar

Molasses Dark residual syrup obtained from refining sugar

Passion fruit Kind of fruit, which contains pulp of acidic taste

Plum pudding Steamed dessert prepared during Christmas

Potato starch Also known as fecule, is the starch obtained from potatoes

Silver service Style of serving food, where the food is served from platter to plate

Tapioca Kind of tuber vegetable rich in starch

Treacle Syrup obtained as a by-product of sugar refining

OBJECTIVE TYPE QUESTIONS

1. What do you understand by cream used in pastry kitchen?
2. What is the difference between a marzipan and persipan?
3. Give at least three uses of marzipan.
4. Name at least two products made by using crème frangipani.
5. What is touille paste and what is it used for?
6. List down at least five types of creams used in pastry kitchen.
7. What is the difference between a pastry cream and crème chiboust?
8. How would you differentiate between crème Chantilly and crème caprice?
9. List down at least three differences between ganache and truffle.
10. What care should be taken whilst whipping the cream?
11. How are sauces used in pastry kitchen different from the ones used in Western kitchen?
12. What is coulis?
13. List the components of a sauce.
14. Describe at least four types of liquids that can be used for making sauces.
15. What thickening agents are used in preparing sauces for pastry?
16. What care should be taken whilst using eggs for thickening the sauces?
17. List a few methods of making chocolate sauce.
18. Differentiate between cream based and custard based sauces.
19. Define Bavarian cream.
20. What factors are considered whilst choosing the sauce as an accompaniment?
21. Define Melba sauce and its usage.
22. What is the difference between caramel sauce, butterscotch sauce, and crepe suzette sauce?
23. What is sabayon and how is it made?
24. What kind of sauce would you serve with extra sweet desserts and why?
25. Why is storage of sauces of utmost importance in pastry kitchen?

ESSAY TYPE QUESTIONS

1. Write a short note on the common faults in sauce making.
2. What different flavourings are used in sauces? What are their effects on sauces?
3. Write a short note on sauces used in pastry kitchen.
4. Describe at least three types of sauces that come under the category of custards along with their uses.
5. What are the steps involved in production of marzipan?
6. How does the service of sauce impact the kind of sauce to be served?
7. Apart from being served along with desserts, what are the other ways in which sauces can be used?

ACTIVITY

1. Visit various pastry shops in your city and write down the types of cakes and pastry products available in them. Now make a list of fillings and creams that were used in creating those products.
2. Make pastry cream and add various flavours to the same. Compare the results and add different textured products to the cream such as roasted chopped nuts, chopped chocolate, broken pieces of meringue and taste the products. Make a creative cake with this cream and compare with each other.
3. In a group of five, prepare chocolate sauce by the listed methods and compare the results.
4. In groups of three, create at least three types of sauces by using a liquid, flavouring, seasoning and a thickening agent. Taste and record your observations. Make standard recipes after making adjustments and share it with the rest of the group.

7 Basic Sponges and Cakes

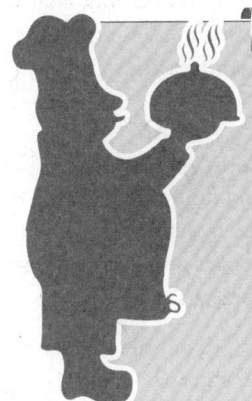

> **LEARNING OBJECTIVES**
>
> After reading this chapter, you should be able to
> - understand the different principles of sponge and cake making
> - know the various steps involved in production of sponge
> - understand the various techniques used in preparing pastry goods and the importance of each with regards to the texture of the product
> - know the role played by different ingredients in sponge making
> - know about various types of international cakes and their usage and serving techniques
> - appreciate the usage of equipment used in making sponges and cakes

INTRODUCTION

In the last chapter, we read in detail about various kinds of creams and sauces used in bakery and pastry. In this chapter, we would deal with basic sponges and classical cakes that use those fillings and bases. Cakes and pastries are one of the most common food items that come to our mind when we talk about bakery and confectionary. The spongy cakes filled with whipped cream and flavours are synonymous to pastries, but we read in the last chapter that in real sense, a pastry is much more than just sponge and filling. In confectionary, a pastry can be referred to as a paste or even dough made with various kinds of ingredients such as flour, sugar, butter, and eggs.

In this chapter, we would discuss various kinds of basic cakes and pastries and their evolution over the period of time. Most of the cakes and pastries that are patented, were made in old hotels and pastry shops and are known as classical cakes; but with experimenting chefs, it is very common to see cakes paired with international flavours. Such category of cakes is known as contemporary cakes.

When a small piece of cake is served individually garnished, it can be sold as a pastry. The pastries can be layered separately to form various shapes such as circles, rectangles, and squares and with new moulds available in the market, one can also make three dimensional shapes such as pyramids and ovals. When cakes are prepared as bite sized, then they are often referred to as *petit four glace*, which is a generic title that covers all small bite sized pastries and cakes that are 'iced'. *Petit four glace* are served with coffee after a meal, particularly in special functions, buffets, etc.

'Cake' in trade terms refers to a cake made from flour, sugar, fat, and eggs. It may also contain milk, baking powder, fruit, and nuts. Cake is usually heavier than sponge. However, 'cakes' have a broader interpretation that includes *gateau* (French) and *torte* (German). These are made of layers of sponge, Genoese, meringues, creams, and pastes, the name given to the cake usually refers to the filling and the main flavour used, for example, lemon cream gateau.

Cakes are the richest and the sweetest of all bakery products. Baking cake is a skill which requires a lot of precision when it comes to the intricate details such as measurement of ingredients and the quality of the ingredients being used. A cake would always have a base which can be either sponge or other ingredients such as crushed biscuits or thin layers of flaky pastry. Sponge cakes are so called because of their texture that resembles a sponge.

Well distributed holes in a cake are a result of the air trapped in eggs, when the cake bakes, the gluten in the flour helps the cake to retain its shape and the air escapes leaving those holes behind. Many sponges can be served on their own but many are used as the basis for various classical cakes and other desserts. In this chapter, we shall first discuss the various types of classical cakes and pastries and then the modern trends.

BASIC SPONGE CAKE

Sponge is a light and airy cake that contains three basic ingredients—eggs, sugar, and flour and is *leavened* solely by aeration which occurs by *beating* or *whisking* the eggs. A basic sponge cake is made by whisking the eggs and sugar until thick and fluffy. Sifted flour is then carefully folded into the eggs to make a sponge which is poured into a greased and lined mould and baked. There are two basic types of sponges.

Fatless sponge This sponge does not contain any fat and therefore, it is important to handle the batter with utmost care. This type of sponge is generally used to make layered cakes and gateaux.

Genoese sponge This sponge is similar to the basic sponge and in addition it has melted fat such as butter incorporated before it is baked. This sponge is richer and less crumbly than the fatless sponge.

Sponge cakes can also be made that are suitable for vegan, lactose intolerant, and low cholesterol diets. Most often this is done by using plant based milk, such as rice or soya, instead of dairy and vegetable oil instead of eggs, although many alternatives to eggs are used such as flax seeds, bananas, and commercial eggless cake powders. Sponges are both high on fat and sugar. Sponges are very versatile and can be used for a number of purposes from the confectioner's point of view. They can be presented in many forms, such as sheets for decorative purposes to be used in making fancy or so called designer cakes and gateaux.

Ingredients Used in Cake Making

The foundation of a good cake begins with the base. Every effort and care needs to be taken in preparing the base, as there is no advantage in decorating poor quality bases in an attempt to make them look better. The purpose of decorating a cake is to make it more appealing to the eye and to the palate. The decoration of a cake is wholly satisfying because it enables you to express yourself in a creative manner. In this chapter, we will consider only basic sponges and cakes, giving you the opportunity to prepare and decorate a variety of basic cakes and pastries.

The main ingredients you require to prepare cakes are eggs, flour, fat, baking powder, and emulsifiers. Many cakes also use flavouring ingredients to create different flavours. Let us understand each of these ingredients individually.

Eggs When using eggs in cake preparation, you should warm the eggs either by placing them in hot water or by warming them along with weighed sugar in gentle heat over a bain marie. The reason for doing this is to produce strong whisked foam that has the stability to withstand the additional mixing of other ingredients. If the foam loses its incorporated air, the result will be a heavier cake. Warming the eggs will also prevent the curdling of mixtures when fat, sugars, and eggs are creamed together. Eggs can be separated and the whites whisked separately to increase the lightness of the cake.

Sugar When preparing a sponge batter, use castor sugar because it readily dissolves in the batter.

Flour All cakes of a light nature need a weaker soft flour (one with low gluten) to obtain a more crumbly result. If this type of flour is not available, an all-purpose flour can be used with the addition of some cornflour to make it softer. Usually, 20% of the cornflour or cocoa powder is replaced with the amount of flour.

Baking powder This is used to aerate the cake. Make sure that it is weighed correctly and sieved several times with the flour to ensure that the cake is not over or under aerated and the distribution is even throughout. Cake mixtures should be cooked immediately or the gases emitted from the baking powder will start to develop and break out of the batter.

Fat Butter is recommended. For creaming, butter should be soft, not oily and the amount of fat that is added to a sponge batter will determine its texture. The more the fat, the heavier will be the sponge.

Emulsifier Commercially prepared stabilisers are used in sponge batters to help keep the batter from breaking down, thus forming a perfect, light emulsion. It is available in powder forms or even gel forms, these types of cake batters have a different recipe as it involves putting everything together into a mixing bowl along with warm water and whisking the entire thing to a stable emulsion, which can be held for a long duration of time.

Flavouring ingredients Many other types of ingredients can be added to the sponge mixes, depending upon the usage that the sponge will be put to. For example, if the sponge is being made for chocolate cake then it is advisable to substitute 20% of the flour with cocoa powder to give a dark rich chocolate flavoured sponge. For a coffee flavoured cake, a paste of coffee with water can be used, for honey and almond cake one could use flaked almonds and honey and so on.

Principles of Sponge Making

The aim of mixing cake batters is to combine all the ingredients into a smooth uniform, stable emulsion, that is, water in fat. It may seem very easy but the process requires a thorough understanding of the principles involved in making a sponge. For example, sometimes an experienced baker becomes too impatient to get on with his tasks and may just increase the speed on the mixer while creaming fat and sugar, thinking that high speed will do the job faster only to later realise that due to the high speed there was no formation of air cells, which resulted in poor texture of the product. So it is very important to be careful even with combining the ingredients, which is the first crucial principle of sponge making.

Combining of ingredients Careful attention has to be given to the mixing process, the sponge mixture has to form a uniform emulsion, so that the water is held in suspension surrounded by fat and other ingredients in the batter, a batter can curdle if the mixture changes to fat in water, with small particles of fat surrounded by water. Curdling can occur due to the following factors.

Incorrect measuring of butter The quantity of butter should be measured accurately in the given recipe, so that the formula has a balance of both fat and water. Whole eggs if ever used will help the batter hold the liquids in the mixture.

Ingredients too cold Ingredients should not be too cold; a temperature of 21°C is best suited to enable an emulsion to form.

Quick mixing of ingredients Mixing of ingredients in the first step too quickly will not be able to incorporate a good quantity of air into the batter.

Quick adding of liquids Adding of liquids too quickly may also cause the batter to curdle hence, they should be added in steps and a little at a time.

Incorrect preparing of moulds Preparing of the moulds prior to baking sponges is of utmost importance and is an art in itself. Many chefs lightly grease the cake tins with oil and fill up the tin with cake flour and pour out the excess whilst tapping it slightly. This ensures a thin film of flour on the cake tin and prevents the batter from sticking to the mould. The other method is to line the cake tin with greaseproof parchment paper.

> **CHEF'S TIP**
> When liquids such as eggs are added to creamed fats, the mixture may curdle. This is caused by the temperature of the liquids or the liquid being added too quickly. If this happens, warm the outside of the bowl a little by placing it in hot water or you can add a small quantity of your measured flour, which will smooth the mixture and return it to an even texture.

Formation of air cells Formation of air cells in a batter is of great importance since they give the sponge its texture and also act as a leavening agent. The air trapped in the batter expands when subjected to heat and this acts as a natural leavener giving the sponge a good raise even if no chemical agent is used.

Correct temperature of ingredients and a suitable mixing process are vital for the formation of good air cells in the batter. In foam cakes, the egg and sugar mixture should be slightly warmed to approximately 38°C. Whipping should be done at high speed first, then at moderate speed to retain the formation of air cells.

Texture Another important principle in sponge making is the texture of the sponge. The development of gluten in the batter is responsible for the texture of the end product. A very little amount of gluten is required in cake making, hence weak flour will be a better choice. In some sponge recipes, corn starch replaces some of the flour requirement, thereby reducing the gluten content even more. On the other hand, certain rich fruit cakes require more gluten to hold the structure and the fruits in the cake.

Since the amount of mixing affects the gluten, the flour in the recipe is always added towards the end of the mixing process after all the ingredients have been added, thus ensuring that there is very little development of gluten. If the batter is mixed for too long after the addition of flour, then the cake is likely to be tough.

Formula balancing Ingredients and quantities can be changed only to a certain extent in a given recipe. For the purpose of balancing, ingredients can be classified into the following four functions.

Tougheners These are the ingredients that provide structure to the cake. For example, flour and eggs help the cake retain its shape and size.

Tenderisers These ingredients must create a soft texture in the cake. Ingredients such as sweeteners, fats, and chemical leavening agents fall under this category.

Driers These are the ingredients that absorb moisture, for example, flours and starches, cocoa powder and milk solids (powder), etc. A sponge may require formula balancing if even after following all the steps it has not come out correctly.

Moisteners These ingredients provide moisture to the batter and include water, milk, liquid sugar, eggs, etc.

The formula would be balanced if tougheners equal tenderisers, and driers equal moisteners. In other words, a balance has to be maintained between the given ingredients. Egg yolks contain fat which is a tenderiser and at the same time contain protein which is a toughener. A common practice in balancing a formula is to decide the flour and sugar ratio, then balance the rest of the ingredients against this ratio.

- If liquid is increased, reduce the eggs and the shortening.
- If eggs are increased, increase the shortening.
- If extra milk powder is added as enrichment, add an equal weight of water.
- If large quantities of moist ingredients such as apple sauce, mashed bananas are added, then the batter may require an increase in the quantity of flour and eggs.

A formula in which the ingredients fall within the aforementioned limits is said to be in balance.

Baking and Cooling of Sponges

After the batter has been made with utmost care, it is important to follow the baking time and temperature guidelines to get a perfect cake. Few of the things that should be kept in mind are:

- Pre-heat the oven. The sponge needs to be given an instant shock of heat as this will help to create the oven spring. Cool ovens will result in dry and crumbly sponges.
- Make sure that the oven shelves are even. The cake batter is very soft and if the shelves are uneven, the batter will tend to flow with the slant, thereby resulting in a thick and thin cake. Whilst the thick will cook, the thin might burn or become crisp.
- Do not let pans, tins, trays, etc., touch each other. There should be even circulation of air as it creates humidity, which helps to bake the products in uniform colour.
- Bake at the correct temperature. Baking at low temperatures will give dry and pale cakes, and baking at high temperature will colour the cake too fast resulting in burning it.
- Do not open the oven door and disturb the sponge, until it has finished rising and is partially browned. Opening the door of the oven might result in the collapse of the sponge, as when the oven is opened, the steam formed in it tends to come out with a force, thereby creating a vacuum in the oven, which results in the collapse of volume.

Test for Doneness

- The sponge will be springy, the centre of the cake on the top will spring back lightly when pressed.
- A cake tester or a wooden skewer/toothpick when inserted into the centre of the cake should come out clean.

Cooling and Removing from the Pan

- Cool the sponge cake for 15 mins in the pan and then take out when slightly warm, if removed from the moulds when just baked the cake will be too hot and will break.
- Place the sponge onto cooling racks for proper circulation of air. If they are not cooled on cooling racks, the moisture will accumulate in the base resulting in a soggy cake.

Important Points for Making Sponges and Cakes

- Weigh and measure ingredients correctly.
- Sieve flour to aerate and remove impurities.
- If using baking or cocoa powder, sieve it several times with the flour to ensure even distribution.
- Tins, frames, hoops, and baking trays should be properly cleaned and prepared. The paper that is used as a liner should be free from creases.
- Dried fruits should be washed and drained well. This is done not only for hygienic reasons but to increase the moisture content in the dried fruits, giving the cake a moist quality. Another way of achieving this is to macerate the dried fruits in spirits or liqueurs.
- Remember to get all the necessary equipment ready (for example, moulds, tins, pre-heating the oven, etc.) before starting to prepare the cake. Whisked mixtures will collapse if left too long before baking.
- Cakes that are large or heavy (such as fruit cakes) require longer cooking time at lower temperatures. Smaller or low density cakes require shorter cooking time at higher temperature.
- To prevent cakes from over-colouring on the top during the baking process, place them under a greaseproof paper and reduce the top heat.
- To check for 'doneness' in small cakes and sponges, press lightly on the surface. The impression made should spring back immediately. For heavy fruit cakes, insert a clean skewer, on withdrawal, it should not have any moist mixture clinging to it.
- Allow cakes to stand in the moulds they were baked in for a few minutes prior to removal.
- Cakes are turned upside down on cooling racks and allowed to cool. Castor or icing sugar or cornflour is sprinkled on the greaseproof or parchment paper to prevent the cake from sticking. Sponge cakes may be cooled in the mould, turned upside down. This will give the cake a flat top and also prevent drying out.
- Do not remove the paper that was used to line the cake until you are ready to use it. This will prevent the cake from drying out.
- Cover cakes properly for storage either in the refrigerator, freezer, or a dry cool place, depending on the cake and your personal needs.
- In the case of frozen decorated cakes, it is advisable to cut and portion the cakes while they are still frozen.

Types of Basic Sponges

Various types of sponges are made by using the aforementioned principles. Each sponge is used for a different purpose. A plain vanilla sponge can be used for making fruit based cakes, such as pineapple, mango, and kiwi, whereas chocolate sponge can be used for making chocolate cakes. Sponges can also be used as bases for mousse cakes and pastries or can be simply crumbled and mixed with fruits such as apples to make apple pie. The sponge in this case helps to absorb the juices coming out of the apple and results in a crisp apple pie. Table 7.1 discusses various types of basic sponges and their uses.

Table 7.1 Basic sponges and their uses

Name	Description	Uses	Method	Storage
Genoese	Genoese is named after its place of origin, Genoa in Italy. It belongs to the family of light and airy sponge cakes. While the technique for making this batter is similar to that of a basic sponge cake, it does differ in that it contains melted unsalted butter. The adding of melted butter produces tenderer and more flavourful sponge cake. The chocolate Genoese is made by adding cocoa powder. Genoese is the basic sponge cake and can be made by omitting the butter. It will then be known as fatless sponge.	Genoese can have a variety of fillings, such as gateau mocha with coffee buttercream from France, wiener orange torte filled with curacao buttercream from Austria. Dobos torte with chocolate buttercream and finished with caramel sugar from Hungary.	**Whisking method**: Whole eggs and sugar are whisked together to a ribbon stage. This is done over a double boiler to get a greater volume. When the temperature reaches 32°C, it is removed from bain marie and continued to be whisked until the temperature reaches 24°C. Flour is carefully folded in melted butter, which is folded in by cut and fold method. The sponge is baked at once in order to retain as much air in it as possible.	The cake if made in sheet should be stored by spreading breakfast sugar on top, before placing another sheet of sponge on top. This prevents the sponges from sticking to one another. The sponge should be wrapped in plastic wrap and stored in a cool and dry environment. If needed to be stored for a longer time, the sponge can be frozen.
Chiffon cake	Chiffon cake is a very light and airy sponge that has the characteristics of both butter cake and sponge. Its texture of a sponge makes it much desirable to a sweet tooth. Though unlike butter cakes, chiffon cakes use oil, and whipped egg whites are used to provide the aeration, along with baking powder that gives it a sponge based texture.	The high oil content in this cake does not allow it to set firm, as oil remains liquid at room temperatures. Therefore, the cake is much more moist than butter cake. This makes it an ideal choice for cakes and gateaux, which need chilling or freezing. Chiffon cakes are also a healthier choice as they do not have saturated fats and rely solely on oil. The disadvantage here is that the cake lacks the real buttery flavour that people often look for when it comes to cakes. It is due to this reason, that these cakes are teamed up with lots of fresh fruits and served with accompanying sauces such as chocolate or fruit based sauces.	**Whisking method**: All the dry ingredients are sifted together. Egg yolks with sugar are whisked until light and creamy. Oil is added and the flour is folded in. A meringue with egg whites and remaining sugar is made and carefully folded in the flour and oil mixture. Traditionally, chiffon cakes are baked in tube shaped round moulds.	The cake if made in sheet should be stored by spreading breakfast sugar on top, before placing another sheet of sponge on top. This prevents the sponges from sticking to one another. The sponge should be wrapped in plastic wrap and stored in a cool and dry environment. If needed to be stored for a longer time, the sponge can be frozen.

(Contd)

Table 7.1 (Contd)

Name	Description	Uses	Method	Storage
Angel food cake	Angel cake is airy and because of its lightness and its pure white colour it is said to be the *food of angels*. This cake has no egg yolks, fat or artificial leavener therefore, it relies totally on stiffly beaten egg whites for leavening. Its sole ingredients are egg whites, cream of tartar, sugar, flour, salt, and flavourings such as fruit extracts and essences. Angel food cake has the highest sugar content of all the sponge cakes and this added sugar is needed to support and stabilise the whipped egg whites. As the egg whites give the cake its volume and structure, care must be taken when adding them to the dry ingredients so that they do not collapse.	Angel food cake is served whole with fruit based sauces or sugar glaze poured on top. It should preferably be sliced with a serrated cake knife as a normal knife would compress the cake as it is very soft.	**Whisking method**: Egg whites are stiffly beaten with sugar. Cream of tartar is sifted with flour and carefully folded in the mixture. This is traditionally baked in tube shaped ring moulds.	The cake should not be stored on top of each other as it can get compressed since it is very light and airy. The cakes should be wrapped individually in plastic wrap and stored in a cool and dry environment. This cake should be made and used fresh, and storing in frozen conditions is not recommended.
Victoria sponge	Victoria sponge is named after Queen Victoria, who popularised this cake in her afternoon teas. Unlike basic sponge, this sponge is made by creaming method and is usually sandwiched with jam and whipped cream. The top is not iced and can be dusted with icing sugar.	It is used as a dry cake in the afternoon tea. The cake is sliced into two halves and sandwiched with jam and whipped cream. It is not iced but can be topped with sifted icing sugar.	**Creaming method**: Butter and sugar are creamed until light and fluffy. Eggs are added one by one until a stable emulsion is formed. Flour is sifted with raising agent and carefully folded in the mixture to form a smooth batter. The mixture is poured in a greased mould lined with paper and baked at 220°C for initial 10 minutes and then at 180°C for 30 minutes.	The cakes should be wrapped individually in plastic and stored in a cool and dry environment. If needed to be stored for a longer period of time, the cake should be stored in freezer. The cake should be allowed to thaw in the refrigerator before serving.

Table 7.1 (Contd)

Name	Description	Uses	Method	Storage
Devil's food cake	This is a rich dark chocolate cake and is made by creaming method, similar to that of Victorian sponge. The only difference is that instead of melted chocolate, this sponge relies upon cocoa powder, which makes it more profound and rich in chocolate flavour. The cake also uses hot boiling water as the main liquid to bind the flour and cocoa powder as it contains less eggs.	This cake is cut into two, layered with rum flavoured sugar syrup and dark chocolate truffle.	**Creaming method**: Butter and sugar are creamed. Eggs and sifted flour and cocoa powder are added. Then hot water is added and mixed with other ingredients. The mixture is then poured in a round cake tin and baked at around 180°C for 40 minutes.	The cakes should be wrapped individually in plastic and stored in a cool and dry environment. If needed to be stored for longer period of time, the cake should be stored in freezer. The cake should be allowed to thaw in the refrigerator before serving.
Swiss roll sponge	This is a very soft sponge and is baked in thin sheets and at high temperatures as low or medium heat will bake it into a biscuit. One could add flavouring depending upon the usage of this sponge. This sponge is also called roulade.	As the name suggests, it is used for making Swiss rolls. Flavoured cream is spread on the sponge sheet and rolled into a tube. If it is difficult to remove the sponge sheet from the paper, then brush water on the back of the paper and let it stand for a couple of minutes. The sheet of paper can then be easily peeled off.	**Whisking method**: Eggs are separated and the egg yolks are whisked with half of the sugar in the recipe. The egg whites are whisked with the remaining sugar to form stiff peaks. Flour is folded in the egg yolk mix and egg whites are also carefully folded in. Melted butter can also be added in this last stage to add richness to the sponge.	The cake if made in sheet should be stored by spreading breakfast sugar on top, before placing another sheet of sponge on top. This prevents the sponges from sticking to one another. The sponge should be wrapped in plastic wrap and stored in a cool and dry environment. If needed to be stored for longer time, the sponge can be frozen.
Madeira sponge	This is slightly different from Victorian sponge. Here the butter and sugar are creamed with egg yolks and the egg whites are stiffly beaten and folded in. The resulting cake has a good volume and a very spongy texture.	It can be served plain as a tea cake or some candied and dry fruits can be added to the same.	**Creaming method**: Butter and some sugar are creamed to form a light and fluffy mixture. Egg yolks are added to the mixture and meanwhile egg whites and the remaining sugar are mixed into a stiff meringue. Flour is folded in the butter and sugar mix and carefully folded in the meringue.	The cakes should be wrapped individually in plastic and stored in a cool and dry environment. If needed to be stored for longer period of time, the cake should be stored in freezer. The cake should be allowed to thaw in the refrigerator before serving.

(Contd)

Table 7.1 (Contd)

Name	Description	Uses	Method	Storage
Joconde sponge	This is a decorative sponge and is mostly used for lining the sides of the cakes. This is quite a modern invention and is made in two stages—stage one is to make deco paste and stage two is to make the sponge.	Various kinds of templates and stencils are available to imprint the designs onto the sponge, which are used as a side collar for cakes and pastries to give them a designer effect.	**Whisking and creaming method**: This is made in two stages. Stage one involves making deco paste by combining egg whites, flour, sugar, and butter in equal parts. It can be coloured to give designer effects. It is spread on a silicon baking mat as it sticks to other surfaces and is then frozen. Stage two involves preparing a sponge by whisking eggs, and then folding in almond flour, flour, and melted butter; then spreading the special sponge mix onto the design in a layer and baking at high temperatures. The resulting sponge gets the design from the deco paste printed on the sponge.	The cake if made in sheet should be stored by spreading breakfast sugar on top, before placing another sheet of sponge on top. This prevents the sponges from sticking to one another. The sponge should be wrapped in plastic wrap and stored in a cool and dry environment. If needed to be stored for longer time, the sponge can be frozen.
Butter cake sponge	Butter cake sponge as known in US and commonly known as an English pound cake around the world is called so because it contains a pound (454 g) of butter, flour, sugar, and eggs.	These cakes are often eaten during afternoon and hi teas. They are usually served sliced and are never iced. At the most they can be topped with sifted icing sugar.	**Creaming method**: Butter with sugar is creamed until light and fluffy. Eggs are added one by one, taking care that the mixture does not curdle. Flour is folded in with hands. Sometimes a small amount of baking powder is added for aeration. Dried candied fruit can be added to make fruit cakes.	The cakes should be wrapped individually in plastic and stored in a cool and dry environment. If needed to be stored for longer period of time, the cake should be stored in freezer. The cake should be allowed to thaw in the refrigerator before serving.

Table 7.1 (Contd)

Name	Description	Uses	Method	Storage
Japonaise	This is a very crunchy base often used for rich cakes and pastries. The combination of flour, almond powder, and eggs, combined with melted butter is used as a base or sponge for preparing cakes.	These cakes are usually used as a base for petit gateaux and petit fours as they are heavy and rich and give a rich taste and feel to the finished product.	**Whisking method**: Japonaise is made by adding 2/3rd of almond powder or hazelnut powder to 1 part of meringue and mixing it well. It can be piped on to a baking mat with round nozzle to form a circle starting from the centre and piping all the way towards the end or it can be spread with a palette knife to form a circular base.	This cake should ideally be used when required and it is not recommended to store it beyond a day. The cake should be wrapped with plastic and stored in a cool and dry environment.
Dacquoise sponge	Dacquoise is a French biscuit that was originally made in Dax, which is in south-western part of France. Dacquoise can be made by using any nut powder and the sponge will get its name from the nut used, for example, almond dacquoise, hazelnut dacquoise, etc.	It can be used only as a base or the entire cake can be made using this sponge. It is a good sponge for people who are allergic to gluten as this does not contain any flour.	**Whisking method**: Dacquoise is made by combining French meringue with powdered hazelnut and/or almond flour. It is then piped in circles and baked until crisp.	This cake should ideally be used when required and it is not recommended to store it beyond a day. The cake should be wrapped with plastic and stored in a cool and dry environment.
Eggless sponge	This is very famous in India because of religious implications. It can be made in any flavour and can be used in place of the regular sponge.	These can be substituted for any regular sponge.	**Creaming or whisking depending on the recipe**: The sponge is made by creaming butter and condensed milk until light and fluffy. Flour, baking powder, and soda water are folded carefully into the mixture and the sponge is baked until cooked. Other recipes use oil, yoghurt, and flour along with baking soda to create a sponge, in which case the cake is made by *whisking method*.	The cakes should be wrapped individually in plastic and stored in a cool and dry environment. If needed to be stored for longer period of time, the cake should be stored in freezer. The cake should be allowed to thaw in the refrigerator before serving.

CLASSICAL CAKES AND PASTRIES

Before we move further to learn different types of classical cakes and pastries, it is important to understand the basic composition of any cake.

Base It is the base of the cake or pastry. It is not necessary that every cake will have a base, but most of the cakes have a base that serves many purposes, such as:

- Adds texture to the cake. For example, black forest cake which is a soft cake layered with whipped cream and sponge with cherries, has a base of sweet paste biscuit, which offers a crunch to the soft textured cake to create an interesting mouth feel.
- Helps to lift up the soft cakes and pastries from the plate for consumption, or else if the cake is too soft it will fall apart.
- Prevents the spongy cake to soak up any odd flavours if refrigerated on a tray.

Sponge This is the body of the cake. Various types of sponges can be used for this purpose. The most basic of all is *Genoese sponge* that is made by whisking eggs and sugar until light and fluffy. Flour is folded in along with melted fat and baked until cooked. A mixture of cocoa powder and flour can also be used to make chocolate sponge, which would be used for making a chocolate flavoured cake. Sometimes other kinds of bases can also be used instead of sponge or with a combination of sponge to layer a cake.

Filling This is the main flavouring of the cake with which it gets its name. For example, a chocolate truffle cake would have the filling of truffle inside. The base of the cake is layered with various kinds of flavoured creams and fillings to prepare the cake or pastry. The fillings and creams discussed in chapter 6 are used in various combinations to create delectable cakes and pastries.

> **CHEF'S TIP**
> All cakes of a light nature need a weaker soft flour (one with low gluten) to obtain a more crumbly result. If this type of flour is not available, an all-purpose flour can be used with the addition of some cornflour to make it softer.

Icing It refers to the topping that is the glaze of the cake, which is given for various reasons, such as:

- To give a decorative appearance to the cake and make it look attractive.
- To form a cover on the cake and prevent it from drying out.
- To add flavour and texture to the cake.

Icings used for cake can be of various kinds. Some cakes are covered only with dusted icing sugar, whereas some can be covered with caramelised sugar or even whipped cream.

Garnish This is one of the most important parts of a cake or pastry. These are put on the cake to decorate it and hence, are known as garnishes. Garnishes can range from fresh fruits to chocolate and sugar garnishes that would complement the flavour and texture of the cake. It is very important to choose the right kind of garnish to finish a cake. It would be odd to garnish a dry fruit cake with chocolate garnish and so on.

Moistening agents The moistening agent in the cake is usually flavoured sugar syrup that adds flavour and moistness to the cake. Each layer of sponge is brushed with a liberal amount of sugar syrup. This is done for the following reasons.

- It helps to add sweetness to the cake.
- It helps to add flavour to the cake.
- Some of the syrups flavoured with liqueurs are traditional for classical cakes. For example, a black forest cake is moistened with kirsch flavoured liqueur.
- Syrups are added to wet the sponge, so that it allows the fillings to stick to the sponge and it does not let the sponge give out its crumbs, whilst spreading the cream with a palette knife.

> **CHEF'S TIP**
> Always spread sugar syrup with a wide painting brush. This helps to spread the syrup equally on the sponge. Do not put too much syrup on the base of the sponge as it will make the cake too soft and difficult to lift.

Now once we have understood the various kinds of bases, they can be layered with various kinds of creams and fillings to make some of the most famous cakes and pastries around the world.

Let us discuss some of the classical cakes and pastries in Table 7.2.

Table 7.2 Classical cakes and pastries

Cake/Pastry	Base & sponge	Filling	Garnish
Sacher torte This cake was patented by Chef Franz Sacher, who was the head pastry chef of Prince Metternich.	The sacher is made from a dark chocolate sponge. The butter is melted along with the chocolate and whipped egg yolks are folded into the mixture. Flour sifted along with cornflour and cocoa powder is then folded in and lastly, whipped meringue is folded in the batter. The sponge is baked, cooled and sliced into two.	The sacher sponge is moistened with sugar syrup and then the two halves are sandwiched with apricot jam. The jam is spread on sides as well as top and is smoothened out to give an even finish.	The cake is usually finished with melted chocolate truffle. Since this is a patented cake, it is customary to write the name *Sacher* on top of the cake.
Dobos torte This cake was created in Budapest by a Hungarian chef Joseph Dobos. This cake became so famous that people from other countries wanted to export it. Chef thought of a nouvelle idea to spread a thin layer of caramel on top of the cake to preserve and package it. Since then the caramel coating on this cake has become synonymous to Dobos torte.	It is a white sponge that is prepared by creaming butter and sugar till fluffy. Whipped egg yolks and lemon zest is added and folded in. After this, meringue is folded along with flour and almond powder, and the sponge is baked until cooked.	The cake is sliced into as many as five layers. Each layer is moistened with vanilla flavoured sugar syrup and layered with caramel flavoured buttercream. Two parts of white butter are whipped along with one part of icing sugar to prepare buttercream.	The sugar is heated over moderate heat until it turns to caramel. This is then spread onto a thin slice of sponge. This facilitates the cutting of the caramel. When the caramel sets, it is divided into equal pieces with a hot knife and arranged on top of the cake like a fan.

(Contd)

Table 7.2 (Contd)

Cake/Pastry	Base & sponge	Filling	Garnish
Malakoff torte This torte is a famous torte that originated in France. It was created during the battle between France and Russia on the Malakoff hill during the Crimean war.	This cake uses a special kind of sponge known as sponge fingers. Egg yolks and whites are whipped along with sugar separately and then combined together with sifted cornflour and flour. This is piped on to the baking trays in finger shapes and then dusted with icing sugar before baking in the oven.	The cake is filled with rum flavoured whipped cream. Layer of sponge fingers are arranged on the base and moistened with rum flavoured sugar syrup. More sponge fingers are arranged on the cream and topped with rum flavoured cream.	The cake is decorated by arranging sponge fingers on the sides of the cake. Swirl of whipped cream is piped on the edges of the cake and garnished with more sponge fingers.
Linzer torte This is a very famous and the oldest tart from the Linz city of Austria and hence the name. Linzer is basically a tart which is eaten as a cake or as a dessert.	A short crust pastry is prepared by creaming butter and sugar with eggs and combining it lightly with flour and hazelnut powder. It is flavoured with lemon zest and left to chill for 30 minutes or until set. This forms the base of the cake. The dough is rolled to 5 mm thickness and lined on a tart or a pie mould.	The lined pie shell is filled with red currant jam or raspberry jam.	The dough is rolled and cut into strips. The strips are arranged in a crisscross fashion on top of the linzer torte and the cake is brushed with egg whites and baked at 180°C for 20 minutes. The cake should be chilled before cutting and is garnished with almond flakes.
Battenberg This cake is believed to be created in 1884 in the honour of the wedding of the granddaughter of Queen Victoria to the prince of Battenberg.	This cake is made with pink and yellow coloured Genoese cake sponge that is cut into bars of square shape. These squares are joined to each other with the help of apricot jam and covered with marzipan.	The cake is not filled but joined with apricot jam.	The cake has no particular garnish but is covered with marzipan and served exposing the chequered sponge.
Black forest gateaux This cake comes from the Swabia region of Germany, which is famous for its black forest. The appearance of the cake represents the forests of this region. In Germany, this cake is also known as *Schwarzwalder Kirsch Torten*.	This cake usually has a base of baked sweet paste biscuit and apricot jam is spread in a thin layer over the biscuit and a slice of chocolate Genoese is put on top. Sugar syrup flavoured with kirsch liquor is used to moisten the sponge.	The cake is layered with fresh whipped cream, chopped dark chocolate chips, and *Morello* cherries. Some recipes also use sour cherries which should be cooked with sugar and corn starch.	Whipped cream covers the top and all the sides of the cake. Dark chocolate flakes are put on top with swirls of whipped cream that is decorated with cherries. The sides can be left plain or can be decorated with chocolate flakes.

Table 7.2 (Contd)

Cake/Pastry	Base & sponge	Filling	Garnish
Napoleon gateau This is one of the classical cakes from France. It is made with baked puff pastry also known as *mille feuille* that translates to thousand layers. It is believed to have been developed in France during the 19th century.	The base for the cake is made by rolling the puff pastry into thin sheets and baking it until crisp and golden brown. This cake is not layered with sponge and hence, it is not moistened with any syrup.	The sheets of baked puff pastry are layered with whipped pastry cream that is flavoured with orange flavoured liquor.	Traditionally, the top of the cake is brushed with hot apricot jam and then warm fondant is poured on the top. Chocolate is piped in straight lines on the fondant and then a tooth pick is used to create a feather design.
Gateau St Honore This is a traditional French gateau that is named after the patron saint of pastry cooks.	This cake utilises a base of puff pastry on which choux pastry is piped all around the rim and the gateau is baked blind.	The dessert is filled with two different types of fillings. ♦ Chiboust cream: One part of pastry cream is mixed with one part of Italian meringue. ♦ Diplomat crème: One part of pastry cream is mixed with one part of melted chocolate and little gelatine. These are piped alternately in the empty space of the gateau.	The cake is decorated and garnished with small profiteroles that are filled with orange flavoured pastry cream and dipped in caramel. The cake can also be garnished with cut fresh fruits and spun sugar.
Charlotte russe This cake was made by French chef Marie Antoine Careme who named it in honour of his employer who was Russian.	This cake is lined with sponge fingers and the base for this cake is also sponge fingers that are soaked in rum flavoured sugar syrup. This cake is usually made in a half sphere shaped mould known as *bombe*.	The lined cake is filled with a mixture of fruits and custard that is prepared by cooking milk and sugar with egg yolks and then cooled down. This is then mixed with whipped cream and gelatine.	The cake is usually garnished with fresh fruits and powdered icing sugar.
Opera gateau This cake is a classical French gateau that was made first in the early 1900s.	The opera sponge is a kind of Japonaise that is made by using almond powder. This cake consists at least five slices of the sponge that are moistened with a strong coffee flavoured sugar syrup, which is flavoured with rum and Kahlua.	The sponge is layered alternately with coffee flavoured buttercream and ganache. The top of the cake is covered with buttercream.	The cake is glazed with melted ganache or chocolate glaze and decorated with gold leaf. It is also customary to write the word *opera* on top of the cake.

(Contd)

Table 7.2 (Contd)

Cake/Pastry	Base & sponge	Filling	Garnish
Devil's food cake This cake was made in America in the early 1900s. There is no historical evidence to the name, but it is believed that since this cake is so rich and moist with chocolate that it is referred to as sinful and hence, devil's food cake.	This cake is made by using dark cocoa powder along with eggs, sugar, and an acidic medium such as sour cream. The acid helps to draw out the rich dark red colour from the cocoa thus giving the cake its characteristic dark colour. The cake is moistened with sugar syrup.	The cake is filled with dark chocolate truffle and covered on all sides with chocolate truffle.	The cake is garnished with chocolate garnishes and dusted with cocoa powder.
Mud cake Mud cake is also referred to as Mississippi mud slice and is believed to have originated in America in late 1970s. The baked cake crumbs are said to look like the sand along the banks of the Mississippi river.	This is a dark chocolate sponge that is quite similar to the brownie, but in this case the eggs are whipped and the cake has the texture of a Genoese cake. It is cut into two and moistened with rum flavoured sugar syrup.	The cake is usually layered with dark chocolate fudge. The sides of the cake are also finished with fudge.	The cake is garnished with dusted cocoa powder and chocolate garnishes.
Walnut brownie The walnut brownies originated in America in the early 1900s. It is a flat type of dark chocolate cake that is somewhat between a cookie and a cake. It is often eaten with tea and can be eaten paired with vanilla ice cream and hot chocolate sauce.	Brownie is a special sponge that is made for various kinds of desserts. The mixing technique here is very important as it decides the texture of the brownie. Chocolate is melted along with butter and kept aside to cool. Eggs and sugar are mixed together, but not whipped as whipping would result in a crumbly texture and the brownie would not get the desired fudgy texture. To the mixture of eggs and sugar, chocolate mixture is added and flour is folded along with walnut powder and crushed walnuts.	This cake is served as it is and is not filled or layered. The rich fudgy texture of the cake acts as a moistening agent for it.	This cake can be served warm, dusted with icing sugar. It can sometimes be covered with chocolate fudge also.
Baked cheesecake This cake comes from America. In order to create the famous Neufchatel cheese from France, the American chefs accidentally stumbled upon a recipe for an unripen cheese which they called as cream cheese. In 1912, a method was developed to pasteurise the cream cheese and thus, the Philadelphia cream cheese was born.	This is a very unique cake as it is not layered like other cakes. In this, a cake ring is lined with biscuit base and baked blind. The cheese is creamed along with sugar, eggs, and cream. The prepared batter is then put into the mould and then baked in a water bath.	This cake does not have any filling.	The cake is served dusted with castor sugar. Sometimes it is spread with castor sugar and caramelised under an equipment called salamander, which emits radiated heat from top only.

Basic Sponges and Cakes 141

Table 7.2 (Contd)

Cake/Pastry	Base & sponge	Filling	Garnish
Chilled cheesecake Chilled cheesecake unlike the baked cheesecake is set in a mould with the help of gelatine. This popular cake from France has a smooth creamy texture that comes from creamy cheese.	The chilled cheesecake traditionally has a base of Genoese sponge, but one can use other bases such as Japonaise, Dacquoise, or even meringue. The sponge used in the base is moistened with sugar syrup. This cake would be prepared in a ring shaped mould which is lined with sponge. The cheese mixture is spread on the sponge and another layer of sponge is placed over it and moistened with sugar syrup. The remaining cheesecake mixture is filled and smoothened on top and the cake is chilled.	The cake is usually filled with a cream cheese mixture, which is made by using a variety of cream cheeses such as Philadelphia, mascarpone, or even yoghurt cheese. Egg yolks are whipped with sugar and folded with cream cheese. The cake can be flavoured with any flavourings such as zest, juice of any citrus fruit, berries, and chocolate. Gelatine is added to the mixture and this mixture is poured into moulds and set.	The cheesecake can be garnished in a variety of ways. Traditionally, it is covered with a fruit gel and garnished with fruits.
Croquembouche This is a very famous cake that originated in France. The name comes from a French word *croque en bouche*, which means crunch in the mouth. This cake is traditionally used as an artistic showpiece and is served on various occasions such as weddings, name christening ceremonies, and baptism ceremonies.	The cake has a base of thick sweet paste biscuit on top of which, small profiteroles made from choux pastry are arranged to form a cone shape.	This cake utilises profiteroles that can be filled with various fillings such as orange flavoured pastry cream and chocolate cream. The profiteroles are then dipped into caramel and stuck to the base and then built on each other to form a cone.	The cake is garnished with spun sugar, roses made with marzipan, and garnishes made with sugar.
Yule log Yule logs are logs of wood that are used to burn in the hearths to keep the house warm. This was traditionally done during the cold winters of Christmas in Europe. French prepared the cake in the shape of a log of wood and the cakes became famous by the name Yule log cake or *Bouche de Noel*.	This cake is made by preparing Genoese sponge in sheets. The sponge can be flavoured with coffee, chocolate or any other flavour corresponding to the flavour of the desired Yule log. The cake is moistened with vanilla flavoured sugar syrup.	The cake was traditionally filled with flavoured buttercream. The cake is then rolled and wrapped in paper and refrigerated until chilled.	The cake is covered with buttercream and groves are made on top to resemble a bark of log of wood. Green coloured buttercream is piped to resemble the ivy vine and meringue mushrooms are placed on the log to give it a natural feel.

(Contd)

Table 7.2 (Contd)

Cake/Pastry	Base & sponge	Filling	Garnish
Christmas cake The Christmas cake originated in Scotland, where it was made with candied fruits and whisky. It was also known as whisky dundee. The Christmas cake is decorated with royal icing to resemble snow and Christmas decorations are placed on top.	It is a dark and moist cake which is enriched with candied fruits and nuts that are macerated in alcohol. It is customary to start the fruit soaking ceremony a couple of months in advance to the Christmas preparations at many places. Eggs, flour, sugar, and butter are combined with molasses and soaked fruits to make this dark, rich, and moist cake.	The cake is not layered as it is served whole.	The Christmas cake can be decorated in many ways. The traditional style is to cover the cake with royal icing or frosting and decorate with Christmas decorations such as holy leaves, Santa Claus face, and stars.
Gateau Pithivier This cake is a kind of pie that is prepared with puff pastry. As the name suggests, this cake originates from the Pithivier region in France.	The cake is made by pinning out the puff pastry to a round circle of 7 mm thickness. Another circle slightly larger than the base is also cut out as it will be placed on top of the cake after being filled.	The cake is traditionally filled with an almond cream mixture that is also known as crème frangipani. It is made by creaming butter, sugar, and eggs along with almond powder and rum.	The sides of the cake are brushed with egg yolks and another disc is placed on top of the mixture. The top of the cake is brushed with egg yolks and then with the tip of the knife, grooves are made on top by starting from the tip of the gateau and working at a slant through to the base. The cake is baked and served dusted with icing sugar.

CAKES SERVED DURING HI TEA

Hi tea is a Western concept which is often confused with afternoon tea. A hi tea was usually an early dinner for children, so that they can eat and go to bed, whilst the parents can go out for dining and celebrating. A hi tea comprises of many kinds of cakes, pastries, and savoury items such as sandwiches and quiches. Most of the cakes served in hi tea are dry cakes. Let us discuss some of the commonly prepared hi tea cakes in Table 7.3.

Table 7.3 Various kinds of hi tea cakes

Name	Description
Tea cake	Butter cake sponge as known in US and commonly known as an English pound cake around the world is called so because it contains a pound (454 g) of butter, flour, sugar, and eggs. This cake can be flavoured with various kinds of ingredients such as citrus fruit zest and juices. It can also be flavoured with artificial flavours and colours. Candied fruits can also be mixed along with the batter to prepare dry fruit cakes.
Victoria sponge	Victoria sponge is named after Queen Victoria, who popularised this cake in her afternoon teas. Unlike basic sponge, this sponge is made by creaming method and is usually sandwiched with jam and whipped cream. The top is not iced and can be dusted with icing sugar.
Madeira cake	This is slightly different from Victoria sponge. Here the butter and sugar are creamed with egg yolks and the egg whites are stiffly beaten and folded in. The resulting cake has a good volume and a very spongy texture. It can be served plain as tea cake or some candied and dry fruits can be added to the same.

Table 7.3 (Contd)

Name	Description
Dundee cake	This is a rich fruit cake from Scotland that is traditionally garnished with almonds on top. The cake is made by the creaming method as in case of pound cake. Spices such as cinnamon and allspice are used along with candied fruits such as raisins, sultanas, black currants, orange and lemon peels, and candied cherries.
Banana bread	Banana bread is also commonly served as a breakfast pastry or even in hi teas. Soft and pulpy bananas that have become black over a period of time are used for preparing this cake. Banana is pureed along with vegetable oil and then mixed with whipped eggs, sugar, and flour and baked in loaf tins. The cake is then sliced and served.
Carrot cake	Carrot cake is a very famous cake from Switzerland and is made by grating carrots and combining them with eggs, sugar, butter, flour, and sometimes almond powder. The cake is usually covered with marzipan and each slice is decorated with carrots made from marzipan.
Fruit loaf	Various kinds of fruits are used for making dry cakes for hi tea. Apples, mangoes, and pineapples are few of the fruits that can be combined in a pureed form or in small chunks to make moist and soft cakes that are often served at hi teas.
Marbled cake	This is same as English pound cake but the batter is divided in two parts. One part is mixed with cocoa powder and the other is flavoured with vanilla. Both the batters are put in a baking tin and randomly stirred with a small rod to intermingle the designs. The resulting baked cake is marbled in texture.

COMMON FAULTS IN CAKE MAKING

Cake baking is a combination of art and science blended with years of experience. Even the most professional bakers sometimes cannot make a product as per the right standard. There can be many faults that may occur during cake making. Some of these can be outside your control and a few you will be able to identify so that either you can rectify them or learn from them so that they are not repeated in the future.

One must also understand that a fault of a cake is identified as fault only when it is unwanted texture of consistency in that particular sponge. As there are sponges with various textures and appeal, it is important to first know the standard product so that any deviation from the standard product can be identified as fault.

Let us discuss some of the most common faults that can occur during the baking process in Table 7.4.

Table 7.4 Faults in cake making

Fault	Reasons
M fault	As the name suggests an M shape is formed in the cake whilst baking. The cake sinks in the middle and does not rise evenly. The cross section of the cake if sliced in half vertically will be in the shape of the alphabet "M" and hence this name.
	Most of the cakes sink in bottom due to recipe imbalance. Some of the things that can go wrong in recipe are:
	• Use of very weak flour
	• Too much of raising agent in the mixture
	• The oven was opened midway resulting in collapse of volume
	• Too much of sugar in the recipe
X fault	This is one of the most common faults that can occur in a sponge. In this fault, the cake rises evenly but the corners of the cake sink inside giving an uneven finish to the top of the cake. Some of the common causes could be:
	• Uneven baking temperature
	• Too much liquid component in the batter
	• Uneven dispersion of raising agent

(Contd)

Table 7.4 (Contd)

Fault	Reasons
Cake does not have good volume	Quite a common problem and can be caused due to various reasons such as: • Eggs not whipped to a good volume • Too much of dry ingredients resulting in a stiff batter • Over mixing of flour in whipped eggs, resulting in loss of volume • Oven temperature too low or too high
Cracked top	This is an undesired appearance in few cakes and in some cakes such as tea cakes, it is important to have a peak resulting in a small crack. Some of the reasons associated with this fault are: • Oven too hot in the initial stage • Less quantity of raising agent
Sugary top	This is a fault in the cake when you see dark coloured spots or specks of sugar on top of the sponge. This fault can occur due to the following reasons. • Recipe imbalance where too much sugar is added • Sugar has not dissolved in the mix due to lack of moisture content • Granular sugar was used in the recipe and it has not dissolved • Cake left too long outside before being put in the oven. Leaving the cake uncovered causes moisture loss and hence, accumulation of sugar patches on top. After the cake is baked, there is a white sugary streak
Curdling of batter	This is a fault that can occur during the batter making process. Many chefs ignore this fault as it can be corrected by adding flour to the batter. But eventually if the mixture is curdled it can impact the final texture of the baked cake. Following could be the reasons why the batter curdles whilst making. • The ingredients are at different temperatures, some are at room temperature whilst others are chilled • The eggs are added too quickly and enough time is not given for emulsification • The batter is being made at a very high speed
Sinking of fruits	This is one of the most common issues that the dry fruits sink to the bottom. This alters the texture of the sponge and also the appearance is not very pleasant. Some of the reasons for this fault could be: • The flour used is a very weak flour • The batter is overbeaten and hence very soft • Too much of raising agent in the recipe • Fruits are not dry and have too much liquid in them

Once you understand these faults you can correct them to make a standard product. For example, in sinking of fruit fault, if the fruit is wet then it sinks to the bottom whilst baking. The chef who understands this fault will rectify by coating these fruits with all the flour mentioned in the recipe. Likewise the faults in temperature can be avoided by following the temperature guidelines mentioned in the recipe.

ICING

Icing is a common English term, also called frosting in America. It is interesting to see that when a mixture such as types of creams discussed in last chapter are used in layering of cake, they are called fillings and when these are used for covering a cake they are known as icings. Icing is done for various reasons. The most important of these are:

- It adds a sweet taste to the cakes and pastries.
- It improves the appearance of the product.
- It helps in preserving cakes as it covers all the sides and top of the cake, thus preventing it from drying out.
- It adds moistness and flavour to cakes and pastries.

Kinds of Icing and its Classical Types

We have discussed various types of creams and fillings used in cakes and pastries in chapter 6. It is important for you to be aware of those basics before we move further to discuss various types of icings. Let us discuss the various kinds of icings that can be done for decorating different types of cakes in Table 7.5.

Table 7.5 Various kinds of icings used in cakes and pastries

Icing	Description
Buttercream	This is a light and fluffy mixture of unsalted butter and icing sugar. The butter is creamed along with the sugar until air is incorporated thereby, making the icing light, creamy, and fluffy. There are various kinds of buttercreams and slight variations could be made to enhance their texture and flavour. They are commonly used for decorating and filling many types of cakes and pastries. Few of the common variations of buttercream are: **Italian buttercream**: In this, half of the buttercream is folded along with Italian meringue. The butter is creamed with less amount of sugar as Italian meringue is already high in sugar content. **French buttercream**: This is made by whipping egg yolks along with boiling sugar syrup until the mixture is thick and creamy. This is then folded along with creamed and fluffy butter. **Swiss buttercream**: In this type of buttercream, the butter is creamed till light and fluffy and then combined with Swiss meringue. Swiss meringue is made by cooking egg whites and sugar over a double boiler until 45°C and then whipping the mixture until a foamy and thick meringue is obtained. The meringue must be cooled down to 30°C before incorporating it into the creamed butter. **American buttercream**: In this buttercream, the ratio of sugar to butter is almost three times. The butter is creamed along with the sugar until air is incorporated thereby, making the icing light, creamy, and fluffy. The consistency of this buttercream is very thick and sometimes the consistency is adjusted by adding a spoonful of milk. **Pastry buttercream**: In this kind of buttercream, one part of buttercream is mixed along with whipped pastry cream. This kind of buttercream can sometimes be very soft and hence, it can be bound with small amounts of melted gelatine. **Fondant buttercream**: This buttercream is made by creaming butter until it is light and fluffy, then fondant is added to the butter and whipped again until it is smooth and creamy. **Flavoured buttercreams**: These kinds of buttercreams are flavoured with various kinds of flavourings and colours to make ornamental cakes and several other types of cakes. Some of the most common flavourings used in buttercreams are vanilla pods, melted chocolate, coffee, nut pastes such as hazelnut, chestnuts, and almond paste, and liqueurs such as rum and grand mariner. Even natural and artificial flavours can be used for flavouring buttercreams.

(Contd)

Table 7.5 (Contd)

Icing	Description
Fondants	Fondant is a sugar based icing that is mostly used on festive cakes and wedding cakes. This icing requires lot of skill and art to be prepared in the kitchen; therefore, it is normally purchased readymade from the market. The consistency of this icing is such that it can be rolled and then used for covering cakes or pastries. The consistency can be regulated by warming the icing over double boiler to make it viscous. It can then be used for dipping petit fours, pastries such as éclairs, and also used as a topping for napoleon pastries and Danish pastries. After setting in this manner it becomes smooth, shiny, and non-sticky. Fondant is prepared by heating sugar and water until it reaches 105°C. Then liquid glucose or acids such as cream of tartar is added and the syrup is cooked until it reaches 118°C. It is then spread on a wet marble table and allowed to cool down until it reaches 45°C. The sugar is then folded and kneaded until a soft dough is obtained. This dough can be rolled and used for covering cakes.
Chocolate icing	Various kinds of chocolate icings are used to cover and decorate cakes and pastries. The two major ones are truffle and ganache. Few other kinds of chocolate icings used on cakes and pastries are: **Chocolate glaze**: It is made by cooking cocoa powder/chocolate, water, fondant, and liquid glucose until the mixture is thick and shiny. Then soaked gelatine leaves are added and the mixture is blended until smooth and shiny. The mixture is allowed to cool down to 32°C before applying on any cake. It can then be used to cover the top of the cakes. The gelatine allows the glaze to set on the cake with a shiny appearance. **Chocolate fudge**: Chocolate truffle is whipped until it becomes fluffy and of matt finish. Softened butter is incorporated into the mixture to create fudge icing. The fudge icings are spread with palette knife and lifted up to form peaks on the top of the cakes.
Foam type icings	These icings are made by whipping egg whites along with boiled sugar syrup. These are often referred to as boiled icings. Italian meringue is an example of foam type icing. The disadvantage of these icings is that it is not a very stable form of icing and should be used on cakes and pastries which would be consumed immediately. To stabilise this icing, another variation of it is made, which is known as *Marshmallow icing*. The Italian meringue is whipped along with melted gelatine and used immediately. The gelatine however stabilises the icing.
Royal icing	Royal icing is prepared by beating egg whites and icing sugar until a thick paste is obtained. The icing should only be beaten with a flat paddle and never whipped. The amount of icing sugar used will guide the consistency of the icing. Royal icing has a unique property of setting to a brittle consistency and this is used by chefs to the best of its ability. Royal icing is used for decorating wedding cakes. It can be piped to make lace structures, etc. It is also used as a glue to stick decorations on the cake. Since this icing is very sweet in nature, it is mostly used for decoration only.
Glazed icings	This category of icings can comprise of various kinds of icings that are used for decorating cakes and pastries. Glazed icings can be of the following types. **Hot and cold gel**: Proprietary cold and hot gels are also available in modern times and they are neutral in flavour. These cold gels can be mixed with flavourings and colours and spread on top of cakes and pastries. The hot gels are required to be heated along with a little quantity of water and flavourings, and then spread over chilled cakes or pastries. Care should be taken whilst spreading the hot gel, as it can melt the top layer of the cake thereby creating an unwanted effect. **Jams and preserves**: Apricot jam is the most commonly used jam in the pastry for various kinds of decorations of cakes and pastries. The Danish pastries are iced with boiled apricot jam. Boiling and applying the jam allows the jam to spread in a thin consistency and it sets like a gel after cooling down. **Hot sugar glaze**: This icing is like a mock fondant. It is the quickest icing to make as icing sugar is combined with very little water and heated over moderate heat until it becomes opaque and of flowing consistency. This can be used to glaze and decorate cakes and pastries.

SUMMARY

Sponges are the base to any cake. A gateau is French for cakes and in Germany they are referred to as tortes. To make any good quality cake, the first step is to make a good sponge and the next step is to layer and ice the cake with good quality filling. Prior to baking sponges, it is very essential to know about various techniques of mixing, as these mixing methods decide the texture of a product. It will be very surprising for you to know that sometimes from the same recipe and ingredients, one could make sponges or cookies and the entire thing will be decided by the method of mixing ingredients involved in making the product.

Unlike bread which relies on yeast or any other raising agent for aeration, the sponge solely relies on trapping of air by physical aeration and this could be achieved mostly by whipping or whisking. In most of the sponge recipes, the flour will be lightly mixed in or folded in and never mixed vigorously as done for bread, as in case of sponges we do not want the gluten to develop and that is the reason that weak flours or cake flours are used for production of sponges. Since the method of sponge making relies mostly on physical aeration, therefore, eggs are often beaten separately and combined together as egg whites have the capacity of incorporating more air in them as compared to egg yolks. Though certain cakes also use the chemical and biological methods of aeration by using raising agents and yeasts, it is mostly done in sponges made without egg.

In this chapter, we also read about the ingredients used in sponge making and understood the role of each ingredient. We saw how eggs formed an integral part of sponge making and how oil or fats affect the texture of the sponge.

We understood the science behind sponge making by understanding the ingredients and how to control curdling or over mixing of the ingredients. We also read about balancing the formulas in a recipe to create sponges with the desired texture. We discussed about various kinds of sponges and their uses in pastry and confectionary.

The method of making the sponges gave us an insight into different methods involved in sponge making and how each method affects the texture of the sponges. Some precautions are to be kept in mind whilst making sponges and in this chapter we also dealt with very basic points that can make a good or poor quality sponge.

We also discussed a few classical cakes and pastries and their icings and classical garnishes. We also read about common faults in cake making and baking and how those can be avoided.

Lastly, we discussed about types of icings and how to apply them on cakes and pastries.

KEY TERMS

Batter Flowy mixture of flour and liquids. The consistency would depend upon the amount of liquid in the batter

Beating Creaming butter and sugar in a mixer using a paddle attachment

Blind baking Usually refers to biscuit shells baked without any filling

Buttercream Creamed unsalted butter and icing sugar in the ratio of 2:1 used for layering and icing cakes

Cocoa powder A residual powder left behind in the production of chocolate

Docking Making small holes in pastry goods to discourage the puffing up

Folding Mixing two ingredients together without losing volume

Gateaux French for cakes. Usually a reference to whole uncut cakes

Icing Layering and decorating a cake

Lazy Suzanne Another name for cake turn table

Leavened The incorporation of air into a dough or batter

Petit fours Bite sized decorative sponges or pastries, served with coffee

Pinning Rolling the dough with a rolling pin

Piping Forcing out the mixture from a bag

Pound cakes Another name for butter cakes

Ribbon stage Whipping of eggs and sugar to a stage where they become thick and pale

Rubbing-in Mixing in flour and butter with fingertips to resemble breadcrumb texture

Short A baked good that snaps when broken, also known as *khasta* in Hindi

Silpats Silicone baking mats

Sponge A light and airy product, made with eggs, flour, and sugar

Torte German for cakes. Sometimes referred to individual slices of cake

Turn table An equipment used for layering and icing cakes

Whipping Incorporating air into liquids, by using wire whisk

OBJECTIVE TYPE QUESTIONS

1. Define a sponge and how is it different from a cake and bread.
2. List down the role of ingredients used in sponge making.
3. What precautions will you take whilst combining the ingredients for sponge making?
4. Why does a sponge batter curdle and how can you fix it?
5. What do you understand about balancing the formula in a sponge or batter?
6. What care should be taken whilst baking sponges?
7. Why is cooling of cakes so crucial?
8. List at least five basic sponges and their uses.
9. What sponge would you use for the following cakes: black forest, pineapple, dark chocolate mousse cake, and dark and white chocolate mousse cake?
10. How is chiffon cake different from angel cake?
11. What is the difference between Victoria sponge and Madeira sponge?
12. What is a silpat and what are its uses?
13. List down at least five points to be kept in mind whilst preparing sponges.
14. How does sieving help in the volume of cake?
15. Describe the various components of a cake.
16. What is the importance of base in a cake?
17. Why is cake moistened whilst layering?
18. Describe at least three types of sponges used for making cakes and pastries.
19. How is a Japonaise different from Dacquoise?
20. How is devil's food cake different from mud cake?

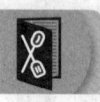

ESSAY TYPE QUESTIONS

1. Define icing and what equipment is used for making it.
2. Explain different types of icings used on cakes and pastries.
3. Write down the procedure of making joconde sponge.
4. What is the history behind the Malakoff torte?
5. Differentiate between chilled cheesecake and baked cheesecake.
6. Why are Yule logs popular during Christmas?
7. Briefly describe at least five types of hi tea cakes and pastries.
8. Critique the common faults in cake making.

ACTIVITY

1. In groups, make at least five different sponge recipes from the recipes provided by your chef instructor. Compare the sponges and write your observation in the given table.
2. In groups, try out the recipes as provided by your chef instructor for the basic Genoese sponge and alter the mixing techniques. One group shall make the sponge with chiffon method whilst two other groups will make the Genoese by Madeira and Victorian methods. Compare the results of the cake and see the difference in the product.

Name of sponge	Texture	Softness	Taste	Colour

3. Visit various pastry shops in your city and write down the different types of cakes and pastry products available. Now do a list of sponges that were used for making those cakes and record your observations.

4. In groups of five, research about at least three cakes from countries such as France, Germany, Spain, America, Austria, India, and China. Share the information with the rest of the team and discuss about the components of each cake.

Cookies and Biscuits

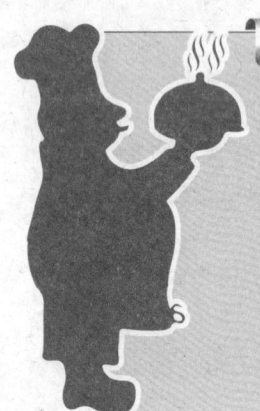

LEARNING OBJECTIVES

After reading this chapter, you should be able to

- understand the basic difference between a cookie and a biscuit
- claim an insight into the different methods used in the preparation of cookies
- analyse the type of cookies and how their baking techniques impact the texture of the final product
- prepare various kinds of classical cookies and biscuits
- Evaluate a cookie and be able to rectify any fault in a cookie

INTRODUCTION

Though the terms 'cookie' and 'biscuit' are used interchangeably and generally substituted for each other, yet there are theories and opinions that tend to differentiate between the two items. A cookie is commonly known so in the USA, while in the UK it is known as a biscuit. Though both are accorded the same significance and served as snacks nowadays, it is quite probable that these were different at one point in time. For instance, the Dutch made small tidbits from leftover cake batters and called them *koekje*, which meant little cake. They mastered the art of making soft as well as crisp *koekjes*. The word 'cookie' is understood to have derived from *koekje* in North America. Biscuit, on the other hand, is understood to have come from the Latin word *panis biscotus*, which meant bread cooked twice. Leftover bread or cakes were baked until crisp and eaten as biscuits. Even the popular *bioscotti* from Italy is prepared in the same manner till date. The dough is shaped into a *roulade* and baked. It is then sliced thinly and baked again until crisp. Even in France, biscuit means to cook twice. Many sponge bases, such as Dacquoise, almond sponge, and hazelnut sponge, are referred to as biscuits. These sponges have been discussed in chapter on sponges—Chapter 7.

For simplifying the classification, a cookie is a product that is soft centred, usually made in the style of preparing cake batter and is traditionally sweet. A biscuit, on the other hand, is crisp and hard like a cheese cracker, which can be savoury. With globalization, increasing awareness, and cross-cultural intermingling, chefs became more creative and cookies and biscuits evolved as separate recipes with the use of creaming butter, sugar, and other ingredients. Earlier, these products were limited to leftover baked products only. With the development of different kinds of flours, sugar, and chemical leavening agents, the production of biscuits and cookies got commercialised and both the products hit the market as separate entities. Like cakes, cookies began to be prepared on festive occasions, especially Christmas. Nowadays, there are a whole range of cookies that are manufactured and distributed on other popular festivals as well, such as Diwali.

PREPARATION OF SIMPLE COOKIES

Nowadays the typical distinction between cookies or biscuits does not hold; these can be sweet or savoury depending upon the choice of the guest. There are various ways of making cookies and biscuits. Some of the common methods of preparing cookies are highlighted in Table 8.1.

Table 8.1 Methods of making cookies

Method	Description	Examples
Straight method	This method is also known as one stage method as it is one of the simplest methods in which all the scaled ingredients are put in a bowl and mixed together until a uniform dough or batter is obtained. This method is apt for cookies that have no or very less moisture in the dough. However, a disadvantage of this method is that it is difficult to regulate the over mixing of ingredients, which can result in chewy cookies and biscuits.	Sweet paste cookies, shortbread cookies, raisin spice bars, gingerbread cookies, macaroons, *biscottis*, *sable*
Creaming method	One of the most common methods for preparing cookies and biscuits, in this method butter and sugar are creamed until fluffy. Liquid ingredients, such as eggs, milk, and cream, are added all at once and then flour is folded into the mixture. The consistency of the dough or batter can be regulated by regulating the moisture content in the mix. One can make a range of cookies with this method.	Piped butter cookies, *Anzac* cookies, chocolate chip cookies, oats and raisin cookies
Sanding method	Also known as *sablage* in French, this method utilises the technique of rubbing-in. The fat is rubbed with flour with fingertips or if making large quantities, the fat and flour can be mixed in a blender. Care should be taken that the mixture is of a sandy texture and does not get over mixed. The liquid ingredients are then mixed to create a dough. Care should be taken not to over mix the dough. This method is usually used for making cookies with short textures.	Sable cookies, *nankhatai*, shortbread biscuits
Sponge method	This method of making cookies is similar to that of cakes. Eggs and sugar are whipped together until light and fluffy and dry ingredients are folded in to prepare batters. Various biscuits and cookies are made by this method.	*Savoiardi*, *amaretti* cookies, anise cookies, chocolate brownie cookies

TYPES OF COOKIES

Cookies are classified on the basis of their method of production and baking technique. Some cookies are piped whereas some are shaped by hands and then baked. The consistency of a piped cookie is softer than the one rolled in hands. The texture of the cookie too largely depends upon the recipe and the style of baking. Some cookies are baked at high temperatures for a short duration to achieve a soft centre and texture, while some are baked at low temperatures for long duration to make crisp cookies. Cookies are made with various ingredients, such as flours (refined, wholewheat, rye), and custard powder; fats such as butter, peanut butter, oil, and margarine; sweeteners such as sugar, honey, brown sugar, and molasses; spices such as ginger powder, cloves, cinnamon, cardamom, caraway, and anise; candied fruits; dried nuts; and chocolates. Moisture in cookies is very rarely given with water. The thinning of batter is done with the help of eggs or butter.

The usage of ingredients is very important when preparing batters and doughs for cookies. Let us discuss some of the salient features of these ingredients.

Flour Unless specified in the recipe, soft flour or a flour with low gluten content is used whilst making cookies as elasticity is not desired in the product. The cookies need to be resilient and brittle.

Apart from refined flour, many other flours such as oats, buckwheat, and millets, can also be used for preparing cookies. Rye flour is traditionally used for making gingerbread cookies for Christmas.

Fats A range of fats—vegetable oils, salted or unsalted butter, and nut butters such as peanut butter and hazelnut butter are used for preparation of cookies. The fat is the most important ingredient in the cookie. It is responsible for the texture of the dough as well as for enriching it. Eggs in the recipe can also add substantial fat in the product. Fats also help in formation of doughs by creaming or sanding methods.

The fat used is usually butter, but margarines also give a good product; however since margarines are trans fats, we should avoid using them.

Sweeteners Many kinds of sweeteners such as sugar, molasses, honey, and brown sugar are used for preparing cookies. Sugar in all its forms such as grain, castor, or icing can be used depending upon the texture and shape required for the cookie. Castor sugar or icing sugar is recommended as they are more readily soluble, which has a softening effect on the gluten in the flour, in turn influencing the shortening properties in the cookie dough. Apart from adding sweetness to the cookie, sugar is also responsible for softness, chewiness, and the spread of the cookie. High content of sugar and fats allows the cookies to spread more whilst baking.

Flavourings Many kinds of flavourings such as essences, chocolates, and spices can be used for preparation of cookies. The flavouring also depends upon the usage of the cookie. For example, a festive cookie prepared for Xmas will be flavoured with sweet spices such as cardamom, cloves, and cinnamon, whereas certain cookies that are the specialty of a country, will use the spice or flavouring of that country, such as, *nankhatai* from India is flavoured with green cardamom seeds and the anise cookies from Switzerland are flavoured with anise seeds.

Various types of cookies along with their examples are described in the following sections.

Drop Cookies

This type of cookie is made from soft dough. The cookie dough or batter is dropped with a spoon or even a piping bag. Dropping through a piping bag would give better control over shape and size which is the most important aspect of baking cookies. When the cookie dough contains ingredients such as chocolate chips, candied fruits and nuts, it is advisable to use a spoon as these ingredients can get stuck in the nozzle of the piping bag. To make some large cookies such as American choco chip cookies, one can also use ice cream scoops to drop the cookie dough onto a baking mat for baking. We should space out the cookies appropriately to allow them to spread. Some common examples of drop cookies are described in Table 8.2.

Table 8.2 Examples of drop cookies

Name	Description
Oatmeal raisin cookie	This is a healthy cookie as it uses oats and raisins in the recipe. The raisins should be soaked in water overnight for softening. It is made by creaming. Butter and brown sugar are creamed together using a flat paddle. Eggs are added one by one until incorporated. Then, dried ingredients such as flour, rolled oats, baking soda, and baking powder are combined together with soaked and drained raisins. If the mixture is not of dropping consistency, milk or egg whites are added to adjust the consistency. The cookie is then dropped on the baking mat with a spoon and baked until crisp.
Chocolate chip cookie	This is a popular cookie that can be made by dropping method or the dough can be refrigerated and rolled in hands before baking. This cookie is also made by creaming method, wherein butter and sugar are creamed together until well blended. They should not be over mixed. Eggs are added and creamed again. All the dry ingredients such as flour, chocolate chips, chopped walnuts, and baking powder are mixed together and folded into the butter and sugar mixture. This mixture is then dropped on baking sheets and baked until still soft as the cookie tends to become crisp when it cools down.
Macaroon	This cookie can be flavoured with chocolate and nuts. Coconut and chocolate macaroons are among the most popular flavours in these cookies. These are made by cooking egg whites, sugar, and desiccated coconut or chocolate until warm. Small quantity of flour is added to the mixture and the mixture is dropped onto a greased tray with the help of a round nozzle. These cookies are baked at 180°C for not more than 15 minutes. These cookies tend to be soft when baked, but they get crisp after cooling. If over-baked, they become hard and chewy.
Crunchy drop	This cookie is made by creaming method. Butter and sugar are creamed until fluffy. Eggs are added one by one until fully incorporated. Dry ingredients such as flour, baking soda, and baking powder are alternately folded in along with milk and mixed together. Chopped walnuts, dates, glazed cherries, and chopped raisins are added into the mixture, which is dropped onto cornflakes and coated with them. It is then baked on a baking sheet. The cookies spread and the cornflakes give a crackled effect to the cookies.
Florentine	These are one of the classical cookies that are finished with a zigzag design of melted chocolate on top. For the mixture, butter and sugar, honey and double cream are cooked to a strong boil at 115°C. Thereafter, the mixture is removed from the heat source and other ingredients such as flour and candied fruits (orange, black currants, cherries, and sliced almond flakes) are added. The batter is then dropped onto a baking sheet while it is hot or else it will become very stiff when cooled.
	After the cookies are baked, they are pulled back together to a round shape with the help of a round cookie cutter and allowed to cool down. Melted chocolate is spread on the flat side of the cookie and given a zigzag design with the help of a comb.

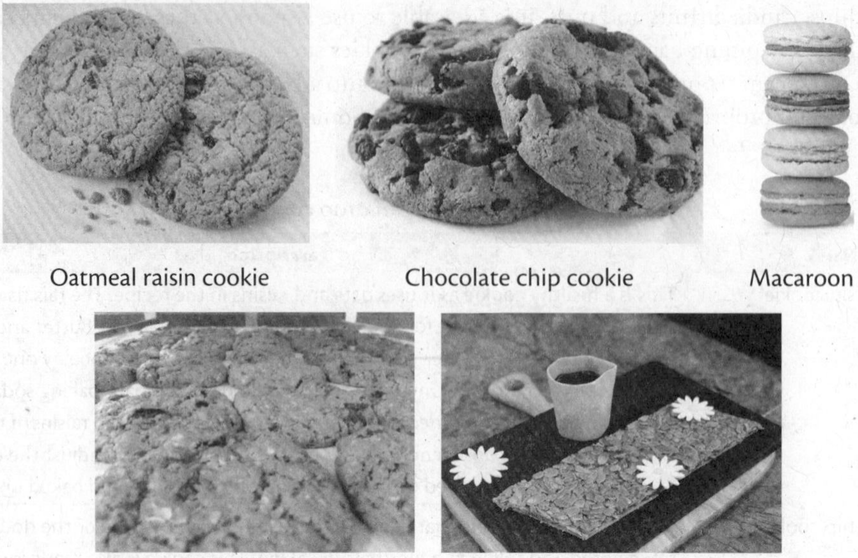

154 Theory of Bakery and Patisserie

Oatmeal raisin cookie   Chocolate chip cookie   Macaroon

Crunchy drop   Florentine

Fig. 8.1 Examples of drop cookies

Piped Cookies

As the name suggests, these cookies are piped through a piping bag or piping tube onto a baking tray. The dough for this cookie has to be of right consistency. If the dough is too thick, then it will be difficult to pipe through a bag and if it is too soft, then it will spread too much while baking. Designs can be given by choosing the kind of nozzle being used. The top of the cookie can be garnished with nuts, candied fruit, etc., before baking. One can pipe stars, rosettes, or straight ridged lines through various kinds of nozzles. Some common piped cookies are described in Table 8.3.

Table 8.3 Examples of piped cookies

Name	Description
Anisette	Also known as anise cookie, this is a famous cookie from Switzerland. It is made by whipping eggs or egg whites with sugar until thick and creamy. Aniseed and flour are folded in and the mixture is piped onto a baking sheet using a plain nozzle. The mixture is then dusted with castor sugar and allowed to dry for an hour. It is then baked at 180°C for around 5 minutes or else the cookie will become hard and chewy.
Butter cookie	This cookie originated from Holland, which is the producer of one of the best quality dairy products. Butter cookie is the most commonly prepared cookie in hotels. It can be piped in various shapes and sizes by choosing the appropriate nozzles. They can also be garnished with various items, such as almond halves, glazed fruit, jam, and seeds such as caraway, fennel, and carom (*ajwain*), before baking. The dough is made by creaming method. Butter and sugar are creamed together until fluffy. Eggs are added one by one and creamed. Flour and flavourings are mixed lightly with hand and the cookie is piped through a nozzle into shapes such as rosettes, swirls, and long sticks. If the mixture is too stiff to force through the piping bag, then one can add egg whites to the batter to make it soft.

Table 8.3 (Contd)

Name	Description
Langues de chat	Also known as cat's tongue, they are often confused with ladyfinger biscuits (see *Savoiardi*). Cat's tongue is prepared by creaming butter and icing sugar until fluffy. Egg whites are incorporated in the mixture and creamed well. Flour is folded in to prepare a thick batter. It is then piped through a round nozzle with an opening of 6–8 mm on a silicon mat. It is piped around 5–6 cm long. When it is baked, the mixture spreads to yield a cookie that is thin, flat, and crisp. The shape resembles the tongue of a cat and hence the name. This cookie can be used as decoration on the sides of cakes and can also be used as a garnish for ice cream sundaes and *coupes*.
Savoiardi	It is also known as ladyfinger biscuit because of its shape, colour, delicate structure, and taste. This cookie is made by sponge method. Egg yolks and whites are stiffly beaten, along with castor sugar until creamy and fluffy. Dry ingredients such as flour and cornflour are sifted together and folded in carefully. The mixture is piped through a round nozzle of 10–12 mm diameter and 5–6 cm long. Icing sugar is dredged over each biscuit before baking. This helps to form a crisp layer on top of the biscuit, which prevents it from becoming soggy. It is baked at 200°C until creamy white colour. *Savoiardis* are used in making the famous Italian dessert *tiramisu* or for decorating cakes or as a garnish for ice creams and sundaes.

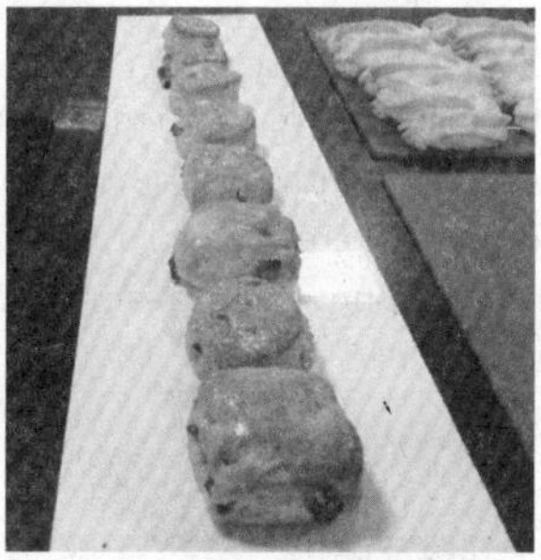

Butter cookie 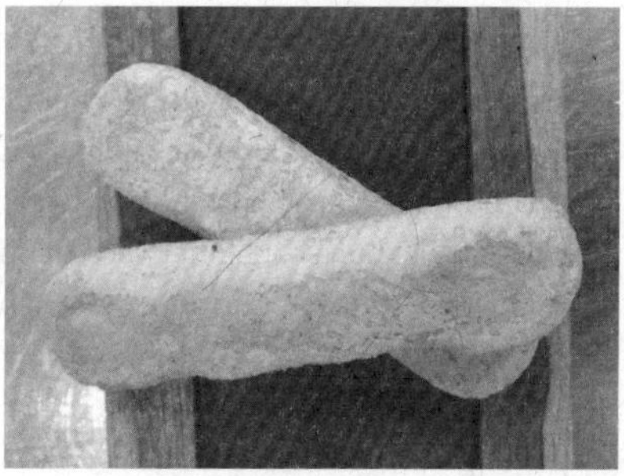   Savoiardi

Fig. 8.2 Examples of piped cookies

Hand-rolled Cookies

These types of cookies are usually made with stiff dough such as sweet paste dough, shortcrust dough, and salt dough. If the cookie dough is soft, then it can be put in the refrigerator to obtain stiffness. Hand-rolled cookies are shaped into rounds between the palms and then put on the baking sheet. These can be pressed further with the help of a fork to add a design as in case of *melting moments* cookies. Table 8.4 highlights some common hand-rolled cookies.

Table 8.4 Examples of hand-rolled cookies

Name	Description
Sweet paste cookies	Sweet paste is one of the most common pastes used for making various types of cookies. The basic dough can be flavoured and coloured as per choice of flavours and moulded into various shapes and baked. Sweet paste can be rolled between palms and flattened before baking. The top surface can be brushed with egg whites and rolled in various toppings, such as granulated sugar, brown sugar, and desiccated coconut, and baked until golden brown.

(Contd)

Table 8.4 (Contd)

Name	Description
Melting moments	Soft and crumbly, melting moments are popular cookies. These are made by combining flour and custard powder with butter and sugar. It is made by creaming method, wherein the fat is creamed along with sugar until fluffy. Dry ingredients such as flour, custard powder, and baking powder are folded in and the dough is rested in the refrigerator for at least one hour. The dough is pinched and rolled between the palms and flattened with the help of a fork. It is baked until light brown in colour. *Note*: These cookies need to be stored carefully as they are very crumbly.
Crescents	These cookies are named after their moon shape. Crescents can be shaped from sweet paste or any other soft dough. The dough is rolled into a small ball and then rolled on a floured surface to form a log that is tapered from both the sides. It is then arranged like a crescent or semi-circle and baked.
Ginger snap	This cookie can also be made by piped method or the dough can be chilled in a refrigerator and then shaped and baked. Classically, ginger snaps are made by creaming butter, molasses, and sugar until a thick paste is obtained. Baking soda is mixed in water or milk and added to the mixture. Lastly, the flour is folded in. The dough can now be piped or left in the refrigerator to cool. The cookie is rolled between hands and then put on a baking tray. The cookies are then flattened before baking at 180°C until golden brown.
Nankhatai	This is a very famous cookie made in India. It is made by creaming equal quantities of vegetable shortening with powdered sugar. Flour is added along with small amount of curd and green cardamom seeds. The flour is very lightly added to the creamed mixture to avoid over mixing. The dough is then shaped between hands and baked until light creamy in colour. This cookie is very soft and crumbly and should be handled carefully.

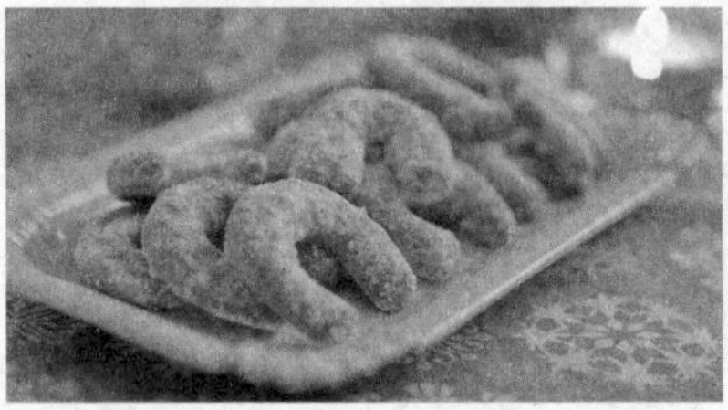

Sweet paste cookies 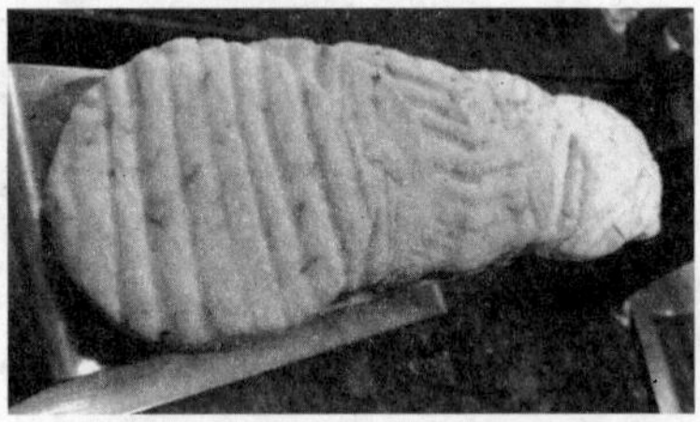   Melting moments

Fig. 8.3 Examples of hand-rolled cookies

Cutter-cut Cookies

These cookies are made by rolling the dough to a desired thickness and then cutting it with cutters of required shape. These cookies are much more symmetric and look neat as they are cut with cutters. The choice of rolling or shaping with hands is purely the chef's choice as it affects the final texture and look of the cookie. Some cookies containing raisins and candied fruits cannot be cut with cutters as it becomes difficult to cut the cookie if the raisin comes in the way. In such cases, the dough is moulded in hands and baked. Some common cutter-cut cookies are described in Table 8.5.

Cookies and Biscuits

Table 8.5 Examples of cutter-cut cookies

Name	Description
Shortbread	Also from Scotland, this cookie is very soft and crumbly. Traditionally, it is made without any eggs. Butter and sugar are creamed and mixed very lightly with flour and cornflour. Since this dough is tough to roll out, it is pressed onto special moulds and then baked. But in modern applications, egg is added to the mixture to form soft dough. It is then rolled out and cut with a rectangle cutter and baked.
Bull's eye	This cookie is made by using sweet paste, which is rolled to 4 mm thickness and cut with a round cutter. Half of the cut cookies are placed on the baking tray and the other half in the refrigerator for 30 minutes. When chilled, the centre is cut out with a smaller cutter to form a ring. Then, these are baked at 180°C till golden brown. The ring is then placed over the flat cookie base and the centre is filled with boiled raspberry jam.
Nice biscuit	This biscuit comes from France and usually comes packaged with an inscription of the word 'nice'. To make the biscuits, dry ingredients such as flour, cornflour, fine desiccated coconut, and soda bicarbonate are sifted together. Ammonium carbonate is dissolved into milk and kept aside. Icing sugar and butter are creamed and dry ingredients, golden syrup, and milk are folded in and combined with sugar and butter mixture to form a smooth dough. The dough is then pinned out and cut into rectangular shape using a fluted cutter. The dough is then placed on the baking tray, washed with eggs and its surface is sprinkled with granulated sugar and then it is baked at 200°C.
Shrewsbury biscuit	This is a famous biscuit from Great Britain. To prepare this cookie, flour and butter are rubbed together to form a texture of bread crumbs. A well in the centre is made and eggs, sugar, and cinnamon are combined in the well using fingers from inside out to incorporate the dry ingredients to form a smooth paste. The paste is refrigerated until it is ready to be rolled out. The dough is rolled out to 4 mm thickness and cut with a 2-inch plain cutter. The cookies are baked at 200°C until creamy white in colour.

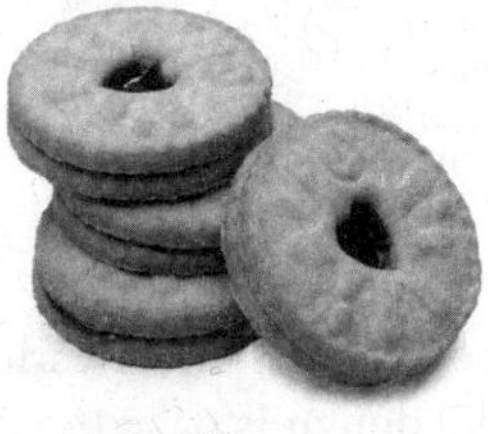

Bull's eye

Fig. 8.4 Example of cutter-cut cookies

Bar Cookies

These types of cookies are shaped in bars or long ropes or pipes and then baked till half done. Then the cookies are sliced to the required thickness while the dough is still warm and placed again on the baking sheets and baked until crisp. This type of baking is also known as baking twice or *biscotti* in Italian. Sometimes, the *biscotti* is frozen and then sliced on a meat slicer to obtain very thin pieces that are baked till crisp and served with coffee or as garnish with ice creams and sundaes. Some common bar cookies are described in Table 8.6.

> **CHEF'S TIP**
> Care has to be taken while rolling, as the gluten in the flour gets stretched and one cannot roll the dough over and over again as the cookie will become rubbery and chewy. Also, the rolling has to be of even thickness or else certain cookies will get burnt and some will be cooked when baked together.

Table 8.6 Examples of bar cookies

Name	Description
Raisin spice bars	This is not a perfectly shaped cookie as the dough is very soft to handle. It is made by combining butter, sugar, eggs, molasses, flour, spices such as cinnamon, cloves, and ginger, baking soda, and soaked and drained raisins. The dough is sticky when made. It should be left in refrigerator to chill and then shaped into long bars and baked for 10 minutes at 180°C. Then, it is removed and cut into 8 mm thick bars and baked again at 180°C for another 7–8 minutes or until golden brown.
Biscotti	This is a broad term used for biscuits baked twice in the earlier times. There can be varieties of flavours and combinations in a *biscotti*, which is popular throughout Europe and North America. In making *biscotti*, the sponge method is followed. Eggs, sugar, and a pinch of salt are mixed over double boiler until all the sugar gets dissolved. The mixture is then whipped until it becomes creamy and light. Thereafter, vanilla, lemon, and orange zest are folded in along with flour, baking powder, and almonds. The mixture is thick and sticky and not flowy as for a sponge. It is then shaped into logs and brushed with eggs. Then it is baked at 160°C for 30 minutes or until golden brown. It is then taken out of the oven and kept aside to cool slightly. The baked *biscotti* is then sliced diagonally to required thickness and length and baked again at 130–140°C until toasted or dry. It should be stored in airtight boxes to retain its crispness.

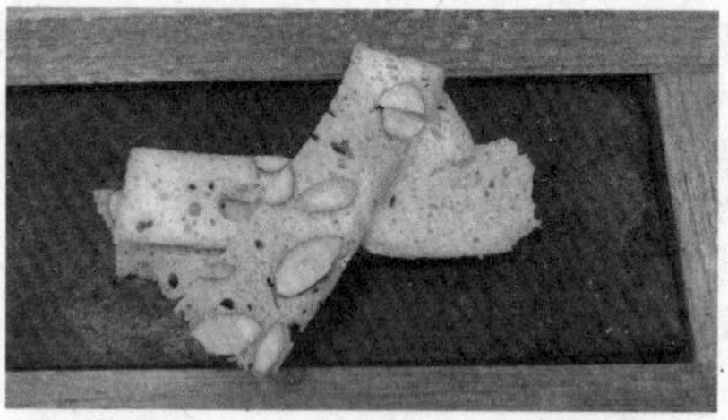

Biscotti

Fig. 8.5 Example of bar cookies

Sheet Cookies

Many chefs confuse these cookies with bar cookies described earlier. There are various methods of preparing this type of cookie. In some cases, the dough is baked in sheets and cut later, while in some cases, they are lined on a tray and the topping is spread onto the base before being baked. Most of the popular sheet cookies are made by this method. Some popular sheet cookies are described in Table 8.7.

Table 8.7 Examples of sheet cookies

Name	Description
Bee sting	It is a very popular cookie from Germany made from yeast leavened dough known as *kuchen* dough. The dough is smooth and is made from flour, sugar, eggs, butter, and milk. It is sheeted to 4 mm thickness and spread on a baking sheet. The bee sting mixture is prepared by cooking butter, sugar, honey, heavy cream, almond flakes, and chopped almonds. The mixture is allowed to cook until it leaves the sides of the pan. It is then poured on top of the prepared *kuchen* dough. It is then allowed to proof for 30 minutes and baked at 180°C for 30 minutes. When it is cool enough, it is cut into squares and served. The bee sting cookies can also be sandwiched along with vanilla flavoured cream.

Table 8.7 (Contd)

Name	Description
Almond bars	This cookie is made by sheeting out the sweet paste to 4 mm thickness and spreading it on a baking sheet. The sweet paste is docked and baked blind. Then cream, sugar, honey, and almond slices are combined in a heavy bottom pan and cooked until the mixture starts to leave the sides of the pan. The mixture is spread on to the prepared sweet paste base and baked for another 10 minutes at 180°C. As soon as the cookie cools down, it is cut into rectangular shapes.
Brownie	Brownie batter is a unique one. It can be baked into a cake or dropped onto a baking sheet to prepare brownie cookies. One method of preparing a brownie cookie is to spread the batter on a baking sheet and bake until fudgy. Then, cut into bars when it cools down.
Honey bee	The procedure for making honey bee cookies is the same as for almond bars. The only difference is that these have candied fruits and black currants in addition to the almond slices.

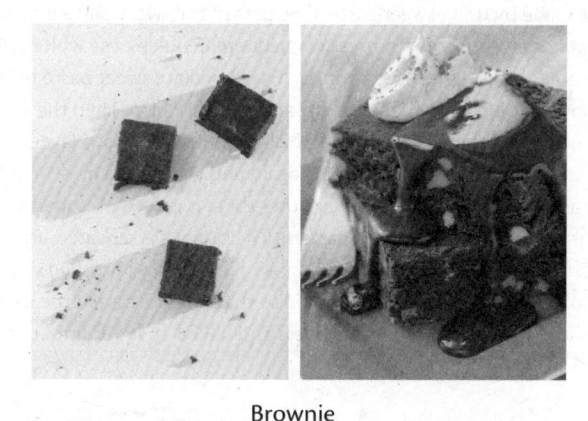

Brownie

Fig. 8.6 Example of sheet cookies

Frozen and Cut Cookies

As the name suggests, this cookie is shaped into logs or square bars and sliced when frozen. Such methods are adopted for various reasons such as the dough is too soft to handle or to give it shape, or to save on time of sheeting the dough when it is chilled, as this facilitates cutting with a cutter. The most common way of preparing such cookies is by using sweet paste. One can mix various nuts and flavourings into the sweet paste and roll it into logs or squares and then freeze them. They are then sliced to 7 mm thickness and arranged on baking sheets. Slicing the cookie in this manner results in evenly sliced nuts which gives it a good appearance. Some commonly prepared cookies with this method are described in Table 8.8.

Festive Cookies

Western festivals or celebrations are incomplete without cookies. These are popular tidbits that have found their way into all cuisines cutting across cultures. Festivals are special occasions that provide an opportunity for traditional cooks and chefs to showcase their culinary skills. Thus, we have a wide variety of cookies being made for Christmas, Easter, Halloween, etc. Some of the classical cookies that are prepared on various festive occasions are described in Table 8.9.

Table 8.8 Examples of frozen and cut cookies

Name	Description
Sable	This popular cookie from Switzerland is prepared by creaming butter, icing sugar, and vegetable shortening until creamy. Flour and egg whites are folded in until a thick paste is obtained. The paste is chilled in a fridge until it can be rolled into logs. After shaping logs of 1 inch diameter, they are frozen for at least an hour or until they are ready to be sliced. The logs are then brushed with egg whites and rolled in castor sugar before being cut into 5 mm thickness. The cookies are baked until golden brown at 200°C.
Pinwheel	This cookie is also made with sweet paste. One part of the sweet paste is mixed with cocoa powder to make chocolate sweet paste. To prepare pinwheel cookies, the white sweet paste is rolled out to 3 mm thickness and brushed with egg whites. The chocolate sweet paste is sheeted to 3 mm thickness and placed on top. The sheet is rolled to form a log of 1 inch diameter. It is frozen for an hour and then sliced to 4 mm thickness and baked at 180°C until cooked.
Chequered	This cookie is made by using sweet paste. One part of the sweet paste is mixed with cocoa powder to make chocolate sweet paste. To prepare chequered cookies, the white sweet paste is rolled out to 1 cm thickness and brushed with egg whites. The chocolate sweet paste is sheeted to 1 cm thickness and placed on top. It is then refrigerated for an hour until firm. Then the sheet is cut into half and sandwiched again with the help of an egg white to yield a sheet of 4 layers alternating with dark and white sweet paste. This sheet is refrigerated again and then sliced into 1 cm thickness and laid flat on a tray. It is brushed with egg whites and another sheet is placed on top in such a way that the white covers the dark to create a chequered pattern. The process is repeated until there are four sheets. Another sweet paste sheet of 1 mm thickness is rolled out and brushed with egg whites. The prepared square log is placed onto the sheet and rolled so that it is encased in the sheet from all sides. It is frozen for an hour and then sliced to 4 mm thickness and baked at 180°C until cooked.

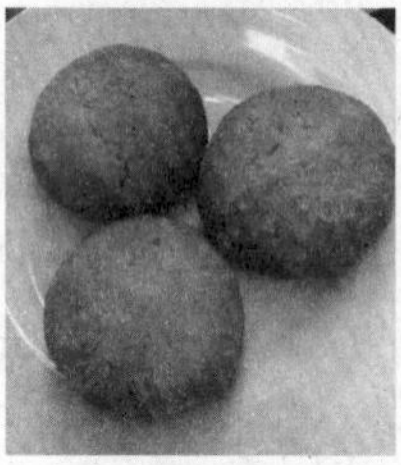

Sable 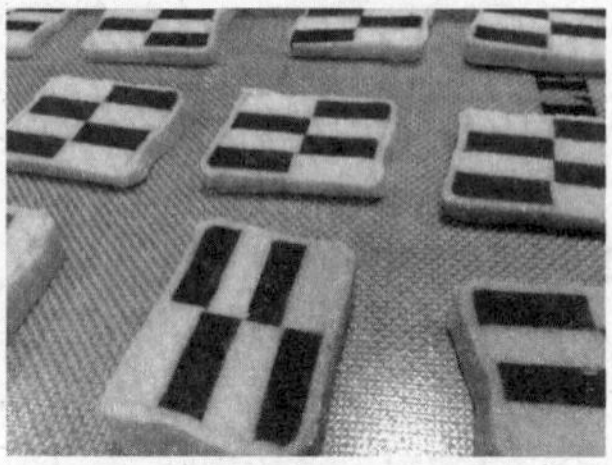   Chequered

Fig. 8.7 Examples of frozen and cut cookies

Table 8.9 Examples of cookies for festive occasions

Name	Description
Basler Läckerli	This Swiss cookie is typically prepared on Christmas. Hot sugar glaze is applied on the cookie while it is hot, with a stiff brush and is worked forward and backward until the glaze gives a grainy appearance. The cookie is cut into rectangles and served.
Pizzelle	This popular Italian cookie is made for celebrating the festival of snakes also known as 'feast day of San Domenico'. The mixture is placed in a mould (like flat pan) that closes like a waffle batter machine. The cookie is cooked on the stove top, until crisp.

Table 8.9 (Contd)

Name	Description
Spekulaas	This popular cookie from Holland is prepared by creaming method. The dough is pressed onto special wooden *spekulaa* moulds and then demoulded and placed on baking sheets.
Gingerbread	This cookie is popularly made during Christmas by warming honey, sugar, and butter and mixing with rye flour, gingerbread spice, eggs, and molasses.
Cinnamon stars	This cookie is a German recipe popularly made during Christmas. The cookie is briefly baked in the oven (180°C for around 6–7 minutes only) or until the meringue turns beige in colour.
Brunsli	It is a popular cookie from Germany made usually on Christmas. The dough is rolled out by dredging with castor sugar to 6 mm thickness and cut with clover shape cutters and baked for 6–7 minutes only.
Pertikus	This popular cookie from Switzerland is also usually made on Christmas. The cookies are piped into horseshoe shape with the help of a star-shaped nozzle and baked until golden brown.

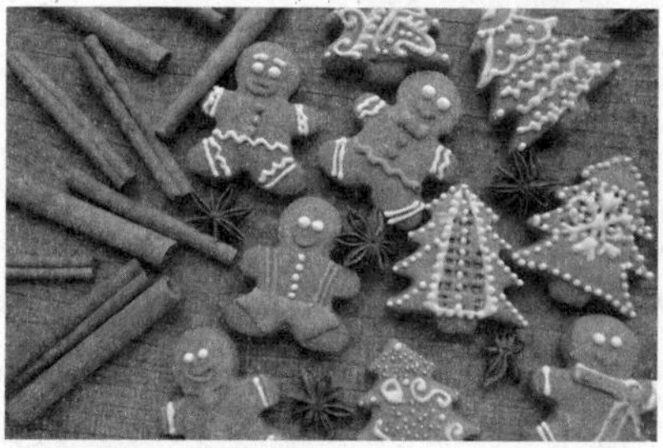

Gingerbread 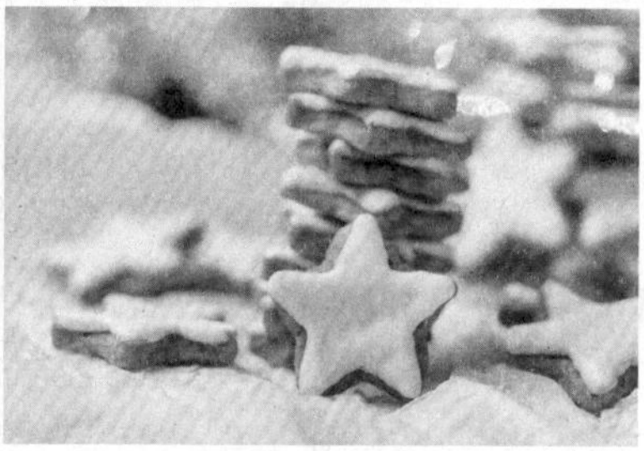   Cinnamon stars

Fig. 8.8 Examples of cookies for festive occasions

USES OF COOKIES

Cookies and biscuits have many uses in the pastry kitchen. They can be used as a base for cakes and pastries or served as an accompaniment with tea and coffee. Cookies are also commonly served as amenities in the guestroom. (Amenities are add-on facilities given to the guests as part of the package.) These could range from shampoo and soaps to arrangement of fruits and canapés in a room. These facilities are not directly charged to the guests but are built in the guest's package. Cookies are the most preferred choice as an amenity, as these do not require any refrigeration and can stay for a few days in the room. Care should be taken to serve cookies that do not get too soggy over a period of time. Cookies are arranged on various kinds of platters and placed as room amenity. Figure 8.9 illustrates some cookie presentations that are served as an amenity.

In large hotels, the room service section is usually responsible for placing the amenities in the guestroom. The front office tips the room service section on the rooms that would be occupied and need to be readied. The latter then coordinates with the pastry kitchen and gets the cookies picked up and placed in the room.

Apart from being placed as an amenity in the guestroom, cookies can also be sold in the hotel's pastry shop. These are usually sold by weight, but some large-size cookies are also sold per piece.

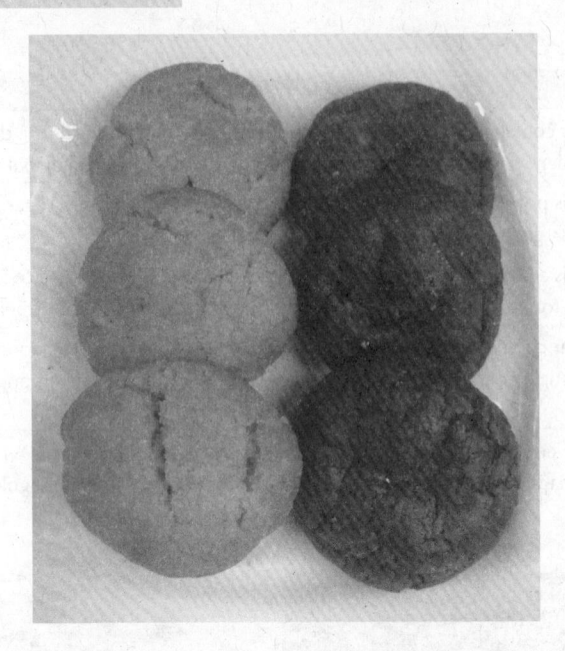

Fig. 8.9 Presentation of cookies as amenities

COMMON FAULTS IN COOKIE PREPARATION

The cookies discussed in this chapter are classical cookies that have unique texture and mouth feel. Some cookies are designed to be crisp, yet some taste good only when they are crumbly. Some cookies require spread, whereas some cookies need to be baked only for a few minutes. Any deviation from the standard product is termed as fault. Chefs can use the knowledge of faults to give a particular texture to the cookie or even correct the texture of a particular cookie. Some of the common faults that crop up in the preparation of cookies are discussed in Table 8.10.

Table 8.10 Common faults in making cookies

Faults	Causes
Cookies stick to pans	• It is important to grease the baking sheets and one has to be careful while doing so as excessive greasing will aid in spreading of the cookie. • Certain cookies need to be taken off the baking sheet while they are hot. If they are left on the pan to cool for a long time, they could stick. On the other hand, soft cookies should be allowed to cool down before they are lifted off. • Too much sugar in the recipe also leads to cookies sticking to the pans. • Improper mixing of the cookie dough or batter could also result in sticking of cookies.
Too crumbly	• Too much sugar in the recipe can make the cookie crumbly. • Improper mixing of the cookie dough or batter could also result in crumbly cookies. • Too much of fat or shortening in the cookie dough can also make it crumbly. If you observe *nankhatai* cookie, you would understand what makes it crumbly. • Too much leavening and eggs could also result in crumbly cookies.

Table 8.10 (Contd)

Faults	Causes
Cookie is very brittle and hard	• Too much flour in the dough could result in tough cookie. • Less quantity of fat in dough could result in hard cookie. • Dough mixed for too long will result in tough cookie as the gluten in the flour would develop hence, the cookie will lose its shortening properties. • There is less liquid. • Low baking temperature also aids in making cookies hard.
Cookie does not get proper colour	• Baking temperature is too low. • Sugar is not enough in the recipe.
Cookie spreads too fast	• Low baking temperature aids in spreading of cookies. • Over greased baking sheets leads to cookie spreading. • There is not enough flour in the dough or batter. • Too much creaming of the dough also leads to spreading of cookies. • Too much liquid in the recipe also leads to spreading of cookies.
Cookie does not spread	• Baking temperature is high. • There is too much flour in the dough or batter. • Less sugar in the recipe also prevents the cookie from spreading. • Insufficient greasing of pans does not allow the cookies to spread.

The information in the Table 8.10 is very important for the budding pastry chefs, as they can alter the texture of cookies by taking care of the faults. If chefs want a particular property in the product (cookie), they can use this knowledge to tailor their product accordingly.

SUMMARY

In this chapter, we discussed the origin of cookies and biscuits and how they have transformed over the years. The earlier cookies were dry and were made from leftover batters or dough of breads. The main purpose of these goodies was to serve as an accompaniment with tea and coffee. Today, cookies are specially made for occasions using various instruments and techniques. Some of the cookies are individually decorated by using various icings and toppings such as fondants, chocolates, or sugar glazes.

In this chapter, we discussed various methods of preparing cookies such as straight method, creaming method, sanding method, and sponge method. Apart from this, we also discussed various types of cookies such as drop cookies, where the moisture in the dough is regulated in such a manner that the batter forms a dropping consistency. The liquid ingredients used in cookie batter are usually eggs, and on rare occasions, milk is used. Piped cookies along with description and examples are explained in brief. Many other cookies, such as hand-rolled cookies, bar cookies, frozen and cut cookies, and festive cookies, are also discussed, along with description and photographs, so that the students can easily identify these products.

Chefs can be creative with preparation of cookies, as long as they are aware of the basic methods of preparing cookies and also have the knowledge of giving the required texture and mouth feel. Common faults that occur while making cookies are discussed along with tips on how the chefs can identify and rectify them.

KEY TERMS

Baking blind A term used for denoting baking of a pastry shell without any filling

Candied fruit Peels of fruits, such as orange, lemon, and ginger, steeped in sugar syrup and then allowed to mature until they are dry and crunchy

Dacquoise A type of sponge made from eggs, sugar, flour, and almond powder

Dock To prick the rolled or sheeted dough with a docker or fork to create small holes which prevent the dough from rising

Fondant An icing that is prepared by cooking sugar and liquid glucose with water to the soft ball stage and kneaded on an oiled marble slab until a smooth dough is obtained

Gingerbread spice A mixture of ground spices, such as cloves, dry ginger, cinnamon, nutmeg, and cardamom, used for flavouring gingerbread dough and other Christmas specialities

Glazed cherries Candied red cherries often used as garnish on cookies before baking

Gluten Protein present in flour that determines its strength

Golden syrup Sweetened corn syrup marketed under various brand names

Koekje Dutch for little cake. It is believed that the term cookie originated from this word

Kuchen dough Yeast-leavened dough from Germany used in preparation of bee sting cookies

Ladyfinger biscuit Another name for Italian *savoiardi* biscuit

Nougat paste A paste obtained by grinding caramelised sugar and almonds. It is also known as nougat praline

Offset spatula A kind of flat palette knife that is bent at an angle

Panis bicotus Latin for bread cooked twice. The word is considered to be the origin of the term biscuit

Rye flour A kind of flour made from rye seeds

Tiramisu An Italian creamy dessert made by using *mascarpone* cheese

Treacle A dark sweetened liquid obtained from sugar refining process

OBJECTIVE TYPE QUESTIONS

1. How did the word cookie originate?
2. What is the difference between a cookie and a biscuit?
3. Describe the straight method of preparing cookies.
4. Describe the creaming method of making cookies with some examples.
5. What is sponge method? What does it do to the cookie?
6. Describe the sanding method of making cookies.
7. Explain the principle of making drop cookies and give three examples.
8. Describe *florentine* cookie and *Anzac* cookie.
9. Explain at least three types of piped classical cookies.
10. What is the difference between *langues de chat* and *savoiardi*?
11. Explain the concept of hand-rolled cookies and give examples of any three cookies made by this method.
12. What are cutter-cut cookies and what precaution should one follow while preparing such cookies?
13. Explain the difference between Shrewsbury biscuit and shortbread cookie.
14. Differentiate between a bar cookie and sheet cookie.
15. Describe *sable* cookie and explain the method of preparing it.
16. Explain the procedure of making chequered cookies.
17. What could be the possible causes if the cookie sticks to the baking sheet?
18. If the cookie is too crumbly, then what could be the possible reasons for the same?

19. How can you prevent the cookies from becoming brittle and hard?
20. If you do not want your cookie to get too much colour, then what should you do?
21. If the cookie does not spread on the baking sheet, what could be the possible causes?
22. If you want your cookie to spread more, what could you do without altering the recipe?

ESSAY TYPE QUESTIONS

1. How have cookies and biscuits evolved over the last few decades?
2. What points must be kept in mind while baking cookies?
3. Explain the procedure of making a *biscotti*.
4. What do you understand by the term festive cookies? Explain at least five kinds of festive cookies.
5. What is the role of cookies in hotels and restaurants?

ACTIVITY

1. In groups of five, conduct a market survey of various pastry shops in the city and make a list of cookies and biscuits sold there. Using the knowledge given in the chapter, classify the cookies on their type and method of preparation. Discuss how you could alter the product to make it more appealing.
2. Divide yourself in groups of three. Select one common recipe amongst yourselves and apply all the faults listed in Table 8.10. Share your observation with the group and see how each fault affects the texture of the cookie.
3. In groups of five, prepare at least three festive cookies and present them to the other groups for tasting and evaluation.

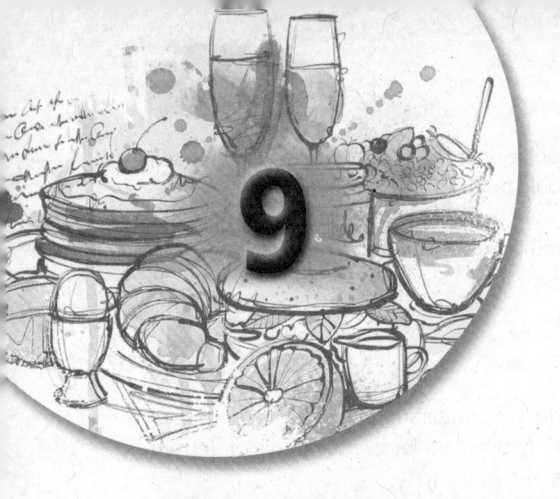

9
Hot and Cold Desserts

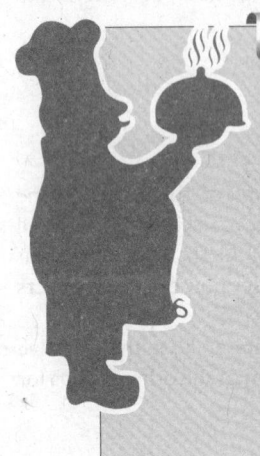

LEARNING OBJECTIVES

After reading this chapter, you should be able to

- understand the various kinds of hot, cold, and frozen desserts
- understand the role of ingredients in preparation of these desserts
- comprehend basic terms such as overrun, churning, and still freezing, used in the production of frozen desserts
- prepare a range of hot, cold, and frozen desserts from crème brûlée to tiramisu to ice creams and sorbets
- utilize sauces and garnishes for various kinds of pre-plated desserts
- analyse the presentation of dessert for buffet as well as à la carte
- prepare a cyclic dessert menu with balanced products
- differentiate among the textures of various desserts and faults associated with them
- use various kinds of equipment in the preparation of frozen desserts

INTRODUCTION

One of the last courses of the French classical menu called 'dessert' goes by the principle of the age-old saying 'all's well that ends well'. This course of meal leaves a long-lasting impression on the guests' mind and satisfies their sweet tooth, thus completing the dining experience. Dessert is usually a sweet food served as the final course of a meal. The use of the term dessert was first recorded in 1600 and it is derived from a French word *desservir*, which means 'to clear the table'. This etymology is reflected in the current table service, where it is customary to remove everything that is not being used (salt/pepper shakers, bread baskets, sometimes even flowers) from the table before serving dessert.

Just as restaurant menus have undergone great changes in recent years, the bakery and pastry kitchen too has undergone many changes from what it once was. This is especially true of presentation, which must meet very high expectations these days. Taste is also important, of course. A good cook must be able to achieve economy in preparation, while maintaining high standards in all aspects of the dessert.

Desserts feature as a display on buffet or are listed on an à la carte menu. The presentation of a dessert changes with the style of service. Modern buffet arrangements have an assortment of desserts presented pre-portioned or whole on display. It would be worthwhile to understand how the desserts on buffet have evolved over a period of time.

Desserts can be of various types and are mostly classified on the basis of their serving temperatures. They can be served hot, cold, or frozen. We will discuss these broad classifications in the chapter and understand how these are further classified. You can refer to Fig. 9.1 for the classification of desserts.

Let us start by discussing hot and cold desserts.

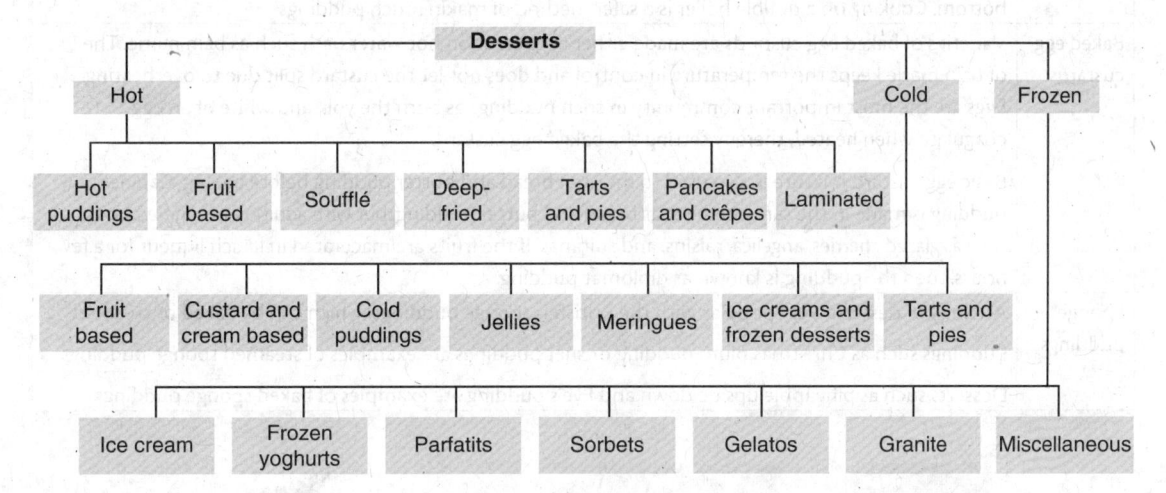

Fig. 9.1 Classification of desserts

HOT AND COLD DESSERTS

Many desserts can be served only hot while some can only be served cold; but there are a range of desserts that can be served either hot or cold. The decision to serve a dessert at a particular temperature is guided by many factors such as guest preference, climate, texture, and flavour of the dessert. Thus, depending on the temperature at which these are served, desserts may be hot or cold (see Fig. 9.1).

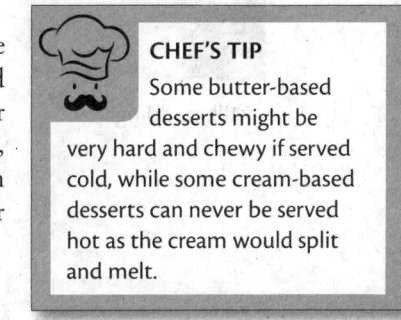

> **CHEF'S TIP**
> Some butter-based desserts might be very hard and chewy if served cold, while some cream-based desserts can never be served hot as the cream would split and melt.

Hot Desserts

Hot desserts are the ones that are served warm or hot in buffets or à la carte. The various types of hot desserts, such as puddings, soufflés, tarts, and pies, are further classified into different types based on the ingredients used for making them.

Puddings

In Western cooking, pudding may also refer to savoury items such as Yorkshire pudding, black pudding, and savoury pudding. But in the pastry kitchen, a pudding is a dessert that is made with milk and sugar and contains starch as a thickening agent. In certain cases, the thickening can also come from eggs. Crème caramel is an example of such a pudding. Puddings can be served hot or cold based on their composition. Table 9.1 discusses some popular puddings along with their features.

Table 9.1 Types of hot puddings

Type	Description
Milk puddings	Milk puddings are made from rice, semolina, tapioca, or sago, or any starch-based cereal. All of them are cooked in sweetened milk. Flavourings, such as vanilla, orange or lemon peel, are optional. They are often served with a fruit or *anglaise* sauce. Both baking and boiling methods are used to prepare such puddings. While cooking milk-based puddings on hot stove, they need to be constantly stirred, so that they do not burn or stick to the bottom. Cooking on a double boiler is a safer method of making such puddings.
Baked egg custards	Varieties of baked egg custards are made either in oven or on hot water bath such as bain marie. The use of bain marie keeps the temperature in control and does not let the custard split due to overheating. Eggs are the most important commodity in such puddings as both the yolk and white of an egg coagulate when heated, thereby setting the baked egg custard. Basic egg custard mixture is also used to moisten bread and butter pudding before baking. Cabinet pudding is made in the same manner as bread and butter pudding, but with addition of candied fruits such as glazed cherries, angelica, raisins, and sultanas. If the fruits are macerated in kirsch liqueur for a few hours, then the pudding is known as diplomat pudding.
Sponge puddings	An array of desserts, very popular with the British is sponge puddings, which can be baked or steamed. Puddings such as Christmas plum pudding or suet puddings are examples of steamed sponge puddings. Desserts such as pineapple upside down and Eve's pudding are examples of baked sponge puddings.

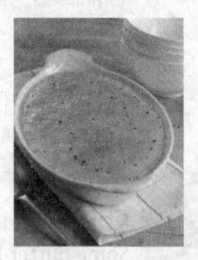

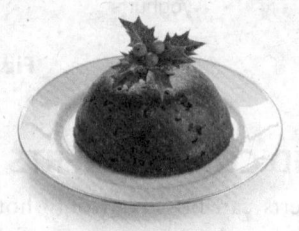

Milk puddings 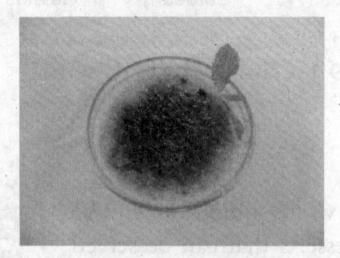   Baked egg custards   Christmas pudding

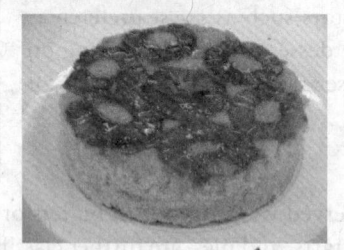

Pineapple upside down pudding

Fig. 9.2 Types of hot puddings

Soufflés

The word soufflé comes from the French word *souffler*, which means to breathe or to puff up. The soufflé is always served as an individual portion to a guest in a special mould called ramekin, which is usually of ceramic, so that it can be presented as it is. It must be presented immediately as the volume of the dessert is created by the eggs in it and it can collapse within a few minutes of being taken out of the oven.

The soufflé is usually classified into two types—hot and cold. These types of puddings originated in France and are very popular there. Earlier, the soufflés were savoury-based such as fish soufflé and cheese soufflé; but with the creativity of chefs, sweet soufflés became a rage. The basic components of the soufflé remain the same, only sugar and flavourings replace the salt and meat products. Soufflé is traditionally starch-based.

In case of savouries, white sauce or béchamel is used as a base, but in pastry, this is replaced with pastry cream or any other milk-based pudding. Whipped yolks, flavourings, and whipped egg whites are folded in and baked until the soufflé rises. The soufflé needs to be served immediately as it can collapse and this would be unacceptable as it will lose its characteristics of being called a soufflé. Classically, any soufflé would have the following three components.

Base The base would be a starch base. It could be a pastry cream, milk-based pudding, or even sweetened white sauce. This starchy thick base is also known as *panada*.

Flavouring A whole range of flavours can be used for dessert soufflés. Chocolate, vanilla, lemon, and cheese are the most commonly used flavourings, but chefs can use their creativity to flavour soufflés.

Eggs Egg white is the most essential ingredient that helps the soufflé to rise in a mould, giving it the traditional name. Yolks are added for enriching soufflé as they have little role in aeration.

The following are some critical factors to be kept in mind while preparing hot soufflés.

- Prepare the base or *panada*. Grease sugar-lined moulds. Set oven to correct temperature.
- Stiffly beaten egg whites are the basis for a successful soufflé. Expansion of air in the egg whites will let the soufflé rise above the rim of the dish as it bakes. This is why it is important to ensure that moulds are properly greased.
- First lighten the *panada* with a quarter of egg white. This will make it much easier to fold in the remaining whites, as beaten egg whites are not sufficiently stable to withstand extensive mixing.
- Do not let the mixture stand or it will collapse.
- Bake at 200°C. Draughts or disturbances during baking will cause the delicate structure to collapse.
- The French tend to favour soufflés with a slightly underdone, creamy centre but well-done soufflés are more stable, and are generally preferred for this reason.
- Dust soufflés with icing sugar, glazed (caramelized under the salamander) or dusted with cocoa powder, if it is a chocolate soufflé.
- Serve the soufflé immediately.

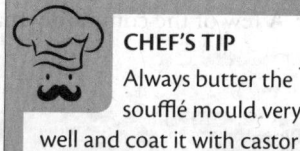

> **CHEF'S TIP**
> Always butter the soufflé mould very well and coat it with castor sugar. This prevents the soufflé from sticking to the base.

Cold soufflés are a recent addition to the pastry kitchens as traditionally these were only prepared and served hot. A cold soufflé is prepared in such a manner that it serves as an imitation to the hot soufflé. In case of a hot soufflé, the mixture rises out of the mould due to the presence of egg and aeration is produced because of the steam generated, but in case of could soufflé, a mould is wrapped with an acetate sheet and the mixture which contains gelatin is poured in the mould and is allowed to set. The sheet is then removed from the mould and the rising of the poured mixture out of the serving bowl, creates an illusion of a soufflé.

There can be many recipes for a good soufflé. But the basic rule is that it must contain around 80% of the base and 20% of French meringue. Let us see the recipe of a basic soufflé.

Basic Soufflé

Ingredients for four portions
Milk 300 ml
Sugar 40 g
Vanilla pod 1 pc
Cornflour 60 g
Egg yolks 80 g
Egg whites 120 g
Sugar 45 g

METHOD
1. Heat milk with sugar and scraped vanilla pod.
2. Mix cornstarch and egg yolks and beat with a whisk until well blended.
3. Add half of the boiled milk into the yolk and starch mix and pour back in the pan and cook for a few minutes, until the sauce is thick and creamy.
4. Remove from heat source and cool.
5. Whip the egg whites and sugar to form a meringue.
6. Fold the meringue into cooled sauce, pour the contents into a greased mould and bake at 180°C for 10-12 minutes.
7. Serve immediately, dredged with icing sugar.

The aforementioned recipe is a basic recipe for vanilla soufflé. If you want to prepare chocolate soufflé, then replace the cornstarch with cocoa powder. In addition to this, any other flavour can be added to the soufflé, for example, coffee, hazelnut, raspberry, strawberry, etc.

Deep-fried Desserts

Deep-fried desserts are another category of desserts that are popular all over the world. As the name suggests, these desserts are served deep-fried. Since these desserts would have sugar added to them, it is important to control the temperature, as they will become brown too quickly because of caramelisation of sugar. A few of the commonly made deep-fried desserts around the world are described in Table 9.2.

Table 9.2 Types of deep-fried desserts

Type	Description
Beignets	Also known as fritters, these are batter-fried fruits. Fruits such as apples, peaches, pears, and figs, are commonly used for this purpose. Some fruits, such as peach halves, prunes, and dates, can be stuffed with rice pudding, marzipan, nuts, etc., and coated with batter and crumbed like à l'anglaise and then deep-fried. Beignets are accompanied with vanilla sauce or ice cream.
Choux fritters	Choux pastry is also served deep-fried. Once fried, it is coated with cinnamon flavoured sugar and served hot.
Helado frito	Deep-fried ice creams are very popular in Mexico, where a chilled ice cream scoop is covered with batter and crumbed before frying.
Oriental desserts	*Toffee fruits* Fruits, such as apple and banana, are batter-fried and coated with sesame flavoured caramelized sugar. *Daarsaan* These are deep-fried flat noodles, tossed in honey flavoured caramelized sugar.

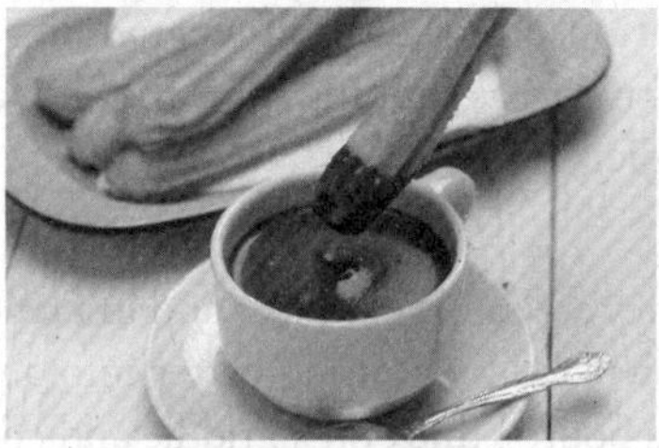

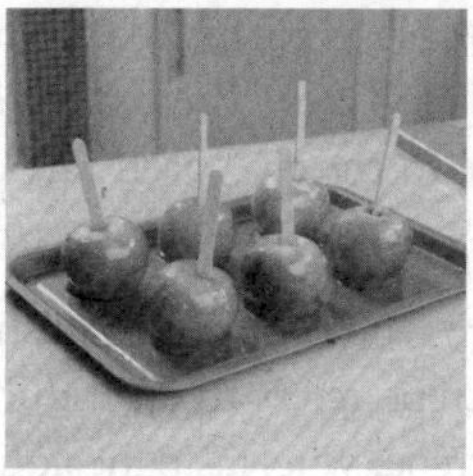

Choux fritters   Toffee apples

Fig. 9.3 Types of deep-fried desserts

Tarts and Pies

This category of desserts can be served hot or cold depending on the type of product. Fruit tarts are served cold, whereas apple pies are served hot. All tarts and pies have the following components.

Base The base of these desserts can be made with various kinds of pastes such as sweet paste, shortcrust paste, and puff pastry. Special moulds called tart moulds having raised edges are lined with the desired dough or pastry and baked with filling inside. The base can also be docked and baked without any filling. This is known as blind baking.

Filling Various kinds of fillings can be used for making hot pies. These fillings could be custard-based, starch-based, or even puree-based. The idea is to allow the filling to set after being baked, so that the tarts and pies can be cut into various portion sizes. Various kinds of fillings and desserts are discussed in Table 9.3.

Table 9.3 Fillings for pies and tarts

Filling	Description
Starch-based	Pastry cream and milk puddings enriched with eggs are commonly used as fillings in tarts and pies. One can add fillings of fruit, berries, jams, etc., on top of the pastry cream and bake the dessert.
Custard-based	Egg custard comprising milk, eggs, and sugar can be used as a filling for tarts and pies. One can also bake plain egg custard in a tart shell like cream pot.
Puree-based	Various vegetable or fruit purees can be combined with eggs and sugar and used as a filling for baked tarts and pies. When fruit purees are poured on top of pastry cream and are baked topped with crumbled flour and butter, it is known as *streusel*.
Nut pastes	Many other fillings such as almond paste also known as *crème frangipani* are commonly used as filling for baked tarts and pies.
Sugar	Mixtures cooked with sugar, liquid glucose, nuts, and butter make sticky fudge like filling, which is also commonly used in baked tarts and pies. *Macaroon* tarts are made by cooking sugar and egg whites with flavourings and adding them into the tart shell.
Cake batters	Various kinds of cake batters, such as brownie and *Genoese* sponge, can also be poured into a tart shell and baked.

Topping Every tart or pie is garnished with various kinds of products ranging from plain dusted icing sugar to various kinds of glazes. These are also known as toppings and they are added to impart a decorative look and texture to the prepared tart or pie.

Crêpes and Pancakes

Crêpes and pancakes are synonyms. In English, they are called pancakes and in French, they are called crêpes. However, in hotels, a crêpe refers to a product prepared by pouring batter into a pan and pouring out the excess to create a thin crêpe, whereas pancakes are poured thick on a griddle and cooked on both the sides.

Pancakes or crêpes are thin, flat cakes that are served rolled or folded around a filling, or infused with a warm sauce or syrup.

The crêpe mixture should be free of lumps, should have a consistency of cream, and should run freely from the spoon. The batter may have to be adjusted with milk. Crêpes should be neatly arranged on plates with the appropriate filling. Keep in mind that the colour combination and the flavour of the sauces used have to complement the dish.

Pancakes are usually served hot and can be garnished and topped with sauces and nuts or gratinated under a salamander.

Laminated Pastries

Laminated pastries such as puff pastry and *phyllo* pastry are commonly used to prepare varieties of hot desserts. Puff pastry can be used to line tarts to make crispy tarts and fruit pies. Some of the commonly made hot desserts using laminated pastries are described in Table 9.4.

Table 9.4 Hot desserts with laminated pastries

Hot desserts	Description
Eccles	This is a sweet snack made from puff pastry and is usually served during afternoon tea. It is dusted with icing sugar and served hot.
Turnovers	The puff is rolled into discs or squares and filled with sweet fillings of fruits mixed with almond cream or pastry cream and turned over or folded over. These are then glazed with egg yolk and baked.
Lebanese baklava	This dessert can be served hot as well as cold. It is commonly made from thin pastry sheets called *phyllo* or *filo*. It is baked till it becomes golden brown and while it is hot, it is dipped in rose flavoured sugar syrup. The cuts help to let the syrup percolate down. It is then served warm or cold.
Strudel	This is a famous dessert from Austria. It is made by stretching the dough very thin and then brushing the surface with melted butter. It is served hot with vanilla sauce.
Tarte tatin	This is a classical French dessert made by using apples and puff pastry.

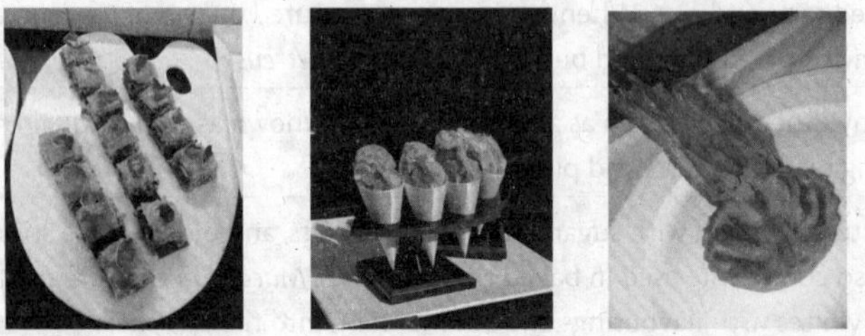

Lebanese baklava   Strudel   Tarte tatin

Fig. 9.4 Hot desserts with laminated pastries

Fruit-based Hot Desserts

Many fruits are also served as hot desserts. They can be served as they are or combined with other ingredients to make fruit pies and tarts as discussed in Table 9.2. Certain fruits, such as Japanese melon, peaches, and pineapple, are grilled on hot plates and served with ice creams. Grilled fruit *brochettes* are also very commonly served in France, along with sauces. Let us read about various kinds of fruit-based desserts served hot in Table 9.5.

Table 9.5 Types of fruit-based desserts

Type	Description
Baked	A variety of fruits can be baked as they are or can be used in fillings for pies, tarts, strudels, etc. Some fruits such as apples and pears are wrapped in puff pastry and baked until cooked. Figs wrapped in filo and baked are a classical dessert served in Greece.
Compote	It is a sweet made from fruit peeled and poached, whole or halved, quartered or diced, and served with syrup. *Compotes* can be served as a sauce or topping or it can be served as a dessert with whipped cream. Some blind baked tart shells are also served filled with fruit compotes.
Flambéed fruit	The fruits are cooked in sauce and then alcohol (such as brandy, vodka, and liqueurs) is poured on top and flamed. The flames rise out of the pan and continue until all the alcohol has evaporated.

Cold Desserts

Cold desserts can be prepared by a variety of methods. We will look at a range of cold desserts, from very simple to more complex types in this section.

Today many of the classical cold sweets are back in vogue, albeit with new flavour combinations and presentation techniques. Many of the classical creations were over-decorated, a style which has now gone out of fashion. We will discuss about the modern plating and presentation of desserts later in this chapter.

Cold Puddings

Cold puddings are the same as hot puddings, the only difference is that these are served cold. All the hot puddings mentioned in Table 9.1 can also be served cold. However, all cold puddings cannot be served hot. One such dessert is blancmange, which is made by heating milk and sugar, and is thickened with cornflour. It is chilled and served demoulded with jam sauce. Custards such as lemon custard are made by cooking lemon juice, egg yolks, sugar, and butter over low heat until a thick custard is formed. This is used for making lemon meringue pies. Some cold puddings are described in Table 9.6.

Fruit-based Cold Desserts

Fruits are a favourite amongst people especially those who are health conscious. Fruits can be prepared in various ways. They can be cut into fancy shapes and arranged to be served as a fruit platter. Beautiful patterns can be created by using colourful fruits on plates. Sauces or puree may be used and often make this an interesting dessert.

Some of the commonly made fruit-based desserts are described in Table 9.7.

> **CHEF'S TIP**
> For best results, leave the peeling and slicing of the fruit until the last possible moment. Once cut, some fruits, such as apples, pears, peaches, and bananas, discolour quickly. To prevent this from happening, they must be immersed in lemon juice and water or in syrup.

Table 9.6 Types of cold puddings

Type	Description
Blancmange	*Blancmange* has an almond-flavoured milk base. It is set with agar-agar, gelatine, or starch (such as cornflour). It is served demoulded with sweet sauce such as berry coulis or jam sauce.
Flummery	*Flummeries* are puddings usually thickened with cornflour, semolina, jelly, or sago. They can be served in the pot or served demoulded with sauce.
Rice conde	These rice desserts are cooked with milk and enriched with egg yolks. If gelatine is added, they should be set in moulds immediately.
Fruit custard	Milk is cooked with sugar and thickened with custard powder. Diced fruits and nuts are mixed and the mixture is then served chilled garnished with jellies.

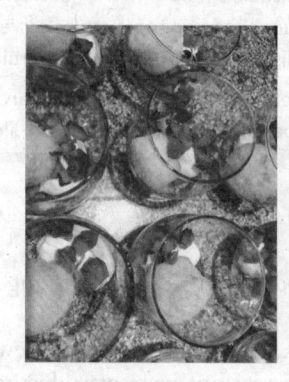

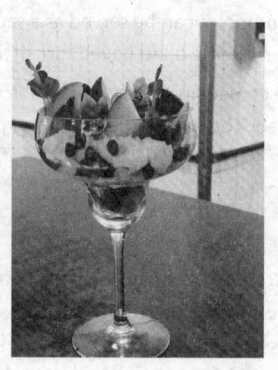

Flummery　　　Fruit custard

Fig. 9.5 Types of cold puddings

Table 9.7 Types of fruit-based cold desserts

Type	Description
Fruit platter	Sliced fruits in various shapes and cuts can be arranged on a platter to create interesting patterns. The important factors to consider when preparing a fruit platter are as follows: *The precision of the layout* *Colour combinations* *Items used in the right proportion*
Fruit salad	Unlike Western salads, a fruit salad is a mix of cut fresh fruits macerated with sugar syrup and flavours. It can be served with a scoop of ice cream or freshly whipped cream. Fruit salad should have a fresh and appetising appearance.
Compotes or poached fruits	These can be served as an accompaniment such as peach Melba and sometimes as a dessert accompanied by sauces and ice creams. Most fruits can be poached without addition of sugar; but some fruits such as apples, plums, and rhubarb, need sugar to develop their full flavour.

Fruit platter	Fruit salad	Compotes or poached fruits

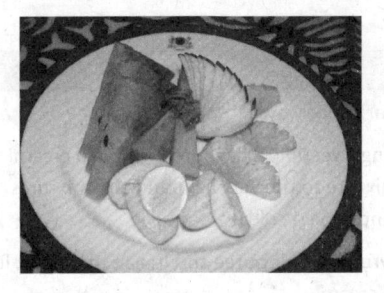

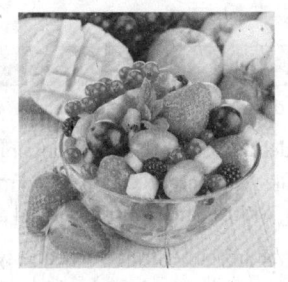

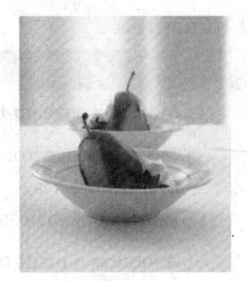

Fig. 9.6 Types of fruit-based cold desserts

Custard and Cream-based Desserts

Custards are generally a mixture of milk, sugar, and eggs heated over a double boiler or hot water bath, so that the eggs thicken the mixture. This mixture is the basic custard and is also known as Bavarian cream or *crème anglaise*. Thickening of a baked egg custard depends on the coagulation of the egg protein. The ratio of eggs to milk controls the firmness of the custard.

When preparing the mixture, always strain your custard for impurities. This will also enhance its quality and smoothness. Using heated milk helps to blend the mixture, and to dissolve the sugar more quickly. Skim off any foam from the surface, because it will result in a porous texture and spoil the appearance of the dessert.

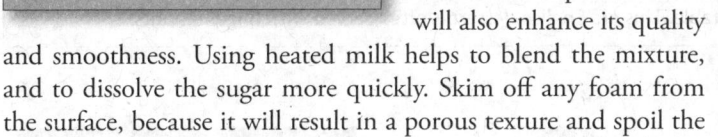

A few of the common desserts using creams and custards are discussed in Table 9.8.

Tarts, Pies, and Flans

As discussed in hot desserts, varieties of tarts, pies, and flans can be prepared and served hot or cold. Some flans are baked and served cold while some are served hot.

Some classical tarts, pies, and flans are discussed in Table 9.9.

> **CHEF'S TIP**
> It is generally accepted that demoulded custards need 8 to 10 eggs for each litre of milk. If there is too much egg, the custard will have a coarse, rubbery texture. Too little egg will produce custard that collapses when it is demoulded.

> **CHEF'S TIP**
> For crème caramel, run a knife around the edge. A *bavarois* can be loosened with your fingers. Gently pull one edge away from the mould, so that the air gets in between the dessert and the mould. This is usually sufficient to release it. Hold the *bavarois* onto your serving plate and give it a few shakes. If it is of the right consistency, it should release nicely from the mould.

Table 9.8 Common cream-based desserts

Name	Description
Bavarois	*Bavarois* is a dessert based on sauce *anglaise*. It is moulded, stabilized with gelatine, and enriched with cream and flavours. Various shapes can be created depending on the moulds used. They can be prepared for buffets or in individual moulds. Bavarian desserts can have several flavours made from the same basic mixture. *Bavarois* may be layered, using a variety of colours and flavours, such as chocolate, vanilla, strawberry. Each layer should be allowed to set before adding the next. Again, varieties are only limited by your imagination.

Table 9.8 (Contd)

Name	Description
Mousse	Mousse is a cream-based dessert that can be made in a variety of ways. Mousses range from the delicate, smooth sweet containing sweetened, flavoured whipped cream, to the more heavy egg yolk, gelatine, and cream-based mixture to the very light and airy mixtures lightened with beaten egg whites. They must be chilled and served cold. A mousse is made by combining either fruit puree and syrup, or fruit puree and Italian meringue. It is stabilized with gelatine and enriched with fresh whipped cream. Mousses can be made by cooking egg yolks and sugar to form a thick *sabayon* to which whipped cream is folded. Bavarian cream listed above can also be classified as a mousse.
Charlotte	This type of cold sweet is usually a *bavarois* encased with Swiss roll slices or finger biscuits, ice wafers, or *Genoese* sponge. *Charlotte* moulds can be fluted or plain. They are lined with slices of Swiss roll placed as closely as possible otherwise there would be gaps created and when the mixture is poured, it will leak from the holes. If you are using finger biscuits, neatly line the base and sides of your charlotte mould, fill the centre, and leave it to set. Trim off the finger biscuits in line with the mould.
Soufflé	These are sweets based on sauce *anglaise*, stabilized with gelatine, enriched with whipped cream, and lightened with beaten egg whites and flavourings such as spirits and liqueurs, and pastes of nuts. These are then set in special soufflé moulds, wrapped in greaseproof paper 2.5 cm higher than the mould. The paper is removed after chilling and the soufflé is decorated.
Fools	A fairly stiff fruit puree is carefully mixed with whipped cream and allowed to set in the refrigerator. Due to the richness of this dessert, fruits which are highly acidic, such as raspberries, gooseberries, and rhubarb, are the most suitable. This old English dessert is often served with finger biscuits.

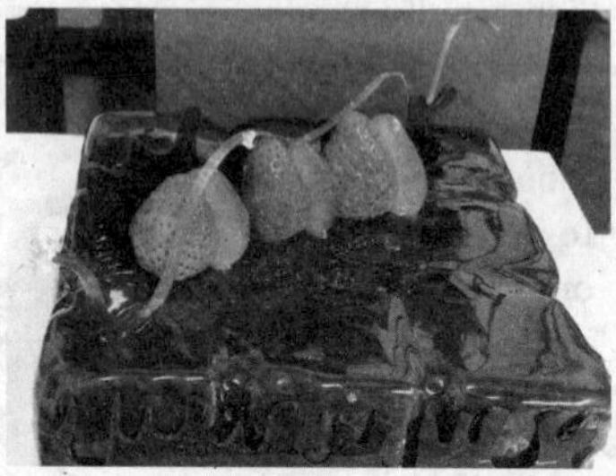

Bavarois 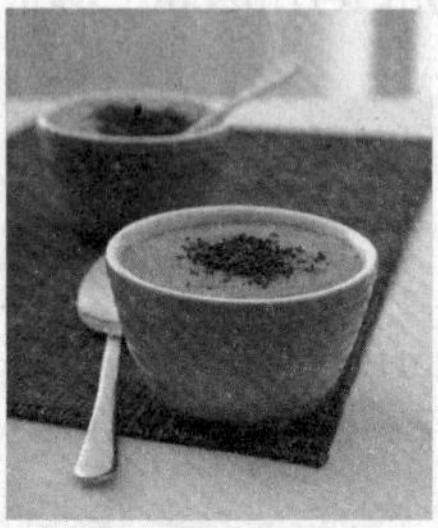 Mousse 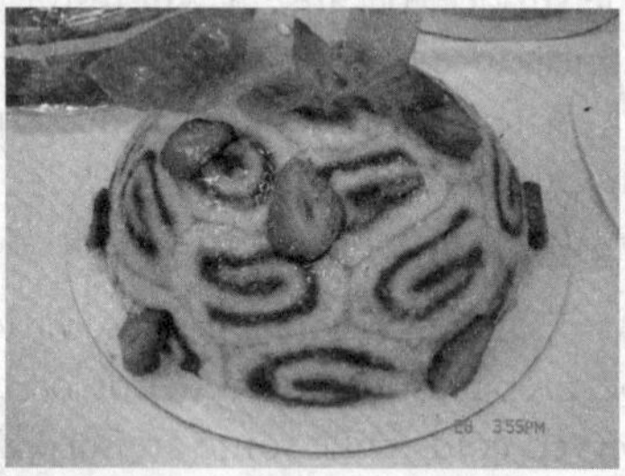 Charlotte

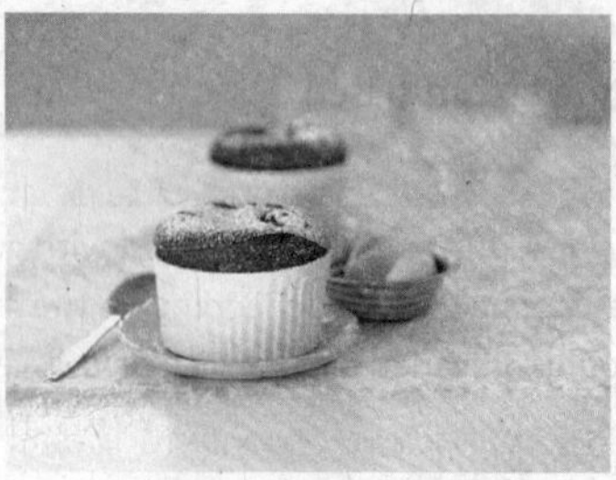

Soufflé 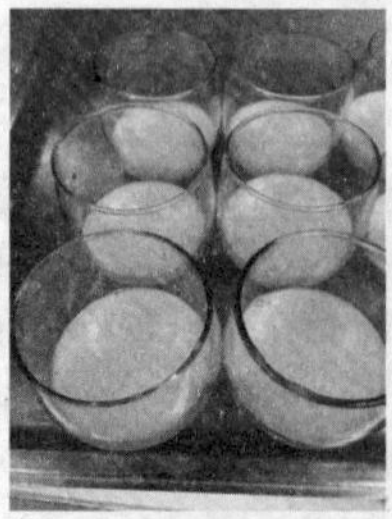 Fools

Fig. 9.7 Common cream-based desserts

Hot and Cold Desserts

Table 9.9 Tarts, pies, and flans served as dessert

Name	Description
Lemon tart	A lemon tart is made by lining the flan or tart mould with sweet paste and baking blind. It is then filled with lemon curd and served either decorated with meringue or as plain.
Fruit tart	Fruit tart and flan can be made by using baked sweet paste tart shells and lining them with melted chocolate.
Bakewell tart	This dessert is prepared by lining the tart mould with sweet paste and filling the centre with raspberry jam and crème frangipani.
Cherry *clafouti*	Cherry *clafouti* is a classical dessert in which cherries are arranged in a tart shell and custard is poured over and baked until set.
Baked custard flan	This dessert is made by pouring basic egg custard into a prepared sweet paste flan and baked at 140°C until cooked.
Chocolate tart	This dessert is made by lining the tart shell with cocoa flavoured sweet paste and baked blind.

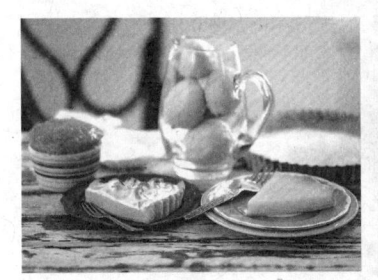

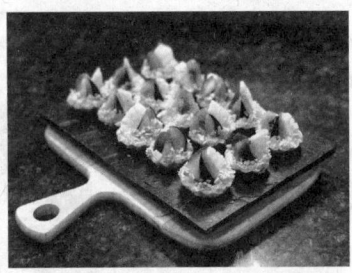

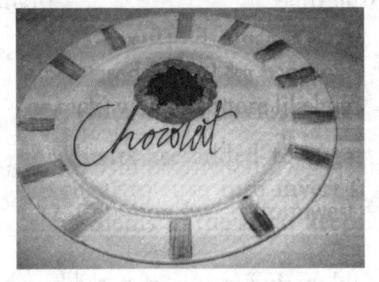

Lemon tart   Fruit tart 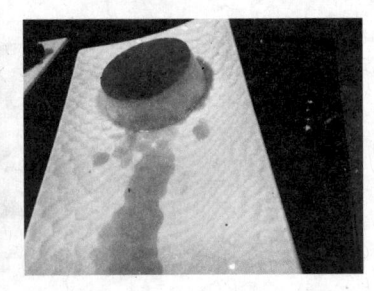   Baked custard flan

Chocolate tart

Fig. 9.8 Tarts, pies, and flans

Jellies

Sweet jellies are made either with liqueur, a dessert wine, or fruit juice combined with sugar and gelatine.

Jellies can be mixed with diced and chopped fruits and herbs to make attractive combinations. Jellies are rarely served as desserts these days, but they form an attractive garnish.

Sponges and Yeast-leavened Desserts

Various other desserts are made by combining sponges with other ingredients such as pastry cream, ganache, and nuts, to make some classical desserts. Yeast-leavened dough, such as brioche and *savarin*, is commonly used for preparing various kinds of desserts. Some of these desserts are described in Table 9.10.

Table 9.10 Sponge and yeast-leavened desserts

Name	Description
Fruit trifle	Fruit trifle is a very popular dessert from England. Fruit trifles are layered in glass bowls to make them look appealing and appetising. The top of the trifle is traditionally iced with a feather icing of jam, cream, and pastry cream.
Zuccotto	*Zuccotto* is a popular dessert from Italy that is made in a bombe mould and filled with chocolate sponge, ricotta cheese, ganache, nuts, and raisins and is served covered with melted ganache.
Tiramisu	This is a very famous Italian dessert that literally means 'pick me up'. It is made by layering a creamy mixture made by combining *mascarpone* cheese, egg yolks, sugar, and whipped egg whites or meringue, with coffee soaked sponge fingers also known as *Savoiardi*. It is a very common dessert served in most five-star hotels around the world.
Baba au rhum	*Babas* and *savarin* are made from yeast dough and are proved and baked in a ring shaped mould known as *savarin* mould or *dariole* mould. To enhance the flavour they are glazed with hot jam glaze and served chilled.

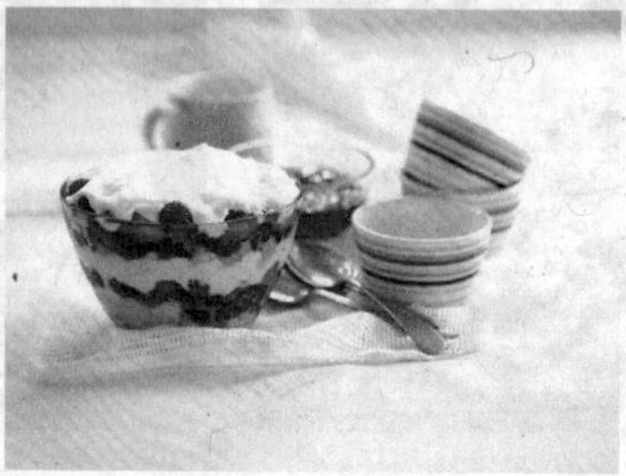

Fruit trifle 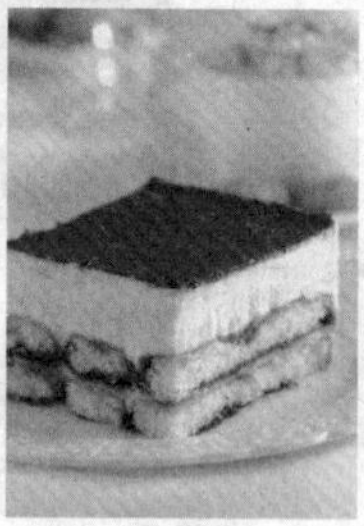   Tiramisu

Fig. 9.9 Sponge and yeast-leavened desserts

Meringues

Meringues are prepared by whipping egg whites with a pinch of salt and sugar. Heavy or light meringue can be made by addition of more or less sugar. Meringues can be divided into three categories as follows:

French meringue Also known as cold meringue, it is prepared by whipping egg whites until frothy and sugar is added in small amounts, whilst whipping continuously. This meringue is supposed to be used instantly as it can separate if it is left outside for a longer period of time.

Swiss meringue This is a hot meringue. Egg whites are whipped on a warm water bath until frothy, sugar is added in smaller amounts and the mixture is whisked over the hot water bath until it is creamy and stands in peaks.

Italian meringue This is the most stable meringue of all. In this method, the egg whites are whipped with small amount of sugar until frothy and then hot melted sugar boiled to 118°C is added whilst continuously whisking the mixture until a thick meringue is obtained.

Meringues can be used in a variety of ways. They can be used as a base for cakes and pastries as well as for garnishes and decorations.

PRESENTATION OF DESSERTS

Chefs in today's world are artists in their own right; only instead of a canvas and palette they deal with plates, sauces, and cut food items laid out in an appealing manner to seduce customers into succumbing to their visual delights and exotic flavours. Even the most delectable dessert dish can be off-putting, if it is badly presented. The variety and combination of ingredients and styles are only limited by one's imagination. However, a sense of balance and subtle blending of flavours must be achieved when working with ingredients. One needs to be aware of the changing trends in all aspects of dessert preparation and presentation to keep up with the modern and changing tastes of guests.

Salient Features of Presenting Desserts

As it is important to present food in such a way that it looks attractive and appealing to the guest, desserts also need to be presented in a manner that they create a lasting impression on the guest. Therefore, one has to keep in mind all aspects of presenting desserts. The following are some of the salient features that guide the presentation of desserts.

Visual appeal Chefs use a range of plates and garnishes to decorate their desserts to impress their guests. For instance, a white coloured dessert will not create the same impact on a white plate, whereas a dark chocolate-based dessert would stand out distinctively on a white background. Sometimes when options for coloured plates are limited, chefs often spray the plates with chocolate spray guns to provide contrasting colours to desserts. Sauces too are selected based on their colours and the flavours they would lend to the dessert. Since all desserts are not presented with sauces, it is important to select the right garnish for the dessert. The whole idea is to make the dessert look appealing, but care should be taken to keep it simple and not clutter the plate.

Balance and harmony It is very important to look at the balance of the dessert or any dish while presenting it. There should be a fine balance in terms of flavours, colours, textures, and taste, which should complement each other rather than create confusion in the guest's mind. For example, sweet meringue *Pavlovas* are served with a tropical fruit salsa. The astringent flavour in the tropical fruits balances the too sweet taste of meringue. Soft-textured desserts, such as mousses and soufflés, are served with crunchy garnishes such as brandy snaps and touilles.

Components of the dessert It is important to be careful in selecting the components of the desserts. The three basic components of a dessert are—the dessert itself, the sauce, and the garnish. Sometimes a dessert can be accompanied with ice cream, sorbet, or even a hot or cold liquid known as *shooter*. The total weight of the pre-plated dessert should be in the range of 80–120 g. However, this also depends on the light texture of the dessert in which case the portion would be determined by the size of the dessert.

Easy to eat and serve Plated desserts should be of the texture that they can be cut with spoon and fork as these are the standard cutlery served with desserts.

Easy to prepare It is important for the presentation to be modern, elegant, yet simple so as to be prepared by the staff in a timely manner.

Fresh and seasonal The best approach to presenting desserts is to use fresh and seasonal items in presentation.

Classical and contemporary It is important to be trendy and modern, but at the same time it is important to have a strong basic foundation. Time-tested classical desserts are always in vogue; only difference is that they are presented in more contemporary styles.

Tips for Presenting Pre-plated Desserts

As food fashions are constantly changing, it is important to be abreast of new tools and techniques that can be used for making desserts more appealing. It is the view of most pastry chefs that a good presentation enhances the impact of a dessert. Whatever dessert you plan to put on plate, always remember to do the following.

Keep the presentation simple Simplicity is the key to success. Simple things are easy to understand, prepare, and serve to the guest. Complicated presentations would involve more handling, clash of flavours, and a messy concoction on a plate.

Use the particular dessert as the visual focus on the plate Many a times the accompaniments or the garnish are bigger than the dessert itself. In such cases, the main dessert gets eclipsed and the rest of the things on the plate dominate the actual dessert. Use garnishes, accompaniments, and sauces that complement the dish and do not take away the individuality of the main dessert itself.

Garnish with a combination of fresh ingredients Always use what is fresh, seasonal, and crisp. Remember dessert is the last meal on the menu and it is important to leave a long lasting impression on the guest's mind.

Use natural products Use natural colours and flavours. It is also important that all garnishes used on the plate must be edible. More emphasis should be laid on the freshness in taste, a balanced appearance and small portions of each dessert, so that the taste can be enjoyed to the last bite.

Desserts are also being served in a combination of flavours, that is, more than one small fresh fruit mousse on a single plate. This is also known as the *assiette* concept. This never leaves a repetitive taste in the mouth as different fruit flavours can be appreciated separately, each one being new to the taste buds. Not only flavours, but different textures, colours, temperatures, and consistencies are being used in unison on a single plate to give an assortment of textures to the taste buds.

More than the visual appeal, where elements might just be added without actually adding to the taste appreciation, desserts now go in for elements, which add to the taste experience, for it is the taste which is remembered. Also, freshly cut fruits or fresh fruit purees or coulis are being used to accompany desserts.

Thus, modern trends call for:

- Smaller portions of the dessert, also presented in small individual platters (a feature for the buffets)
- Multiple elements with varying textures, colours, temperatures, etc., on a single plate
- Extra emphasis on freshness (freshly cut fruits and freshly made purees and coulis used instead of readymade crushes and synthetic products) and taste with minimum decoration
- Making desserts simpler with tastes that can be appreciated and are not confusing the taste buds

BUFFET DESSERTS

Buffet has always been a very interesting concept of serving as well as having food.

A buffet includes different courses starting from the appetizers, salads, main courses, and desserts. Desserts form a very important part of the buffet. Also, it is that part of the buffet which is most elegantly presented.

The concept of buffet has changed a lot over the years, mainly in terms of the presentation and techniques of preparing the desserts. Buffet desserts always have a variety of textures and flavours which are presented beautifully in a highlighted part of the buffet. A good and balanced buffet should be carefully planned as the selection of desserts plays a large role in successful buffet presentations.

In Table 9.11, a sample rotational menu classified under various sub-headings is shown.

Table 9.11 Buffet matrix for dessert buffet

Items	Monday	Tuesday	Wednesday	Thursday	Friday	Saturday	Sunday
Puddings	Cherry *clafoutis*	Cabinet pudding	Diplomat pudding	Ginger and wild honey pudding	Coconut and cinnamon pudding	English bread and butter pudding	Queen's pudding
Mousse cakes (individual portions)	Cappuccino slice	Bailey's Irish mousse	Black forest slice	Nougatine mousse cake	Apple mousse	Charlotte russe	Blueberry mousse
Eggless cheesecakes	Lemon-scented cheesecake	Mango cheesecake	Pandana cheesecake	Vanilla bean cheesecake	Strawberry cheesecake	New York cheesecake	Choco banana mousse cake
Tarts	Almond frangipani tart	Mix fruit dutch tart	Tarte tatin	Citron tart	Peach frangipani tart	Walnut frangipani tart	Tangerine pine nut tart
Chocolate cakes	Hazelnut truffle torte	Devil's food cake	The Opera	Pistachio truffle torte	Sacher	Dobos	Alhambra
Cream cakes	Rose and fig cream cake	Oregon cherry cream cake	Panna cotta cream cake	Kiwi cream cake	Strawberry cream cake	Raspberry cream cake	Lamingtons
Eggless desserts in glass	Raspberry fool	Kir royal	Summer berry compote	Hazelnut cream	Pistachio and praline fool	Pineapple panna cotta	Butterscotch cream cake
Classical dessert	Tiramisu	Cream caramel	Cardinal schnitten	Fruit trifle	St Honore	Napoleon gateau	Gateau pithivier
Low-calorie desserts	Fruit compote	Apple crumble pie	Grilled pineapple skewers	Almond blancmange	Baked yoghurt	Bitter chocolate tart	Crêpe with banana

Classifying deserts in this manner will help chefs to design better buffet menus and at a glance, one would be able to see the balance in colour, taste, texture, and flavour of the dessert. Creating categories helps chefs to plan the dessert menus in better and creative ways. A matrix ensures that you are not repeating the flavours or the ingredient more than once on a given day.

In a buffet, there have to be different types of desserts, such as soufflés, mousses, pastries, eggless, sugar free, cheesecake based, as well as quite a handful of regional desserts. Among all these desserts, there have to be one or two hot desserts.

This kind of service definitely requires proper planning and execution of the plans, but it cuts down on the time of service during the meal period and makes it efficient and faster.

FROZEN DESSERTS

Now that we have discussed the hot and cold desserts, let us take a look at the frozen desserts. The most common frozen dessert known to any child is an ice cream. Ice creams are favourite among people of all age groups. Be it summer or bone-chilling winter, frozen desserts never lose their popularity. In the pastry kitchen, a range of frozen desserts are prepared and served in à la carte and buffet operations all over the world. Ice creams do not need any introduction as they are easily available commercially.

Frozen desserts are further classified into the following types.

- Churn-frozen desserts
- Still-frozen desserts

Table 9.12 provides an overview of the various types of frozen desserts. There are various kinds of frozen desserts that are mainly classified on the basis of the method employed for preparing them. The two most commonly adopted methods for preparing frozen desserts are churn freeze and still freeze. In case of churn freeze, the mixture is allowed to freeze while being churned constantly. This method helps in producing a product that is smooth on the palate because of very small ice particles. Churning also incorporates air into the mixture, thereby making it light and foamy. Ice creams and sorbets are made by this method. Still-frozen desserts, on the other hand, are mixed and frozen without churning; they also give a smooth texture and soft mouth feel. Depending upon the kind of dessert, the mixture is churned prior to freezing or air is incorporated in many other ways such as by adding whipped eggs and cream.

Let us now look at the two methods of preparation.

Churn-frozen Desserts

As the name suggests, these desserts are churned constantly during the freezing cycle. The process of churning and freezing at the same time does not allow water crystals to form and the resulting desserts are smooth and creamy. There are many types of churn-frozen desserts, ice creams being among the most common ones. An ice cream can be defined as a smooth frozen mixture of milk, cream, sweeteners, and flavours with some amount of air incorporated in it as described earlier. There are many kinds of ice creams, each of which has a typical texture or mouth feel because of the kinds of ingredients used in its making. All the ingredients play a very important role in the production of ice creams and especially sorbets. Sugar is the most crucial of them all. The texture or the mouth feel of churn-frozen desserts depends upon several factors such as:

- Type of the churn-frozen dessert
- Ingredients used in its preparation
- Process of making the mixture
- Equipment used in churning

Table 9.12 Types of frozen desserts

Churn-frozen	Still-frozen	Others	Classical frozen
French ice cream	Granita	Bombe	Baked Alaska
American ice cream	Kulfi	Frozen mousse and soufflé	Cassata
Ice milk	Parfait	Iced Charlotte (Charlotte glace)	Fried ice cream
Frozen yoghurt		Iced gateaux (torte glace)	Sundaes and coupes
Gelato			
Basic ice creams			
Sorbet			

Types of Churn-frozen Desserts

All churn-frozen desserts have one thing in common—the method of preparation, in which the mixture is churned while it is being frozen. The two most common churn-frozen desserts are ice creams and sorbets. The basic difference between the two is that an ice cream is smooth and creamy and has a dairy base, such as milk and cream, whereas a sorbet is made with liquids such as juices, paired with sugar. Some common types of churn-frozen desserts are described in Table 9.13.

Table 9.13 Common types of churn-frozen desserts

Type	Description
French ice cream	This type of ice cream is commonly enriched with egg yolks and butter. Full-cream milk is combined with dairy cream and sugar and is cooked with whipped egg yolks until a thick sauce is formed. Thereafter, flavours and stabilizers are added and the mixture is allowed to cool in the refrigerator for at least 24 hours before it can be churned. Refrigerating the mix overnight develops flavours and matures the ice cream mixture.
American ice cream	American ice cream is made in the same manner as French ice cream, but without the addition of eggs. Eggs have an ability to stabilize the mixture and make it creamier because of their emulsifying properties. Since American ice creams do not have eggs, it is necessary that some ice cream stabilisers (refer Table 9.18) are added to the mixture.
Ice milk	These are ice creams made with dairy products that have low butterfat content. These are very popular among people who are conscious of their calorie intake and have dietary restrictions. Eggs and butter are never added to these ice creams.
Frozen yoghurt	This ice cream can be made in French, American, or ice milk style. It contains yoghurt in addition to the milk and cream. The recipes are always adjusted for milk and cream when the yoghurt is added. The total proportions of fat, liquid, and emulsifiers need to be constant for a standard product. Too much fat, for example, will precipitate out while churning and give the ice cream a curdled appearance. The preparation of frozen yoghurt can yield a better product when regular ice cream mixture is set with a culture of yoghurt and then churned as a normal ice cream. This method results in a smooth and creamy product.
Gelato	*Gelato* (plural: *gelati*) is the Italian version of ice cream. It is generally made with very low fat content and is often made using only milk and no dairy cream. Some fruit-based *gelati* are made by combining fruit puree, sugar, stabilisers, and cream and churned until smooth. Though there is cream in fruit *gelati*, yet it is low in fat content as compared to conventional ice creams. Also, fruit puree content comprises a large percentage of the ingredients. Since most of the *gelati* are made without cream, fat, and other emulsifiers and stabilisers, the resulting product does not have too much of overrun. This gives the ice cream rich mouth feel, since it easily melts in the mouth.
Sorbet	Sorbet is derived from the Persian word, *sherbet*. In English, the term 'water ice' is commonly used in place of sorbet. In Italian, these are called *sorbetto*. Sorbets are used as one of the courses in the French classical menu and are usually served in the middle of the meal before the main course is served. They are used as an interval in the gastronomic fare. It is because of this reason that sorbets are usually made using citrus fruits, such as lemon, orange, and berries, that aid in digestion as well as cleanse the mouth for other courses to follow.

Methods of Preparing Churn-frozen Desserts

In this section, we will discuss the steps of preparing the two most common churn-frozen desserts—ice cream and sorbets.

Preparing the ice cream mix There are two kinds of ice creams: eggless or the ones enriched with eggs. The method of preparing the mix will follow the same process in both cases. The steps for preparation of basic ice creams are as follows:

Step 1   Heat milk in a clean pan and bring to a boil. Meanwhile, whisk egg yolks and sugar in a bowl until creamy and thick.

Step 2   Add the whisked egg yolks to the milk and cook until the mixture thickens or coats the back of a spoon. Cool the mixture and add the desired flavours at this stage. If an eggless ice cream mix is being prepared, then add the desired stabilisers at this stage and cook the mix until it comes to a temperature of 80°C.

Step 3   Remove the mixture from the fire and add cream and mix well. This will also help to bring the temperature down. Chill the ice cream mixture in the refrigerator overnight to mature the mix.

Step 4   Churn the mixture in a churning machine until smooth and creamy.

Step 5   Transfer the mixture to a clean container immediately and freeze in a freezer at a temperature of −20°C.

> **CHEF'S TIP**
> Maturing the mix in the refrigerator helps in bonding the proteins of milk, cream, and eggs with water molecules. This in turn helps in making smoother ice creams as the resulting mixture becomes homogenous, thereby not allowing the water molecules to form ice crystals.

Let us now take a look at the recipe of making a basic vanilla flavoured ice cream with egg.

Vanilla Ice Cream

Ingredients
Milk 1 l with 3.5% fat content
Cream 400 ml with 35% fat content
Sugar 300 g
Egg yolks 6
Ice cream stabiliser 10 g
Vanilla pod 1 pc

METHOD
1. Mix yolk and half the sugar and whisk until dissolved.
2. Heat the remaining sugar with milk and scraped vanilla pod to 85°C.
3. Pour the hot milk into the egg mixture and cook again until the mixture coats the back of a spoon. Remove from fire and cool down to 50°C.
4. Heat the cream to 85°C and cool it down to 50°C.
5. Mix the cream with the milk and egg mixture now and keep it covered in fridge for at least 12 hours.
6. Churn in ice cream machine and freeze until service.

To prepare an eggless ice cream, you would require an ice cream stabiliser, which is sold as a proprietary ingredient. Following is the recipe for making basic vanilla flavoured ice cream without egg.

Eggless Vanilla Ice Cream

Ingredients
Milk 1 l with 3.5% fat content
Cream 200 ml with 35% fat content
Sugar 300 g
Ice cream stabiliser 30 g
Vanilla pod 1 pc

METHOD
1. Heat sugar with milk and scraped vanilla pod to 85°C.
2. Hold the milk at this temperature for at least 4 minutes and cool down to 60°C.
3. Heat the cream to 85°C and cool it down to 60°C.
4. Mix the cream with the milk and dissolve the ice cream stabiliser and keep the mixture covered in fridge for at least 12 hours.
5. Churn in ice cream machine and freeze until service.

The aforementioned recipes are basic recipes and one can add various flavourings to prepare flavoured ice creams.

Preparing sorbets Sorbets in the modern times have also replaced ice creams, as they are made without any cream and fat and are thus, light and healthy. They are a combination of water, fruit juice, and sugar and are commonly known as water ice. Sugar plays an important role in sorbets and one has to be careful about the density of sugar in the syrup. Since this is the only ingredient that has to play an important part in deciding the texture of the final product, equipment such as saccharometer and baumanometer is used to measure the density of sugar. The production of sorbets becomes trickier as the density of sorbet mixture would change with the type of fruit being used in the mixture as concentration of sugar in each fruit or juice varies. For freezing, the density of the sorbet mixture must be between 18°–20° Baume. If on measuring, one finds that sugar density is too high, the mixture can be diluted with water and vice versa. Many recipes also add 1–2 percent of egg whites to the mixture before churning. The egg white helps in giving a smooth and airy texture to the sorbet. In many Italian sorbets, a part of sugar is whipped with egg whites to make an Italian meringue, which is then mixed along with water and flavours. The resulting sorbets are smooth and airy and many a time, a customer can get confused between a *gelato* and a *sorbetto*.

The following are some precautions that need to be taken while making sorbets.

- The density of the sugar should be measured.
- Sorbets should be rapidly frozen while being churned.

There could be many recipes of a sorbet depending upon the kind of ingredient used. Let's see the basic recipe of a lime sorbet.

Lime Sorbet

Ingredients
Water 1350 g
Sugar 300 g
Stabiliser 10 g
Liquid glucose 40 g
Lime juice 200 ml

METHOD
1. Mix sugar, water, and liquid glucose and bring to a boil.
2. Cool the mix to 65°C, add stabiliser and mix well.
3. Mix in the lime juice, cool the mixture and then churn in an ice cream machine.

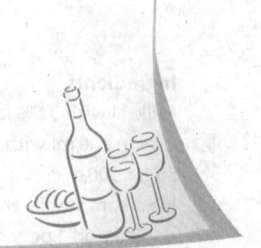

You can add various flavours by omitting the lime juice and replacing it in the same quantity with other juices to give the desired flavour to the sorbet.

Factors Affecting Overrun in Churn-frozen Desserts

There are four major factors that affect the overrun in churn-frozen desserts, namely freezing equipment, fat content in the mix, mixture, and the amount of liquid in the freezer.

Type of freezing equipment Modern freezing equipment works on the same principle as the age-old churning machines, which were also known as hand-cranked freezers. These machines consisted of a drum that was filled with ice, chilled water, and salt. A tub containing the ice cream mixture was placed in the drum containing the freezing mixture (ice and salt). The tub was placed in such a way that the ice covered the entire tub, thereby allowing the freezing of the ice cream mixture on the sides of the tub. To the tub was attached a scraper device called paddle or a dasher, which was used to constantly stir the ice cream manually. This scraped the freezing mixture from the walls of the tub into the ice cream mixture. The churning was carried out till the mixture attained the desired smooth and creamy texture with air incorporated into it.

Modern ice cream freezers operate on the same principle; the only difference being that the refrigeration is provided with electricity and not with ice and salt as the freezing agent as in case of the age-old churning machines. There are two kinds of freezers available in the market: vertical and horizontal. Vertical freezers are similar to older machines where the paddle moves in the tub vertically. This produces a lower overrun in the ice cream mixture as compared to the horizontal ice cream churners which incorporate more air into the ice cream mix and give a bigger overrun. These, however, are more suited for home-kitchens. On a commercial scale, which entails bulk production, there are many more kinds of freezers, also known as continuous ice cream freezers. These freezers produce almost 100% overrun and sometimes more. As the name suggests, the mixture continuously runs from one end to the other and is extruded as ice cream from the other end.

Fat content in the mix The fat content in the mixture also influences the amount of air that can be incorporated in the ice cream mixture. The more the fat content, the lower the overrun and vice versa.

Mixture The overrun of the churn-frozen desserts also depends upon the texture and consistency of the ice cream mixture. The more the solids, the lower the overrun and vice versa.

Amount of ice cream mixture in the freezer The amount of ice cream mixture put in the freezing tub is another factor that affects the overrun of the frozen dessert. If more mixture is added to the churning machine, then very little space will be left for the air to get incorporated in the mix, which would yield heavy and dense ice creams. Ideally, the ice cream freezers should be half filled with the ice cream mixture to get a good overrun.

Still-frozen Desserts

As the name suggests, this range of frozen desserts is not churned or stirred but allowed to freeze as it is. Some examples of still-frozen desserts are *granitas*, *kulfi*, *parfait*, etc., which have their own unique taste and texture. These are frozen without any further mixing or agitation. The resulting mixture is not airy or fluffy as it does not have any overrun. Nonetheless, it is important that still-frozen desserts too have a smooth mouth feel and texture. Therefore, a range of ingredients and methods are involved in making different types of still-frozen desserts.

Types of Still-frozen Desserts

Just like churn-frozen desserts, still-frozen desserts too are of various types depending on the process involved and the ingredients used for preparing the same. Some common still-frozen desserts are described in Table 9.14.

Table 9.14 Types of still-frozen desserts

Type	Description
Granitas	*Granitas* or *granita* is an Italian frozen dessert that is similar to sorbet with regards to ingredients. *Granitas*, however, have low concentration of sugar. This is so because large ice crystal formation is the desired texture for this dessert. *Granitas* can also be called shaved ice in English. This is made by combining fruit juices and sugar and allowing it to still-freeze in a large flat container such as gastronome trays. When the mixture is frozen, the *granita* is shaved off and served with additional syrups or as they are. It often replaces sorbet in a course.
Kulfi	*Kulfi* is among the most common still-frozen desserts in India. In this, the milk is reduced to thick sauce-like consistency which is known as *rabri*. The *rabri* is then flavoured with sugar, chopped nuts, saffron, and other flavourings as required and poured into small conical moulds made of clay or metal. The traditional way to quickly freeze this dessert was to put the mixture in a clay pot with ice water and salt and shake the pot to and fro to allow it to freeze. Nowadays, the moulds are kept in freezers and served along with cornstarch vermicelli known as *falooda*, which is commonly flavoured with rose syrup.
Parfait	*Parfait* in French means perfect and that is kind of true for this still-frozen dessert. It has a creamy texture that is not a result of churning. A *parfait* in the USA would mean scoops of ice cream with different flavourings and toppings in a tall glass, but in France, where the dessert originated, it is a mixture of creamed egg yolks combined with whipped cream and flavourings frozen in tall moulds, which are unmoulded at the time of service. The *parfait* can be flavoured with a range of ingredients but flavours such as coffee, vanilla, chocolate, liqueurs such as kirsch and orange are most commonly used for flavouring them.

Methods of Preparing Still-frozen Desserts

The methods of preparing still-frozen desserts differ from one type to another. Since these desserts are not churned, their texture is decided by the ingredients used and the way these are prepared and frozen. Let us discuss the preparation of these still-frozen desserts.

Preparing granitas *Granitas* are fairly easy to make as they are made by combining liquids such as fruit juice with sugar syrup. The mixture is prepared in the same manner as for sorbets, the only difference is that it is not churned like a sorbet and is allowed to freeze in a shallow utensil and then shaved. The shavings of the frozen dessert are shaped into a scoop and served as *granitas*.

Preparing parfaits The basic ingredients used for making *parfait* are sugar, eggs, and cream. There is more than one method of preparing the basic *parfait* mix. Let us discuss the most commonly followed method in hotels in simple steps.

Step 1 Bring sugar and water to a boil and then cook the syrup to a temperature of 118°C. Remove from fire and dip the bottom of the pan in cold water to arrest the cooking.

Step 2 Whisk egg yolks until creamy and whisk them further by adding hot syrup into the egg yolks. The whipping process should be carried out until the egg yolks become thick and creamy and double in volume.

Step 3 Add any flavouring at this stage and incorporate well. Fold in whipped cream.

Step 4 Put the prepared mixture in a long mould and freeze until required.

Preparing kulfis *Kulfi* is a famous Indian dessert that is quite popular across the world. The texture of *kulfi* is very important and depends on the degree to which the milk and sugar are cooked. *Kulfis* are available in many flavours and shapes. Some people set it in a clay pot, while the most traditional way is to freeze it in aluminium conical moulds that are put into a pot with ice and salt and shaken periodically to freeze the *kulfi*.

The stepwise preparation of *kulfi* is as follows:

Step 1 Bring milk to a boil; reduce the heat and cook it stirring continuously until it is reduced to one-third of its original volume. At this stage it is known as *rabri*.

Step 2 Remove from the flame and add sugar and condensed milk. One can add flavourings and other ingredients at this stage and cool the mixture over ice.

Step 3 Pour the *kulfi* into desired moulds and freeze until required.

Other Types of Frozen Desserts

There is another category of desserts that neither falls in the category of still-frozen nor churn-frozen desserts. These desserts are also referred to as miscellaneous frozen desserts. Some of them are made in their own unique style, whereas most of them are a combination of churn-frozen and still-frozen desserts, for example, *bombe*. It is one dessert that can be made with various combinations of ice creams, sorbets, and *parfaits* layered together in a mould with or without cake sponge. Sometimes mousses are prepared and frozen, though one can say that those are kinds of *parfaits* which can be categorized into still-frozen desserts, but sometimes a mousse might not be prepared with eggs as all *parfaits* are. Some of these desserts are also classical and still feature on the menus of many hotels. Common desserts in this category are described in this section.

Bombe

Bombe is a dessert made with a combination of churn-frozen desserts such as ice creams or sorbets and *parfaits*. It is due to this reason that at times, the *parfait* mixture is also known as *bombe* as it is used for making this classical dessert in a spherical-shaped dome mould. A few classical bombes are discussed in Table 9.15.

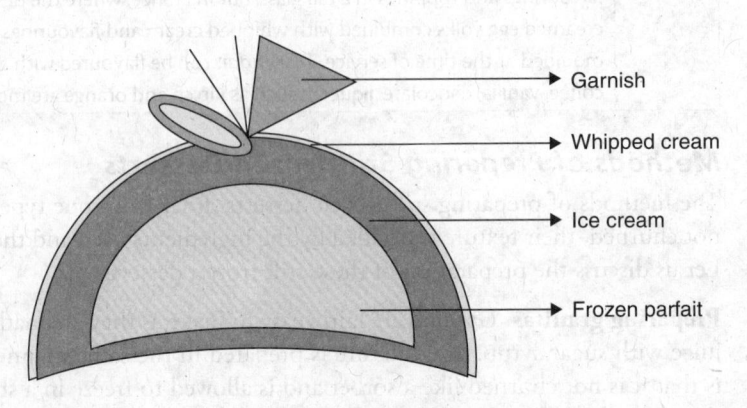

Fig. 9.10 Representation of a bombe

Table 9.15 Classical bombes

Classical bombe	Covering ice cream/sorbet	Parfait filling
Africaine	Dark chocolate ice cream	Vanilla and apricot
Aida	Strawberry ice cream	Kirsch liqueur
Alhambra	Vanilla bean	Fresh strawberry
Bresilienne	Pineapple sorbet	Vanilla, Caribbean rum, and chopped pineapple
Cardinale	Fresh raspberry sorbet	Vanilla bean and crushed praline
Ceylon	Coffee ice cream	Dark rum
Copella	Coffee ice cream	Praline
Diplomat	Vanilla bean	Maraschino liqueur and candied fruits
Florentine	Raspberry sorbet	Crushed praline
Formosa	Vanilla bean	Strawberry with chopped strawberries
Zamora	Coffee ice cream	Curaçao liqueur

Frozen Mousses and Soufflés

Mousses and soufflés are classical French desserts that are served chilled or used as a filling for various cakes and pastries. A whole range of desserts can be prepared by still-freezing mousses and soufflés to impart a different texture altogether to the final product. The concept is similar to that of a *parfait* as mousses are also made with various bases, such as *sabayon* and *crème anglaise*, and are folded along with whipped creams and flavours. There are no different ingredients for soufflés, but it is only the look of the dessert that gives an impression as if it has risen out of a mould. This effect can be given in a variety of ways.

Iced Charlottes (Charlottes Glaces)

Charlottes are usually made in shapes of cakes or they can be made in spherical dome shaped mould known as charlotte mould as used for *bombes*. The mould can be lined with sponge fingers or with slices of Swiss roll pastry. It should be kept frozen until required and served with fruit pulp or sauce. There are as many varieties of iced charlottes available as ice cream combinations are possible.

Iced Gateaux (Tortes Glaces)

This frozen dessert is inspired from various cakes and gateaux. To prepare an ice cream cake, a cake ring of the required size is set onto greaseproof paper, lined with a layer of sponge, and filled with 3 cm thick layers of ice cream (same or different flavours) and finally covered with a layer of sponge. Fruit or nuts can be added to the ice creams and the sponge may be splashed with liqueurs. Figure 9.11 shows a cross-section of an ice cream cake.

Classical Frozen Desserts

Some of the classical frozen desserts have been discussed in this section.

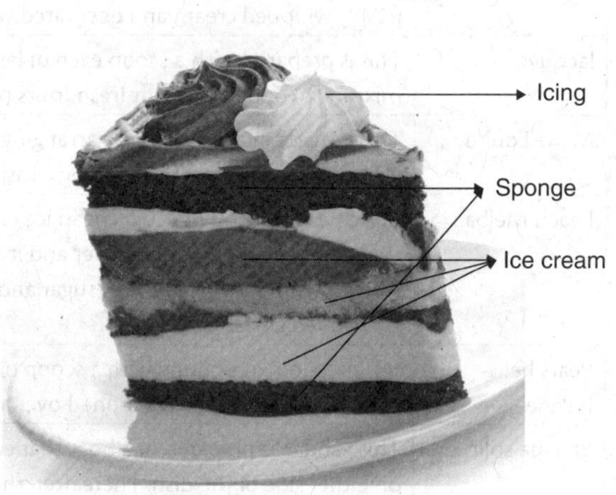

Fig. 9.11 Cross-section of an ice cream cake

Baked Alaska

It is also known as *soufflé omelette surpris* because of the baked look of whipped egg whites on the outside and frozen ice cream inside. Baked Alaska is also commonly known as *Norwegian omelette* and is made by lining a mould with *Genoese* sponge. Layers of ice creams, depending upon the choice, are put on the sponge and the base is also sealed with a layer of sponge. The dessert is frozen again until set. It can be garnished with cut fresh fruits.

Cassata

Cassata is almost like *bombe* but the filling is not of *parfait*. This dessert popularly comes from Italy and is made by layering three different kinds of ice creams and sorbets lined with a layer of *Genoese* sponge. Some cassatas are also made by layering the moulds with ice creams and filling with a mixture of Italian meringue, whipped cream, and candied nuts. One such classical *cassata* is *Cassata Napoletana*.

Fried Ice Cream

This dessert hails from Mexico where it is commonly known as *helado frito*. It is also commonly seen in China. A scoop of ice cream is wrapped in a covering such as pancake or sponge and allowed to freeze again until it is hard. The covered ice cream is then dipped into a sweetened batter of flour sugar and milk and usually covered with varieties of coatings ranging from crushed nuts to corn flakes.

Sundaes and Coupes

Assorted ice creams and sorbets are combined in small metal cups known as *coupes* and hence the name. Sundaes are combined in shallow dishes allowing the coupes to be decorated liberally with fresh whipped cream, fruits, and nuts. When the same is layered in long glasses, they are commonly known as *parfaits* in America, as discussed earlier. Some of the classical combinations for coupes and sundaes are described in Table 9.16.

Table 9.16 Classical coupes and sundaes

Name	Description
Arlesienne	This is prepared by putting diced candied fruits soaked in kirsch liqueur in a cup and a scoop of vanilla bean ice cream over them. The ice cream is topped with half of poached pear and apricot them sauce.
Black Forest	This is chocolate ice cream garnished with dark cherries soaked in cherry brandy. It is topped with freshly whipped cream and decorated with large shavings of dark chocolate.
Jacques	This is prepared with a scoop each of lemon sorbet and strawberry ice cream in a shallow dish. The mixture is topped with cut fresh fruits marinated in cherry liqueur.
Marie Louise	This is made in a long glass by arranging fresh raspberries in the glass with a scoop of vanilla bean ice cream over them. The topping consists of raspberry sauce and whipped cream.
Peach Melba	In a coupe, a scoop of vanilla bean ice cream is put and topped with half of poached peach. Then the Melba sauce is spooned over and it is garnished with slivered almonds. Melba sauce is made by stewing fresh raspberries with sugar and making a puree of the same. The puree is combined with stewed red currants.
Pears belle helene	It is prepared in a coupe with a scoop of vanilla bean ice cream and topping of half of poached pear. Chocolate sauce is spooned over and it is garnished with slivered almonds.
Banana split	This sundae is prepared in a boat shaped shallow dish. A banana is split lengthwise and arranged on either side of the dish. Thereafter, three kinds of ice creams are arranged in between the split banana and topped with syrups, nuts, and freshly whipped cream.

Ingredients Used in Frozen Desserts

Various kinds of ingredients are used in the preparation of frozen desserts. Every ingredient has a role and contributes in making the dessert unique in texture as well as taste. Thus, it is very important to understand the role of ingredients in the making of desserts. Sugar, for example, plays a significant part in churn-frozen desserts. If it is less, then there will be large water crystals in the resulting dessert and if the sugar is too much, then the dessert will not freeze well. Apart from sugar, several other ingredients such as starches, eggs, and even stabilisers play a major role, which needs to be understood well so as to be able to make the desserts as per the standards. Table 9.17 highlights the role of various ingredients in a frozen dessert.

Table 9.17 Role of ingredients in frozen desserts

Ingredient	Role
Sugar	Sugar is the most crucial of all ingredients in frozen desserts as the ratio of sugar to the overall mix determines the texture and the consistency of the preparation. Too much sugar in the mix will prevent freezing and the mixture will not become firm whereas low concentration of sugar will result in a product that is not very smooth and has large ice crystals. Sugar is responsible for smoothness of the frozen dessert.
	Usually 18 to 20 percent of the weight of the mixture should be sugar, but this can change with the addition of other ingredients in the mixture that also would contain certain amount of sugar. In case of sorbets, the amount of sugar is even more crucial as there is no cream or milk. In those cases, it is important to determine the density of the sugar in the mixture, which is measured with the help of a *saccharometer*. Density of sugar syrup is measured in *Brix* or *Baume*.
Eggs	Eggs are used in various forms in frozen desserts. Egg yolks are commonly used in ice creams, whereas egg whites are used in the preparation of sorbets and some other frozen desserts. Egg whites are sometimes whipped with sugar to form meringues that give a smooth texture to sorbets. Eggs also help in emulsifying the mixture, thereby producing smooth texture in ice creams. Egg whites in sorbets trap water molecules by forming a thin film around them thereby preventing the crystals from being formed in the mixture.
Milk and other dairy products	Usually milk of high fat content is used in making ice creams and desserts, unless the ice creams are specific to certain dietary requirements. Other kinds of dairy products such as skimmed milk, buttermilk, and yoghurts are also used to produce frozen desserts. Each of these dairy products yields a product with a characteristic texture and flavour.
	Cream of rather high fat content is used in frozen desserts and should never be boiled along with milk. Boiling the cream would result in melting of fat which will surface out during the cooling process and would precipitate out when churned in the freezer. The proportion of cream to milk is usually 25 to 30 percent.
Starch	Many kinds of starch are sometimes used for adding base and texture to frozen desserts. The most commonly used starch is custard powder but it can vary with the type of ice cream. In some cases, rice powder is also used to thicken the mixture. Starch works on the same principle that it binds all the water molecules together to form a homogeneous mass which produces a smooth textured ice cream. One has to be careful in adding starch to the mixture as too much of starch will make the ice cream bulky and heavy.

(Contd)

Table 9.17 (Contd)

Ingredient	Role
Stabilisers	Stabilisers play a pivotal role, especially in the making of ice creams on a commercial scale. Though products such as fat and eggs act as natural stabilisers, there are a range of chemicals that are used as stabilisers in the commercial production of frozen desserts. The main function of stabilisers is that they hold the dessert molecules together and do not let them melt away easily. The ice cream thus retains its shape and texture for longer duration as compared to those without any. Many natural ingredients such as *xanthin*, *guar* gum, and gelatine, are used as stabilisers in ice cream production.
Emulsifiers	As the name suggests, an emulsifier is an agent that helps the mix to come together and impart homogeneity to the product by preventing the formation of ice crystals during the freezing process. Apart from the range of natural stabilisers, such as eggs and starch, chemical emulsifiers are used in combination with stabilisers to obtain a smooth and airy product. Home-churned ice creams lack volume, but the taste and mouth feel is rich and flavoursome; that is the reason many fine dining establishments serve a range of home-churned ice creams and frozen desserts. However, there are many people who find home-made ice creams not up to the mark because of their comparison with commercially made ice creams that use stabilisers and emulsifiers to create foamy and airy product.
Butter	Unsalted fresh dairy butter is sometimes used in French ice creams. The fat in ice creams is responsible for giving it smoothness and a rich mouth feel. One has to be careful in adding fat to recipes because even cream has an amount of fat that surfaces as butter fat from the churning process. Too much fat in an ice cream would congeal up together during the churning process to form tiny lumps, which would make the ice cream granular and spoil its texture. On the other hand, the right amount of fat in ice cream prevents water molecules from coming together, thereby resulting in a smooth texture.
Flavours	Many kinds of flavours can be added to the basic ice cream mixture (refer steps involved in preparing basic ice cream). Flavours in frozen desserts should be added in adequate large quantities, otherwise, one would feel very little taste because when frozen desserts are consumed they numb the taste buds on the tongue. On the contrary, too much flavour would spoil the taste of the frozen dessert. Scrapings of vanilla pods, melted chocolate, chocolate chips, cookie dough, caramel drops, fudges, fruits, and purees are the most common flavourings added to frozen desserts. Creativity and style of menu is the key to flavouring a frozen dessert. Many a speciality restaurants have taken a step further and made a combination of ice creams such as bacon ice cream and smoked salmon ice cream.

Equipment Used in the Production of Frozen Desserts

Apart from the ice cream churning machine, there are many more tools and equipment that are used in the production of frozen desserts. As desserts are highly prone to bacterial contamination, it is of utmost importance that health and hygienic standards are maintained while preparing ice creams. It is also extremely necessary that each equipment is properly washed and sanitized before use. Various kinds of equipment used in preparing frozen desserts are as follows:

- Hand-crank ice cream machines
- Vertical freezing machines
- Horizontal freezing machines

- Continuous freezing machines
- Bombe mould
- Saccharometer
- Vermicelli press
- Ice cream containers
- Ice cream scooper

Smaller models of vertical freezing machines for home use are also available in the market where the machine can be hand cranked or it can work on automatic principle, wherein the jar is placed inside a cavity where ice is filled and the jar moves whilst the surrounding ice helps in freezing the ice cream. Models of hand-crank ice cream machine for domestic use are also available in the market.

Storage and Service of Frozen Desserts

Storage and service of frozen desserts is of prime importance. Water freezes at 0°C. Thus, freezing temperatures start from −1°C. But ice creams and other frozen desserts must be stored at much lower temperatures to get the right texture and consistency. Once a frozen dessert is prepared, it should be rapidly frozen to avoid melting otherwise ice crystals would form in the frozen dessert. Ice creams and sorbets are stored at a temperature between −18°C and −20°C. However, before serving it is important to move the ice cream to a temperature of −10°C to −11°C. This temperature will ensure that the ice creams and sorbets are soft to serve.

One must always use an ice cream scoop to serve an ice cream or a sorbet. A scoop is used for scraping the ice cream until the mixture rolls to a ball in the scoop. For large banquet operations, ice creams can be scooped in advance, put on a base such as a small piece of sponge to secure the ice cream in its place. The batch can then be frozen and removed just before service. Sorbets also can be pre-portioned in chilled glasses and stored in the freezer.

> **CHEF'S TIP**
> Never refreeze a melted or soft ice cream, as it can form large crystals. Instead, use this ice cream to prepare cold milkshakes and smoothies.

SUMMARY

Dessert is an integral part of any meal and it is, thus, very important to focus on its presentation as well as taste. Since it is the last meal on the menu, it is important for chefs to create an everlasting impression on the guest's mind. In this chapter, the primary objective was to let the students have a thorough understanding about various kinds of desserts. Though the broader classification is hot, cold and frozen desserts, each of these categories have further classifications based on the ingredients used.

The classification of desserts is explained with the help of tables so that it is easy for students to see the difference at a glance. Each of these categories have been discussed in detail under various sub-headings.

In this chapter, we also emphasised on presentation of the desserts, both in à la carte as well on the buffet. Factors important for presenting desserts were also listed and explained in detail so that students can understand why a dessert is presented in a particular way.

The modern approach to buffet dessert was also given in detail. Earlier, the desserts on buffet were presented in large platters and bowls with a whole range of decorative items on the buffet. The modern style is to be minimalistic and yet classy. The desserts are presented in individual platters and the guests can choose what they want to have. When the desserts are presented whole, it tends to look messy after a few guests have selected their portions. Individually presented dessert, thus, helps to keep the appeal of the buffet clean and fresh at all times.

We also discussed about creating a buffet matrix that would help the chefs to plan balanced cyclic menus for their buffets.

Various kinds of ice creams such as French ice cream, American ice cream, *gelato*, ice milk, and frozen yoghurt were also discussed. The various steps involved in the production of ice creams and factors that need to be kept in mind while preparing them were explained as well.

A whole range of still-frozen desserts, such as *parfaits* and *bombes* were discussed in detail. The concept of American and French *parfait* and the difference between the two were also briefly explained. Step-by-step production of *parfait* was also discussed.

Various kinds of classical bombes are illustrated in tabular form for easy understanding. This chapter also discussed various kinds of other classical frozen desserts such as baked Alaska, *cassata*, *kulfi*, fried ice cream, and various classical sundaes and coupes. Lastly, equipment and instruments used in the production of frozen desserts were also listed.

KEY TERMS

Almond touille Garnish made from touille paste

American ice cream An ice cream made without the addition of eggs

Angelica Candied stems of angelica plant used commonly in desserts

Assiette French for a plate

Bailey's Irish cream A kind of liqueur, often used in confectionery

Baked Alaska A frozen dessert made by covering assorted ice cream in sponge and then covering it with meringue prior to baking, also known as Norwegian omelette or *soufflé omelette surprise*

Baume See Brix

Blow torch An equipment attached to a butane cylinder or any gas source, which emits a sharp narrow flame often used for spot colouring of sugar as in case of crème brûlée

Bombe A kind of multi-layered still-frozen dessert set in a dome-shaped mould

Brioche Yeast-leavened dough enriched with butter and eggs

Brix A unit of measuring density of sugar, it is measured in percentage

Buttermilk The liquid obtained after butter is churned out or separated from cream

Candied fruit A term used for commercially available dried fruits candied in sugar

Caribbean rum A white-coloured rum from Caribbean islands

Cassata Napoletana A classical cassata from Italy

Continuous freezers Ice cream freezers put to commercial use

Crème anglaise Made by cooking milk, sugar, and egg yolks in a bain-marie until the sauce coats the back of the spoon

Crème frangipani Made by creaming butter, sugar, eggs, and almond powder to a paste like consistency, also known as almond paste

Curaçao A blue-coloured orange-flavoured liqueur from France

Dariole mould Another name for savarin or a ring-shaped mould

Docked A term used to denote the pricking of lined tart or pie with a docker or a fork to prevent the pastry from shrinking

Emulsifiers Natural and chemical ingredients used to help frozen desserts attain a smooth and creamy texture and retain homogeneity

Falooda Noodle-shaped vermicelli made with a paste of cornflour and water cooked until transparent. The paste is passed through a press to obtain strands of desired thickness, it is a common accompaniment with *kulfi* in India

Feather icing A kind of design created with the help of a toothpick

Hot and Cold Desserts

Finger biscuit A sponge batter that is piped like fingers and baked in oven until crisp, also known as sponge fingers or *savoiardi*

French ice cream Ice cream made with egg yolks

Gelato Italian ice cream made with little or no cream at all

Guar gum Gum obtained from the endosperm of *guar* beans, used as a stabiliser

Helado frito Fried ice cream from Mexico

Horizontal freezer An ice cream freezer in which the tube moves horizontally while being frozen

Hydrometer An instrument used to measure the specific gravity (or relative density) of liquids, i.e., the ratio of the density of the liquid to the density of water

Ice milk A term used for ice creams made with low fat content

Key lime A kind of lime usually found in America

Kirsch Liqueur obtained from cherries

Kirsch liqueur Cherry-flavoured liqueur

Liquid glucose A kind of sweet sticky and viscous liquid obtained by treating corn syrup with acid

Maple syrup A sweet syrup obtained from maple trees often served as an accompaniment with pancakes and waffles

Maraschino A type of red cherry

Mascarpone cheese Creamy cheese from Italy often used for desserts

Maturing A term in ice-cream making that involves allowing the ice cream mixture to rest in a freezer for at least 24 hours, so that the proteins mix homogeneously with liquid ingredients

Meringue A type of dessert in which egg whites are whipped along with sugar until a thick creamy product is obtained

Norwegian omelette See Baked Alaska

Overrun A term used to denote the amount of air incorporated into the frozen desserts while churning

Panada A thick starchy paste of milk or any liquid with starch cooked together

Parfait A still-frozen dessert made by whipping eggs and combining with whipped cream and various flavours

Peruvian cream Another name for baked custard served in the pot itself

Phyllo pastry A Greek preparation comprising thin sheets of flour dough, it is used in preparation of both sweet and savoury products and also known as filo

Pineapple upside down Dessert made by lining a cake mould with pineapple slices dredged in sugar and filled up with a cake sponge mix and baked. This dessert is served upside down to display the pineapple, hence the name

Praline Caramelized sugar and almonds, crushed into a coarse texture

Rabri An Indian dessert obtained by reducing milk until it becomes thick and coats the back of a spoon

Red currants Small red berries with a sweet and sour taste

Rhubarb A plant, the stems of which are used in desserts as they have a sweet and sour taste

Ricotta cheese A type of soft cheese from Italy, resembles fresh cottage cheese

Sabayon A sauce based on a foamy mixture of egg yolks whipped with small amounts of sugar and liquid over a bain-marie

Saccharometer Tool used to measure the density of the sugar in a liquid

Salamander An equipment that radiates heat from above, commonly used for gratinating

Sherbet Water and flavourings sweetened with sugar

Shooter A liquid served as drink along with desserts in small quantities

Sorbet Served as a course in French classical menu, it is churned water and sugar with flavourings, also known as *sorbetto* in Italian

Soufflé omelette surpris See Baked Alaska

Stabilisers Natural and chemical ingredients that prevent the ice creams from melting away rapidly

Swiss roll Dessert made by spreading a sponge sheet with filling and then tightly rolling the sheets to form a roulade. When sliced, the slices depict a pinwheel design

Tapioca A kind of tuber, the starch of which is commonly used for culinary purposes

Vertical freezer An ice cream freezer in which the tube moves vertically while being frozen

Water ice See sorbet

Xanthan gum A kind of polysaccharide made by fermenting glucose or sucrose with bacteria

Yorkshire pudding A savoury product made with flour batter, baked and served with roast beef

OBJECTIVE TYPE QUESTIONS

1. What do you understand by the term overrun? How does it impact the texture of the ice cream?
2. What is the principle behind the churn-freeze method?
3. What is the difference between gelato and sorbet?
4. What factors would you keep in mind while preparing the basic ice cream mixture?
5. What do you understand by the term pudding? Give a few examples.
6. Explain the use of saccharometer while preparing frozen desserts.
7. Differentiate between the following.
   a. Sorbet and granita
   b. Parfait and kulfi
   c. Cassata and bombe
8. What is Baked Alaska?
9. What is the difference between cabinet pudding and queen's pudding?
10. What are sponge-based puddings? Give a few examples.
11. How are hot soufflés different from cold soufflés?
12. What are pre-plated desserts?
13. What factors guide the presentation of pre-plated desserts?
14. Describe Peach Melba and pears belle helene.

ESSAY TYPE QUESTIONS

1. What are the two most common methods involved in production of frozen desserts? Explain.
2. Explain the role of sugar in frozen desserts. Why is it so crucial, especially in case of sorbets?
3. What is the role of eggs in frozen desserts?
4. Name and describe at least five classical bombes and their components.
5. How are desserts classified?
6. Describe at least three different kinds of puddings made with different bases.
7. Explain the components of hot soufflé and the role played by each of these.
8. List at least five critical factors that should be kept in mind while making hot soufflés.
9. Describe at least three deep-fried desserts and their methods of preparation.
10. List and describe the components of flans, pies, or tarts.
11. Describe custard-based desserts and their applications.
12. Describe the components of a plated dessert.
13. What is the importance of classical desserts? Give examples of how you can present at least three classical desserts in modern style.
14. What is a buffet matrix? How does it help in making balanced menus?

ACTIVITY

1. In groups of five, conduct a market survey of hotels and speciality restaurants and make a list of various kinds of frozen desserts served by them. Further, make a note of commercially available and home-churned ice creams and share with the rest of the group.
2. In groups of three or four, make at least two sundaes or coupes with sauces, garnish, and accompaniments. Present the dishes to other groups and get your product evaluated and critiqued. Make standard recipes of the same and distribute to everybody.
3. In groups of five, undertake a market survey of hotels and speciality restaurants and note the components of a dessert buffet. Observe how the desserts are balanced with regard to textures, temperatures, etc. Record your observations and share your findings with other groups.
4. Divide the class into groups and prepare a range of hot puddings using different bases as explained in Table 9.1. Compare the taste, textures, and flavours and observe what desserts can be served hot or cold. Share your learnings with other groups and record them.

5. In groups of three to four, prepare a rotational menu for 10 days with a total of 12 desserts in each. Devise your own category and place desserts under the same. Critique each other's menu with regard to balance in flavours, colours, textures, shapes, and taste.
6. In groups of three or four, use the information from the book and prepare health ice creams with dietary requirements. Present to the other groups and get your product evaluated and critiqued. Make standard recipes of the same and distribute to everybody.
7. Take a field trip to an ice cream factory in your area and make a report on the processing of the various kinds of ice creams and other frozen desserts.

10 Sugar Confections

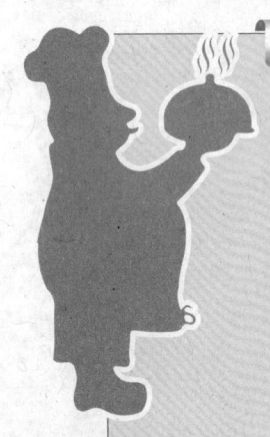

LEARNING OBJECTIVES

After reading this chapter, you should be able to
- understand the range of uses of sugar for making showpieces
- cook sugar to its various stages and be able to differentiate one stage from another
- boil the sugar following the salient features to create clear sugar syrup for sugar work and other uses
- differentiate between marshmallows, gum paste, caramels, toffees, and fudges
- prepare sugar products such as nougatine, honeycomb, rock sugar, and candies
- prepare the basic sugar showpiece by using the techniques mentioned in the book

INTRODUCTION

There are two broad sections in confectionary. One that prepares cakes and pastries and the other that prepares chocolates and candies. The former is also known as *bakers confections* and the latter is referred to as *sugar confections*. Since we have already discussed chocolate in Chapter 2, in this chapter, we will discuss confections prepared from sugar and its by-products.

A range of confections are prepared by sugar and its by-products, which will be discussed in detail in this chapter. Confections are prepared by boiling different types of sugar to produce transparent and brittle products that are classified under boiled or pulled sweets, whilst the same boiled sugar can be mixed and kneaded to prepare fondants which are yet another type of sugar confections. The sugar can also be combined with other products such as milk solids to prepare caramels, toffee, and fudges, or whisked to incorporate air and be stabilised with gelatin to make marshmallows. Thick sugar syrups can be jellified with gelatin or pectin to create sweet candies such as *pate de fruits*. Thus, we can see that a simple ingredient like sugar can be used in a variety of ways to create a range of sugar confections in pastry kitchen.

The art of sugar confectionary dates back to 3,500 years ago and was popularised by the Egyptians. Most of the sugar confectionary in those times was prepared using honey and in later centuries, sugar cane that was used popularly in India and China was being used by various confectioners around the world.

Sugar in pastry and bakery is the most important ingredient. It not only adds taste to the product, but also plays a very important role in textures and is used as an ingredient to make decorations and sculptures. These days it is a dying art as it requires a lot of skill and time apart from the environmental conditions. The sugar is cooked to a particular temperature and then it is pulled, casted, and even blown to create spectacular showpieces that are used as decorations and props on buffet (Fig. 10.1). These days this art is limited to pastry competitions and only a few festive occasions. It takes many years of practice, patience, and dedication to master this art. We will discuss the usage of sugar for creating these masterpieces in the chapter.

In Chapter 2, we read about different kinds of sweetening agents and sugars used in bakery and confectionary and that for making sugar sculptures and other clear candies, it is important to use breakfast sugar as it does not contain impurities and yields a clear solution. When the art of sugar refining was not so advanced, chefs used granulated sugar but clarified it with a mixture of acid and milk. The protein present in milk would curdle because of the acid present and would form a scum, which was carefully skimmed out resulting in a clear solution. However, these days chefs commonly use isomalt sugar to make sugar showpieces as it is easier to work with and also gives a clearer product.

STAGES OF SUGAR AND ITS USES

Working with sugar is a combination of art and science. We could say more of science unless the chef is creatively assembling a sugar sculpture. The boiling of sugar is very crucial to making products in confectionary as with a change in every two degrees of boiling sugar, the texture of the sugar mixture changes, which may or may not be suitable for a particular usage. If a recipe calls for sugar syrup to be at 103°C, then it cannot be less or more as it will impact the final product. For example, whilst making a French macaroon, the temperature of the sugar has to be around 121°C. If it is less than that, the macaroons will have a sticky base and if the temperature is more than that, the base of the macaroons will become hollow and chewy.

Not only does the temperature of the sugar impact a product, but even the density of the sugar syrup can play a major role in textures of certain pastry products such as ice creams, sorbets, jellies, and jams. For this purpose, the density of the sugar is measured in a unit called *baume or brix*, by using a hand held device called *refractometer*. The device is also known as saccharometer.

Let us look at the various stages of sugar as used in confectionary and how to test them in Table 10.1.

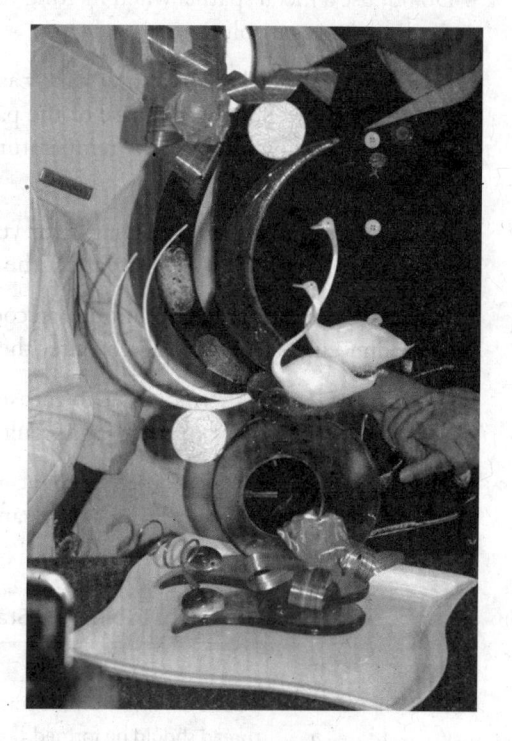

Fig. 10.1 A sugar showpiece

Above the temperature of 165°C, the sugar will start to attain a caramel colour and at 170-175°C, it will burn to a black colour, often referred to as *black jack* in confectionary terms. It was customary to use the black jack in bakery and pastry goods to give a dark colour to the products, but with more developed research and findings, it was established that burnt sugar can be harmful to health and can be carcinogenic.

We will discuss each sugar stage when we discuss the products made with sugar in the coming sections of the chapter. Sugar can thus be used for creating a number of products such as artistic showpieces, syrups, sauces, and bases for many desserts depending on the degree of temperature that it is cooked to. It is very important to treat sugar in the most appropriate manner for desired results. Whilst cooking sugar, the below mentioned precautions should be followed.

> **CHEF'S TIP**
> The density of the sugar changes with the temperature, therefore, the density of the sugar solution must be checked at 20°C for best results.

- Always use a clean pot of substantial depth as this will allow the expansion of sugar syrup, especially if the recipe calls for addition of any ingredient such as baking soda as in case of making honeycombs, discussed in the later part of this chapter.

- Preferably use a copper pan as it is a good conductor of heat and will help in evenly cooking the sugar.

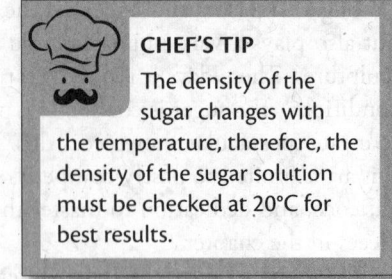

- Always start by cooking sugar on a low temperature and then increase the heat. The sugar syrup is best boiled at high heat.

- Always use a brush, dipped in water to wipe off any sugar crystals that accumulate on the side of the pan as it will colour the sugar.

- Do not use a metal spatula when melting sugar as this can allow the sugar crystals to crystalize thereby spoiling the sugar solution.

- Keep a shallow bowl of cold water handy as this will help you to arrest the cooking temperature of the sugar syrup, by allowing the base of the pan to be submerged in water. If this is not done, then the carry over cooking can raise the temperature by a few degrees, which can make the sugar unusable for a particular product.

- Always use breakfast or castor sugar for your sugar solutions as grain sugar contains impurities and icing sugar has starch which can affect the final texture of the syrup.

- Usage of electric hot plates or induction cook tops is preferred as the heat source from gas burners can cause uneven heating and thereby alter the texture of the sugar syrup.

- Always use a sugar thermometer to measure the exact degree of sugar temperature especially when working with sugar for making sugar sculptures as one needs sugar at a particular temperature.

- Heating sugar below a specified degree can make the sugar soft and pliable and not suitable for the intended use, while overheating of the same can result in hardening of the sugar, again not suitable for the intended use.

Table 10.1 Stages of sugar and ways to test

Stage of sugar	Way to test
107°C, Thread	Place a dry finger on the surface of the syrup and when you join the finger with the thumb, a thread should be formed.
112°C, Strong thread	Follow the aforementioned steps and this time the thread will be thicker.
118°C, Soft ball	Chill your fingers by placing in cold water, and place the finger on the surface of the syrup. When you join the fingers and roll them together, the syrup should set into a soft ball shape. One has to be very careful whilst doing this as the syrup is very hot. The other way is to pour a few drops of sugar syrup into cold water and then pick up the sugar ball and roll between fingers.
125°C, Hard ball	The syrup sets more firmly when dipped into cold water. The method of testing is the same as in case of soft ball and the only difference is that here the syrup will be harder than the soft ball.

Table 10.1 (Contd)

Stage of sugar	Way to test
140°C, Soft crack	The syrup will harden when dipped in cold water. When the dipped sugar syrup is rolled between fingers, you will feel that the sugar is harder than the hard ball and is almost solid to touch.
150°C, Crack	When the solution is cold, the sugar will break and crumble.
155°C, Hard crack	When the solution is cold, the sugar will crumble and have a very slight tinge (amber).

PRODUCTS MADE FROM SUGAR

A range of products are made by using sugar. Since such products are sweeter than usual, most of these are used on festivities and special occasions. Let us discuss a few products made from sugar in detail.

Sugar Syrup

One of the most crucial things of pastry kitchen and yet one of the most complicated to prepare is sugar syrup. Good sugar syrup must be at a density of 30 B°. If you do not have a saccharometer, then the thumb rule is to follow the given recipe for making sugar syrup.

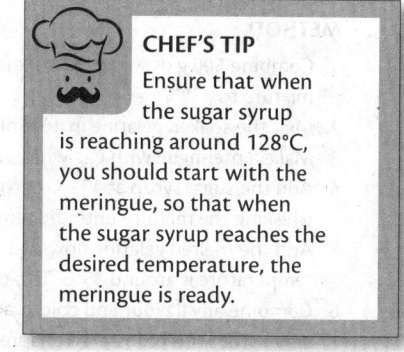

> **CHEF'S TIP**
> Ensure that when the sugar syrup is reaching around 128°C, you should start with the meringue, so that when the sugar syrup reaches the desired temperature, the meringue is ready.

Simple sugar syrups are used as moistening agents in cakes and pastries and are also used for preparing sorbets and other products.

Sugar Syrup

Ingredients
Sugar 1350 g
Water 1 kg

METHOD
1. Mix water and sugar and slowly heat the mixture until it comes to a boil.
2. Skim it if it contains any impurities and then store it at room temperature.
3. Add a few lime wedges or slices of whole orange to give it a flavour, if required.

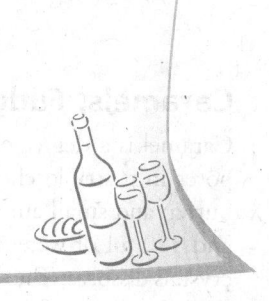

Marshmallows

Marshmallows are sugar confections that are produced and eaten mostly during Christmas. These are loved by children and can be eaten as they are or can be roasted over fire to give them that melting and charred flavour. Mallow is a kind of plant that is native to Europe and North Africa and often grows in marsh lands. The Egyptians used to use the sap from the mallow plants as medicine for curing throat infections. The French pastry chefs transformed this syrup into a delectable confection, popularly known as marshmallow.

Marshmallows are prepared by whipping sugar, gelatin, and egg whites until foamy and then either piping the mixture or setting it in a tray dusted with cornstarch. After 12-14 hours, it is cut into desired shapes and coated with a mixture of icing sugar, cornflour, and flavours. Marshmallows are very popular in US and are eaten with ice creams, in desserts, or as they are. Some recipes utilize only sugar syrup and gelatin and no egg whites. It is important to focus on the temperature of the sugar syrup when making marshmallows. Let us now look at a basic recipe of preparing marshmallow.

Marshmallow

Ingredients
Water 150 ml
Castor sugar 500 g
Liquid glucose 75 g
Gelatin 25 g (soaked in 150 ml water)
Egg whites 175 g
Castor sugar 25 g
Colour and flavour As desired

METHOD

1. Combine 500 g of sugar, 150 ml of water, and 75 g of liquid glucose in a clean pot and cook the mixture to 138°C.
2. Melt the soaked gelatine in 150 ml of water over a double boiler until clear.
3. Make a meringue with egg whites and 25 g sugar in a clean bowl.
4. Add the sugar syrup at 138°C in the meringue, pouring slowly from the sides, whilst continuously whisking the mixture until the temperature of the mixture comes down to 60°C.
5. Add the melted gelatine now and continue whisking until the mixture is white in colour and the temperature is around 35°C. This can approximately take 10-15 mins.
6. Combine any flavour and colour at this stage and either pipe with a round nozzle on to trays that are dusted with cornstarch or spread them in a mould dusted with cornstarch, and allow to rest overnight.
7. Cut into desired shapes and coat with a mixture of icing sugar and cornstarch, in equal proportions, when it has dried up and does not stick to fingers when touched.
8. Keep them covered in an airtight box and use as required.

Caramels, Fudges, and Toffee

Caramel is a degree of cooking of sugar to 170°C, however this stage of sugar is used for many purposes in pastry kitchen. It can be used for making caramelized sauces by adding a mixture of cream, butter, and small amount of cornstarch. For making caramel, 240 g of sugar, 120 g of liquid glucose, and 120 ml of water is combined and heated until all the sugar crystals dissolve. The sugar is then boiled; one should keep wiping the sides down of the pan with a brush dipped in water. As soon as the temperature is 170°C, the mixture is removed from the heat and the base of the pan is dipped in cold water to arrest the temperature.

The syrup can now be used for making various garnishes such as spun sugar or can be drizzled on a silpat in a criss cross fashion to yield sugar nest. The creativity will depend on your usage and ideas. At this stage, a few nuts such as almonds, hazelnuts, or pistachios can be dipped in the caramel and pulled out slowly yielding a long thin thread that can be trimmed at any length. These sugar pulled nuts can be used as a fancy garnish in desserts. The caramel can also be used for glazing éclairs and cakes such as *dobos torte* and even a few fruits can be glazed with it.

> **CHEF'S TIP**
> Whilst making toffee, arrange a ring shaped mould or a tray that is lined with cellophane paper. Allow the toffee to set overnight. Then invert the tray and peel of the cellophane. The toffee can now be cut with a slightly oiled knife into desired shapes. Once cut, it can be wrapped in cellophane paper.

If this caramel needs to be transformed into a sauce, boiled cream should be added to it as it will not cause the caramel to seize and thereby, result in the caramel frothing out of the pan. It should then be whisked with a whisk and butter should be blended in two to three stages, until a creamy and shiny sauce is obtained.

Toffees and fudges are created by cooking sugar, liquid glucose, cream, butter, and condensed milk to form a sticky and chewy product known as toffee. For toffee the mixture is cooked till 121°C and if it is cooked to around 128°C, then the resulting toffee is known as *stick jaws* as it clings to the teeth, when chewed.

Toffee can be transformed into fudge by adding extra fat such as peanut butter or by agitating the mixture with a whisk.

Candies

Candy is a term associated with sugar confections and refers to all the products made with boiled sugar, which is heated to a hard crack stage and beyond and then allowed to set with different flavours. The sugar can also be heated to 160°C and then allowed to cool down to 150°C, and then pulled and stretched and pulled again to make a shiny candy. Candies can be made in individual silicone moulds or can be pulled and stretched and woven over sticks. Items such as lollypops and caramelitos are all examples of sugar candies.

Fondant

Fondant is used for icing wedding cakes and many other confectionary products and is used as drizzling on top of Danish pastries and other pastries such as *mille feuille*. The handmade fondant is not as white as the readymade fondant commonly known as RTR, which is an abbreviation for *ready-to-roll fondant*.

Sugar when heated undergoes a chemical reaction. The sugar that is commonly used in confectionary is *sucrose*. Upon constant heating, the sucrose breaks down into simpler sugar compounds and this act is called *inversion of sugar*. The addition of an acid into sugar acts as a catalyst and increases the rate of inversion. It is because of this reason acids such as cream of tartar, citric acid, or lime juice are commonly used in sugar whilst boiling it. Let us look at the basic recipe for making fondant.

Fondant

Ingredients
Sugar 500 g
Liquid glucose 72 g or Cream of tartar 1 tsp
Water 178 ml

METHOD
1. Bring sugar and water to a boil and when the temperature reaches 105°C, add liquid glucose or cream of tartar and bring to boil on high temperature until the temperature comes to 115°C.
2. Grease a marble table lightly with around 2-3 ml of oil and pour the sugar syrup on to the greased marble table.
3. Sprinkle little cold water on it to prevent crystallization.
4. Allow the mixture to cool down to around 38-40°C.
5. Start to mix the syrup with a spatula once it cools down to the desired temperature. Make the shape of 8, whilst mixing until a thick mixture is obtained.
6. Knead the paste now until it comes together like dough and attains a shine.
7. Place it in a plastic wrap and store in a cool place until further use.

Gum Paste

Gum paste also commonly known as *pastillage* in French is made by combining icing sugar and gelatin to the consistency of a dough. Even though this dough is made from edible ingredients, it is rarely used for direct consumption. Instead, this paste is used for decoration purposes such as making showpieces, flowers, leaves, or any other geometrical structure that can be used in a display. The unique quality of this paste is that it dries out in a few hours to a brittle structure that can be joined to a sculpture or with each other with the help of royal icing (refer to Table 7.5 in Chapter 7).

The gum paste was traditionally made with a vegetable gum called *gum tragacanth* but nowadays, it is common to see gelatin being used for the same. Since this paste is used for making showpieces, it is important to keep it sparkling white in colour. In order to achieve this, one must work on a clean marble or stainless steel surface. Metals such as aluminium can cause a greying effect. Also, addition of lime juice or vinegar will help to bleach the sugar. After the paste is made, it must be used immediately or can be stored in a plastic wrap or damp cloth for up to a few hours.

Let us look at the basic recipe of gum paste.

Gum Paste

Ingredients
Icing sugar 1 kg
Cornflour 120 g
Gelatin powder 12 g / Soaked Gum tragacanth
Water 110 ml
Vinegar 10 ml

METHOD
1. Combine water and gelatine and allow the gelatine to swell. This process is often known as blooming.
2. Melt the mixture over double boiler, add vinegar and keep aside.
3. Sift icing sugar and cornflour together and combine with the liquid ingredients.
4. Knead the paste until it forms into dough. Keep kneading until the mixture is whitish in colour.
5. Remove from the dough mixer and use immediately. If you need to store the mixture, cover it with a damp cloth and use within a few hours.

Nougatine

Nougatine is a fairly easy product made with sugar and sliced almonds. The art is to caramelize the sugar to a clear amber colour and then add sliced almonds. Nougatine often resembles a peanut candy in India called *chick*. Nougatine finds its usage in many preparations in confectionary. It can be shaped to prepare sugar sculptures or can be used for decorating and garnishing a cake or pastry. Thinly rolled nougatine can be wrapped around a metal cone to make ice cream cones. The usage completely depends on the artistic skills of the chef. The nougat, when warm is pliable and can be moulded into various shapes. When cold, it turns brittle and then it can be crushed to a coarse texture and used on cakes and pastries. It can be even grounded into a paste often known as *praline paste*. Though one can use any kind of nut to make nougatine, almonds are used traditionally. Now, let us look at a simple recipe of making nougatine.

Nougatine

Ingredients
Castor sugar 700 g
Liquid glucose 250 g
Water 180 g
Sliced almonds 350 g

METHOD

1. Heat sugar and water and when it comes to a boil, add liquid glucose and heat until the sugar turns light amber in colour.
2. Remove from fire and add sliced almonds.
3. Mix well and pour onto a greased marble slab or on a silicone mat.
4. Allow it to come to a temperature of 50-60°C and then place another sheet of silicone mat on top and roll with a rolling pin. Alternately, the rolling pin can be oiled before use. The nougat is now ready to be moulded or cut into desired shapes.

Rock Sugar

As the name suggests, this product is so called as it looks like a porous rock or a coral. Rock sugar is commonly used in sugar sculptures and can also be broken into smaller pieces and used as a garnish for desserts. The technique of making rock sugar is very simple. The sugar syrup is heated to almost soft crack and then a small amount of royal icing is mixed into the sugar syrup. The mixing of royal icing in hot sugar syrup causes the mixture to rise up like lava from a volcano. The mix is immediately poured into a mould lined with aluminium foil and allowed to set for 30 minutes to 1 hour. The rock sugar can now be taken out and broken into pieces and used as desired. Please find below the basic recipe of rock sugar.

CHEF'S TIP
The bowl is lined with aluminium foil for easy removal. If you have silicone mould, it can also be used and in that case you do not have to use aluminium foil.
To make coloured rock sugar, use coloured royal icing.

Rock Sugar

Ingredients
Sugar 500 g
Water 185 g
Royal icing 25 g

METHOD

1. Combine sugar and water in a pot and boil the syrup, until a temperature of 138°C can be seen on the sugar thermometer.
2. Remove the pan from the heat source and immerse the base of the pan in cold water to stop the temperature from rising.
3. Add the royal icing and mix thoroughly and quickly with a spatula and immediately pour this mixture into a mould. The mixture will continue to rise in the mould.
4. Allow it to set and when cool, break it into desired shapes and size.

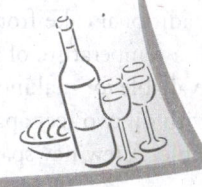

Honeycomb

Honeycomb is very similar to rock sugar as it resembles a sponge with many air bubbles trapped inside, but the texture is crunchy and brittle thereby making it a great snack. It can also be used as a garnish on desserts. In this case the mixture of sugar, honey, water is heated up to 148°C, which is hard crack stage. When the mixture reaches the temperature, the base of the pot is immediately lowered in cold water for a couple of seconds to arrest the temperature. Then, baking soda is added and the mixture is whisked immediately with a whisk. As the mixture starts to foam up, it is quickly poured into a mould lined with parchment paper and allowed to set for an hour. After that, it can be cut into desired pieces. Honeycomb is used immediately or stored in airtight containers.

Jam

Also known as *confiture* in French, it is a product made with fresh fruits and sugar. Pectin, a natural enzyme present in a citrus fruit, helps in setting the fruit to a jelly consistency. Pectin is also available in powdered form and must be mixed with an equal amount of castor sugar, and this mixture should be added to the fruit mix, only when the mixture reaches 50°C. Certain fruits such as strawberry, apples, and guava are rich in pectin and hence, good for making jams and jellies.

When pectin is added to the mixture, the jam is ready when the temperature reaches around 103°C. Following is a basic recipe of making jam.

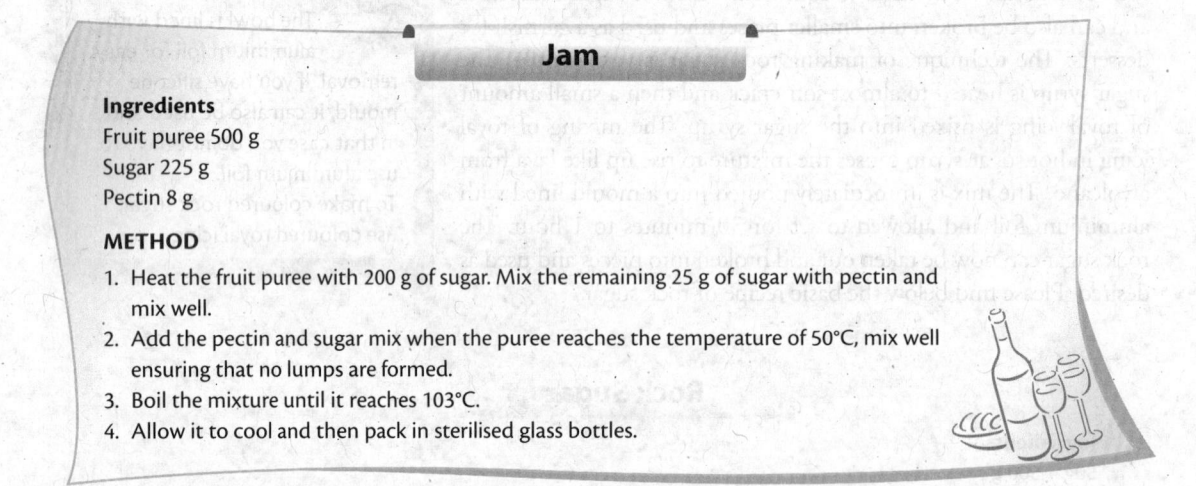

Jam

Ingredients
Fruit puree 500 g
Sugar 225 g
Pectin 8 g

METHOD

1. Heat the fruit puree with 200 g of sugar. Mix the remaining 25 g of sugar with pectin and mix well.
2. Add the pectin and sugar mix when the puree reaches the temperature of 50°C, mix well ensuring that no lumps are formed.
3. Boil the mixture until it reaches 103°C.
4. Allow it to cool and then pack in sterilised glass bottles.

Spun Sugar

As the name suggests, the sugar has an appearance of small threads that look like as if a yarn has been spun. It is a very commonly used garnish on desserts and cakes, especially croquembouche, which is a traditional cake from France. One has to be very careful whilst making this garnish as very hot sugar at a temperature of nearly 160°C is used for making it. Though these days table top machines are also available for making spun sugar, traditionally it was made by fixing two wooden or metal sticks greased with oil two feet apart on a table in such a manner that a feet and a half of the stick pointed out of the table. A few newspapers were kept on the floor to collect any dripping from the hot sugar syrup.

The sugar is boiled to around 165°C and then removed from the heat source. The base of the pan is then dipped immediately in cold water to arrest the temperature. A wire tool, maybe an old whisk which has its front cut and looks like a broom is dipped in the sugar and flicked on the wooded rods in a fast and quick motion, allowing the sugar to form many thread like structures. When enough sugar has been spun, the spun sugar is carefully removed and used immediately. Unfortunately, this garnish cannot be stored for long as it absorbs moisture and becomes soft and sticky.

Pate De Fruits

A French term for paste of fruits, *pate de fruits* is a sugar and jelly confection that allows the fruit puree to set into a firm jelly, which can be eaten as a sweet snack or served as petit fours. Pate de fruits are commonly eaten on festive occasions such as Christmas and are popular amongst people of all ages. These utilize natural pectin present in fruits and also extra pectin is added to the fruit puree, which is mixed with sugar and cooked to 106°C. This mixture is then poured into a slightly greased container or silicone moulds to make pate de fruits. It takes around a couple of hours to set and when it cools down, it is cut into assorted shapes and dredged in granulated sugar. Let us now look at a basic recipe of pate de fruits.

Pate De Fruits

Ingredients
Fruit puree 390 g
Citric acid 4 g
Water 5 ml
Sugar 525 g
Pectin powder 10 g
Liquid glucose 150 g
Granulated sugar for coating As required

METHOD
1. Combine around 50 g of sugar and pectin and mix together until well blended.
2. Mix the remaining sugar along with liquid glucose and fruit puree and heat until the temperature reaches 50°C. Now add the pectin and continue boiling until the temperature reads 106°C on the sugar thermometer.
3. Remove from the heat source and add citric acid dissolved in water.
4. Pour the mixture into a silicone mould or individual pate de fruit moulds and allow it to cool.
5. Cut into desired shapes, when it sets firm and roll in granulated sugar.

ART OF SUGAR WORK

Sugar sculpturing was a much practiced art a few decades ago, but it soon began to die owing to the immense labour, technique, and patience involved, also its usage on buffets reduced due to its shorter shelf life because of the hygroscopic nature of sugar, wherein it can absorb moisture and deteriorate easily. Then it became a piece of art that was only produced on very special occasions or in pastry competitions, which allowed the pastry chefs to display their creativity and passion for bakery and pastry.

Today this art has revived due to technological advancement and types of sugar available. One such sugar is isomalt. This sugar is invert in nature and hence, does not crystalize easily. There are many types of isomalts available in the market, and if you want to use it for edible garnishes, then you must use the food grade quality only.

It takes years of dedication and perseverance to master this art, not to mention a few burns along the way. In this chapter, we will read about the basic techniques involved in sugar work. It is important to follow the salient features listed about boiling sugar in the early part of this chapter.

Now let us discuss the role of sugar in making sugar sculptures and other decorations. Making artistic showpieces is an art that is practiced for a number of years by budding pastry chefs. It requires an eye for creating artistic visions and a huge amount of patience and understanding of sugar and how it reacts to heat. In the following sections, we will discuss the basic techniques such as sugar boiling, casting, pulled sugar, and blown sugar along with a few garnishes that can be made by using these techniques.

Preparation Prior to Commencing Sugar Work

Making an artistic showpiece of sugar is an art and requires a methodical approach. Each and every step in this methodical process is crucial to producing a quality product. Selection of sugar, selection of right utensils and even the work surfaces will play a pivotal role in your product. Whilst working with sugar, the temperature of the syrup will be as high as 160°C and hence it is crucial to be safe to avoid any sugar burns. One has to make certain important preparations before starting to make sugar art. It is therefore important to do a few preparations beforehand so that when the sugar syrup reaches 160°C, we do not waste time in arranging things as the syrup will become hard and the process of cooking sugar will have to be repeated all over again.

This section discusses the preparations to be made in this regard.

Pans for boiling sugar Although it is recommended that copper pans be used for boiling sugar, but in case of non-availability, one must ensure that a pan is of high quality and thick bottom. Thin bottom pans may result in burning of the sugar at the base. The pan could be of stainless steel, enamel, or even brass. It is important that the pan should be such that it can be cleaned and maintained easily. The use of aluminium pans should be avoided, as they can cause discolouration of sugar crystals. The pans must be scrupulously cleaned before being used to boil sugar.

Marble slab A marble slab or a table top with light coloured granite is important for sugar work. The slab must be very clean and free from any dirt particles that will hamper the clarity of sugar work. The marble must be cleaned, wiped, and very lightly greased with vegetable oil. It should always be ensured that the slab is cold as warm marble slab will aid in sticking of the sugar to its surface.

Other equipment Other necessary equipment includes a metal scraper for turning the sugar syrup in order to cool it down to required consistency. Sugar thermometers, scissors, knife, brush, and cold water are also required to wipe the sides of the sugar syrup whilst it boils. Spirit or gas burner may also be needed, if an alternative heat source such as a gas stove or blow torch is not available.

Leaf moulds These come in many shapes and sizes and are useful for producing neat looking leaves quickly. However, moulds are not fundamental equipment as many leaves are made without moulds.

Silicone mould Silicone rubber in liquid form is available from modelling or craft shops, can be used for making leaf, face, bottle, or various other shapes of your choice. Also there is a range of readymade silicone moulds available in stores for preparing sugar showpieces.

Storage containers Containers are used to store sugar work until ready for use and should be of good quality plastic. Before using, a little silica gel or lime crystals should be placed at the bottom of the containers, and then they should be lined with foil paper.

Heat lamp This is essential if you want to create pulled sugar as it will help to maintain the temperature of the sugar required for the desired texture. They are available in almost all culinary stores across the world, but in case of non-availability you could use an infra-red lamp from one of the medical stores, which is often used for providing heat during physiotherapy. It should be ensured that the bulb has a minimum wattage of 250 Watts so that it can help to keep the sugar temperature at 70-75°C.

Blowing pump Also known as sugar pump, it is an apparatus which has a metal tube attached to a hand operated pump, quite similar to the blood pressure measuring apparatus. It is an art to blow sugar to create hollow structures to make fish, fruits, and other figures. These figures can then be sprayed with a spray colour machine to give more artistic effects.

Blow fan A small air blowing fan is used to constantly cool the sugar especially when it is blown to create figures. It can be a small table top fan that does not have too much of pressure.

Silicone mats Silicone mats are used to hold on the sugar whilst it is being worked upon. Care must be taken to keep these clean and a silpat should be kept separately to be used for sugar work only and not for any other bakery purpose.

Ingredients for Sugar Work

Now that we have established the need for basic pre-preparation for sugar syrup, it is important for us to understand about the different ingredients that will be used in preparing the sugar showpiece from sugar. The sugar as an ingredient is the most basic thing and it is important to select the type of sugar that one would use for getting the most clear and shiny piece of sugar art.

Let us discuss below the ingredients that will be used in making sugar art and also the reason as to why these should be used.

Sugar The best type of sugar to use is cane sugar as it is considered purer than beet sugar. It was commonly quoted that lump sugar is the best form of sugar to use. This stems from the days of loaf sugar when it was the purest variety available. Granulated sugar is currently considered as the variety that gives the best results consistently. It is best used from 1 kg bags, opened and used at one boiling. This is preferable to using sugar from a bin or sack, which is more likely to have foreign bodies in it.

Anti-crystalizing agents These ingredients are added to sugar to help prevent the sugar from crystallizing. They cause some of the sugar to turn into invert sugar, which will not revert to the crystal form. The presence of these ingredients in the sugar keeps it malleable and soft as long as it is kept warm. Sugar should be kept warm either in an oven or under a heat lamp once it has been pulled. Many anti-crystalizing agents are used for sugar work. Some of the common ones are as follows:

Glucose Best variety to use is the one which is very thick. Normally, it is used in the ratio of 200 g glucose per 1 kg of sugar. Liquid glucose is a kind of invert sugar. One must always use wet hands to remove liquid glucose or else it will stick to the hands.

Tartaric acid solution This is the strongest of all the anti-crystalizing agents and hence, must be used with great care. It is normally added with the help of an eyedropper to ensure that only the correct quantity is used. Tartaric acid is available in both powdered and liquid forms. An acid slows down the crystallization process. Acids such as tartaric acid make the sugar more elastic and soft and hence, easier to pull and stretch. If too much of it is added then the sugar will be too soft to hold on in showpieces and if it is too less, then the sugar will be too hard to create blown figures.

Cream of tartar This is of medium strength and can be used on its own or with glucose or tartaric acid solution. It is always diluted before adding to the sugar—one level teaspoon if it is used with glucose or two level teaspoons if it is used on its own.

Fondant As fondant contains a large percentage of glucose, it can be used in place of glucose if no glucose is available. Simply add a large lump to the boiling sugar.

Lemon juice This is the weakest acid used in sugar work and is not strong enough to be used on its own. It can only be used as back up to other anti-crystalizing agents. Lemon juice also has a bleaching effect on the colours of the sugar keeping them clear and bright.

Colours Any food colour can be used. But the best types are powder or gel forms as they do not contain water, which might hamper the texture of the final syrup. Also powder colours give you an advantage to decide the shade of the colour. Spray colours are also used on the sugar after it has been pulled or casted. To be successful at sugar work, it is necessary not only to know how to cook and pull sugar but also how to colour it correctly. It is also important to remember that the base colour of the sugar will have an effect on the colour added. For example, if red is added to sugar it will give a different colour depending on the degree to which the sugar has been cooked. For better understanding, see Table 10.2 which shows that if bright red colour is added to a pot of cooked sugar, then how it changes.

Table 10.2 Change in colour of pulled sugar

Stage	Effect on sugar colour
At hard crack stage	Light red pulled sugar
At light caramel stage	Bright red pulled sugar
At mid caramel stage	Deep red pulled sugar
At dark caramel stage	Very deep red pulled sugar

Sugar always looks better if colours are mixed and not used in their pure form. This applies particularly to greens when making leaves. To make bright green, combine green with a hint of yellow to give a natural leaf green colour. Also find below some tips for adding colours.

- To obtain white pulled sugar, add a small touch of blue to clear sugar.
- To obtain silver pulled sugar, add a small touch of mauve to clear sugar.
- To obtain gold pulled sugar, cook sugar as dark as possible.

Silica gel It is used for storing and protecting sugar from humidity. The advantage of silica gel is that it changes its colour from blue to pink, when it is humid and can be regenerated once dried in oven to get rid of the moisture.

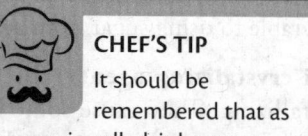

> **CHEF'S TIP**
> It should be remembered that as sugar is pulled, it becomes lighter, so more colour should be added to obtain the required shade.

Food lacquer/Deco spray It is commonly known as confectioners' varnish or food varnish. It gives shine and protects the sugar structure from humidity and thus, helps in extending the life of the sugar showpiece.

Cooking Sugar

Let us now read about boiling basic sugar for sugar work and all the points mentioned in the salient features in earlier part of this chapter must be taken into account whilst starting to boil the sugar. All the ingredients and equipment mentioned earlier should be ready to use and the area should be spotlessly clean. Following is the basic recipe of cooking sugar.

Cooking Sugar

Ingredients
Castor sugar or isomalt 1 kg
Water 350 ml
Glucose 200 g
Tartaric acid solution 12-14 drops

METHOD
1. Combine sugar, water, and liquid glucose and heat over moderate heat until the sugar has dissolved.
2. Boil briskly, as a lengthy boil will encourage graining.
3. Keep sides of pan clean during boiling.
4. Cook to 158°C and add tartaric acid.
5. Continue cooking until sugar reaches 160°C.
6. Stop the cooking process by plunging the pan in a bowl of cold water.
7. Pour the sugar onto the lightly oiled marble slab or a silpat when the sugar has cooled down slightly.
8. Fold the sugar syrup into the centre as soon as it settles and allow it to settle again. Repeat this process until the sugar is cool enough to pick up.
9. Pull as quickly as possible and then mould the sugar into a ball. Sugar must now be kept warm until it is used. If all the sugar is not used, it can be stored in an airtight box with silica gel and reheated in a microwave at a later date and used again.

The sugar prepared in this manner is now ready for various usages such as casting, blown, and pulled, and each of these techniques yields a different result and appearance. This unique ability of these sugar techniques gives an artistic impression to a showpiece structure or a garnish. Let us now discuss these techniques in detail.

Sugar for Casting

Whilst using sugar for casting, no acid is added into the syrup whilst boiling as we need a brittle and a fairly hard structure for it. Sugar with no acid is poured into various shapes cut from modelling clay or steel rings, which have been lightly oiled to prevent the sugar syrup from sticking. When the sugar is poured into a prepared mould, it should be allowed to set without being disturbed and when it solidifies, the prepared pieces should be handled with gloves so that no finger marks are transferred onto the showpiece. The rings can also be placed on top of a textured silicone mat and then when the sugar is poured, the texture design will be printed on the sugar structure as shown in Fig. 10.2.

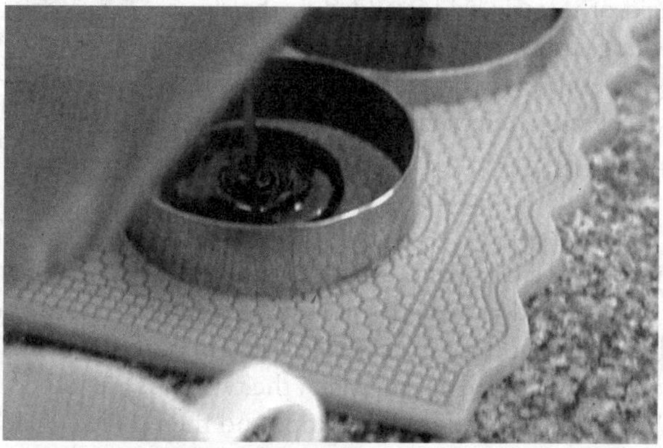

Fig. 10.2 Pouring sugar onto a textured mat

One can also use granulated sugar or castor sugar in a deep tray and form a figure in the sugar with fingers. Now one can pour the sugar syrup in the design and allow it to set. The sugar will stick to the sugar structure giving it a unique texture as shown in Fig. 10.3.

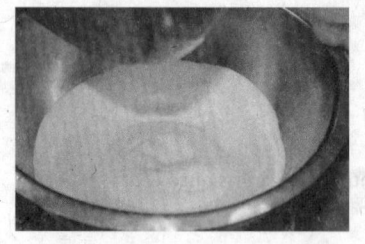

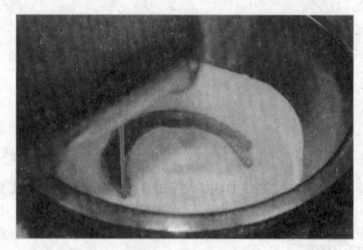

Step 1 Pour sugar in a bowl   Step 2 Make a well and pour sugar syrup   Step 3 Cover the syrup with more sugar and allow the mixture to cool

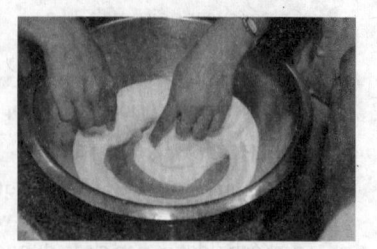

Fig. 10.3 Steps for casting sugar syrup in grain/castor sugar mould

Casted sugar structures can be used as a base to create figurines by pouring the sugar into the desired moulds. Silicone moulds are good for this purpose. Figure 10.4 shows the steps of casting sugar.

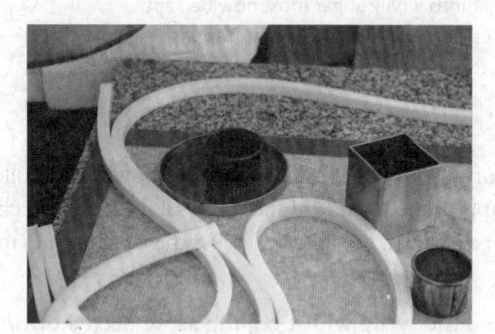

Step 1 Arrange the desired moulds   Step 2 Pour the sugar syrup in the moulds and allow to set

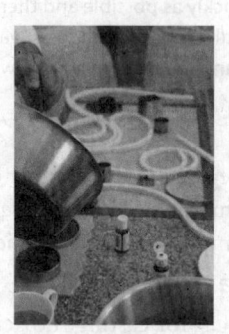

Fig. 10.4 Steps for pouring sugar into moulds for casting

Pulled Sugar

Cooking of sugar for the pulled sugar is similar to the casting sugar except that citric acid or tartaric acid is added to the sugar to make it softer for pulling and stretching. In case of pulled sugar, the sugar is allowed to boil to 158°C and then tartaric acid is added and the sugar is heated to a temperature of 160°C. Once it reaches the temperature, it is removed from the heat source and the base of the pan is plunged into cold water to stop further cooking of sugar.

> **CHEF'S TIP**
> When pouring sugar in a ring, pour slowly as it may cause bubbles in the figure. In case bubbles are there, just use a blow torch to remove them.

The syrup is then poured over a clean and lightly oiled marble slab or silicone mat. When the sugar cools down to around 85°C, it is folded from the sides in an inward motion, and this is done a couple of times until the sugar collects into a soft mass. It is then lifted in both the hands and stretched to around 10-12 inches and the two ends are folded apart. When the two ends are joined, it should be tried to coil them together, then they should be pulled up like a rope and then pulled again. The more you pull, the shinier and more opaque the sugar will become. Figure 10.5 shows the steps of making pulled sugar.

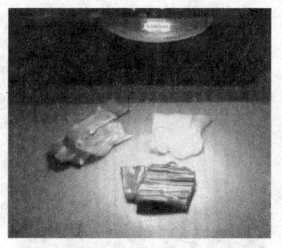

Step 1 Arrange the coloured pieces of sugar

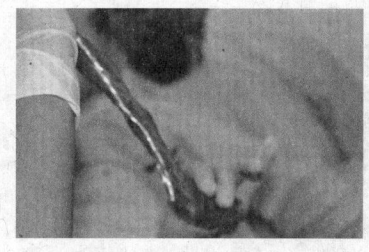

Step 2 Start to pull the edges to form a rope

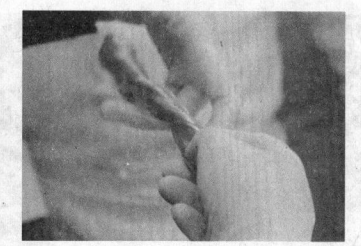

Step 3 Twist and pull again to form a rope

Fig. 10.5 Steps of making pulled sugar

It is very important to keep the focus on the temperature because if the temperature falls below 70°C, it will be difficult to pull the sugar. It is important to use latex gloves when pulling sugar because it is fairly at a hot temperature to handle. If the temperature of the sugar drops, then you must allow reheating under a sugar lamp. The sugar when pulled and stretched can be put to many uses. It can either be used immediately to make pulled flowers as shown in Fig. 10.6 or it can be cooled down and stored in an airtight container until further usage. Let us take a look at the various uses of pulled sugar.

Pulled sugar flower In this case, each petal is pulled and cut with scissor and shaped around thumb. The edges are curled with fingers. After all the petals have been pulled, they are then carefully joined with the help of a spirit burner or blow torch. A lot of care has to be taken while making pulled sugar flowers as one is working with latex gloves and the fire at the same time. The gloves should be kept away from fire because latex is inflammable. The flower can be sprayed with colour later or colour can be added whilst pulling the sugar. Figure 10.6 shows the steps of making pulled sugar flower.

Pulled sugar ribbons This is a very unique usage of pulled sugar and chefs make colourful ribbons, which become the centre point of any sugar showpiece. You can make ribbons of many colours and various widths. The choice of colour and its combinations is purely based on the aesthetic appeal or the theme of the sugar showpiece. As shown in Fig. 10.7, a coloured pulled sugar is chosen as per what the chef would like to incorporate into the band. For example, in Fig. 10.7 we have chosen red, blue, and green.

The pulled sugar pieces are placed horizontally in such a way that they touch each other. The ribbon is then pulled to around 6-8 inches, which results in a ribbon of three colours. The ribbon is then folded again in such a manner that two long ends meet each other; in this manner a ribbon with six colours is created. You can pull again and repeat the process until the number of desired colours in the ribbon is achieved. Whilst pulling if the ribbon becomes hard to pull, allow it to warm under the heat lamp for a few seconds. Now the final ribbon can be pulled to a thin sheet and the required width. The flattened ribbon should be placed on the marble table and cut at the desired length with a sharp knife whose cutting edge has been heated by a blow torch. Each cut piece of the ribbon can now be softened under the heat lamp and curled to make bows, curls, and other deigns depending on the showpiece.

Pulled sugar garnish The pulled sugar can be used for making various other garnishes such as pulled threads that can be coiled over a tube to make a spiral. Sugar can be pulled to make individual chards or flames that can be used as a garnish for desserts.

214 *Theory of Bakery and Patisserie*

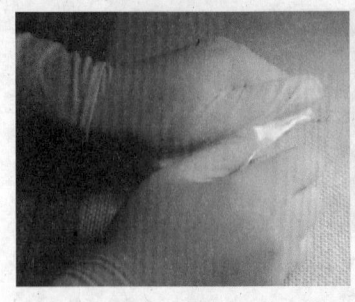

Step 1 Flatten the pulled sugar and pinch out a small piece from the side

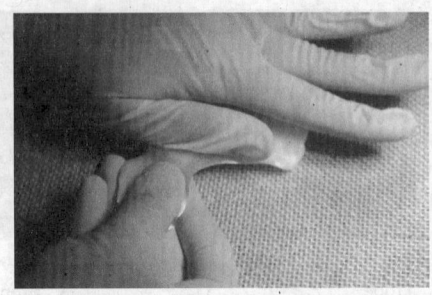

Step 2 Pull the pinched piece to form a petal and cut with scissor

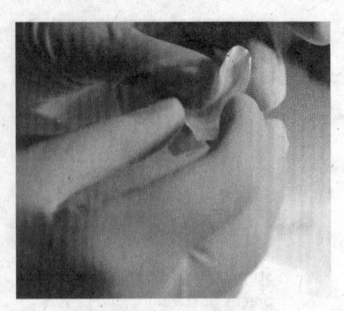

Step 3 Fold the petal to form the centre part of the flower

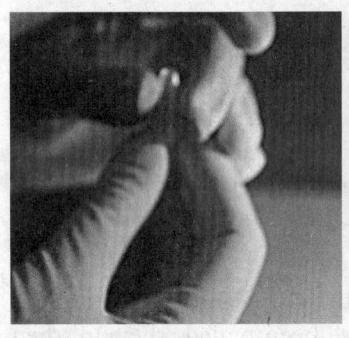

Step 4 Shape it under the sugar lamp so that it is still pliable

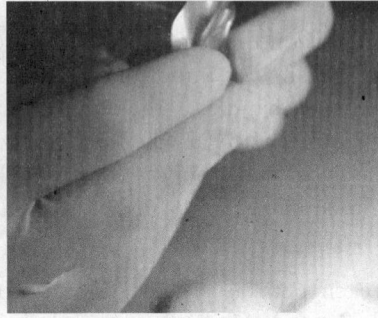

Step 5(a) Make another petal and arrange on the first one

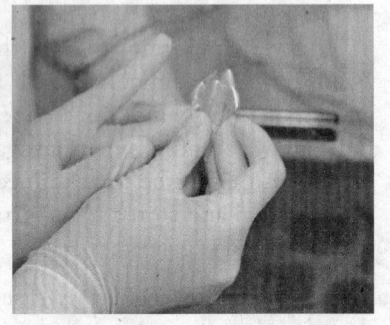

Step 5(b) Make sure that the shape of the flower is formed as and when we arrange the next petal

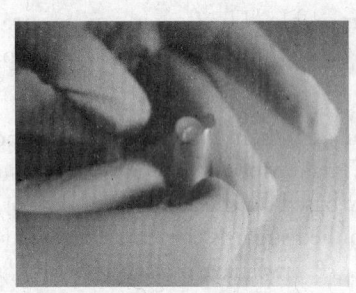

Step 6 Curl the third petal in a way that the earlier two petals are visible distinctively

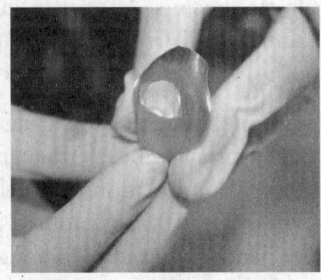

Step 7 Repeat the steps to form the flower

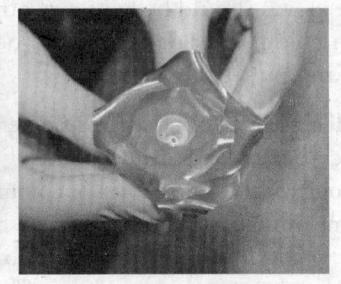

Step 8 Keep arranging the petals to the size you wish to prepare

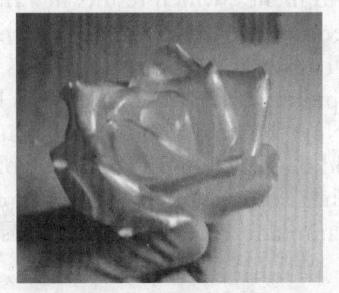

Step 9 Rose flower ready after arranging all the petals

Fig. 10.6 Steps of making pulled sugar flower

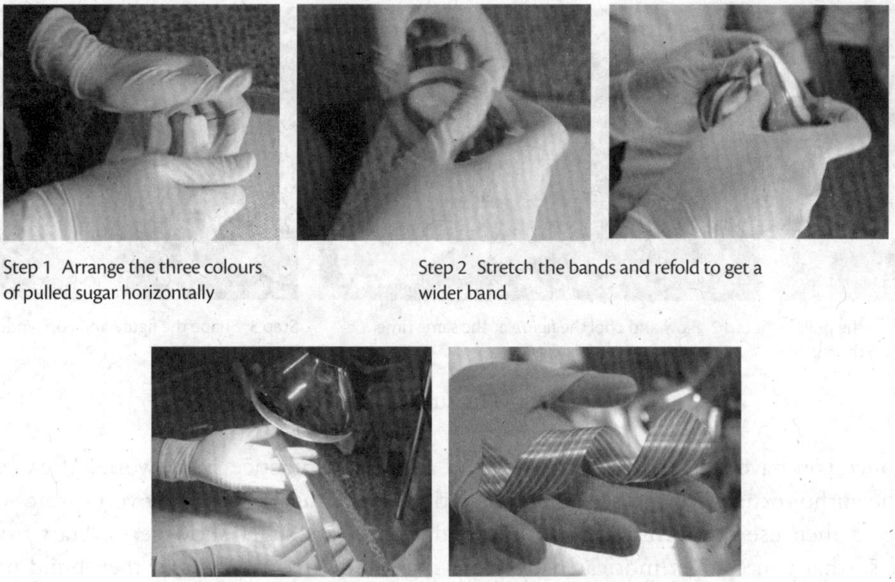

Step 1 Arrange the three colours of pulled sugar horizontally

Step 2 Stretch the bands and refold to get a wider band

Step 3 Stretch and pull to desired length

Step 4 Cut the ribbon and shape into desired shapes

Fig. 10.7 Pulling sugar for ribbons

Pulled sugar can also be used for making other parts of the figure such as eyes, nose, and other body parts. For example, whilst making a fish, its body is prepared by the sugar blowing technique, but other details such as fins and gills are made by pulled sugar.

Blown Sugar

This is one of the most interesting elements of sugar work and requires a great deal of practice and understanding of sugar temperature. The sugar is cooked and pulled as per the pulling sugar technique and then the pulled sugar is allowed to soften before it is blown into figures of desired shape and size. After the sugar is pulled it is allowed to slightly soften under the heat lamp. It is then made into a small ball and flattened to create a cup like structure. The metal part of the sugar blowing apparatus is slightly oiled and inserted in the cup in such a manner that the sugar covers the metal tip completely with a small gap in the middle and in the space around the metal tube.

After this, air is blown into the sugar with the help of the pump. As you do this, it is important to keep cooling the sugar under a fan. At first you will find it difficult as right pressure has to be provided when blowing into the sugar figure. Care has to be taken that the sugar is being blown evenly or the figure will crack if more pressure is exerted onto it. The blown structure is then removed from the metal tip by either pulling it away slowly from the tube or by heating the tube with a blow torch so that the sugar structure releases easily. The blown sugar technique can be used for blowing thin and hollow structures of fruits such as peaches, apples, and cherries. Figure 10.8 shows the blowing of the duck which is used in the final sugar showpiece as depicted in Fig. 10.1.

> **CHEF'S TIP**
> Adding a band of black colour between each colour, makes the ribbon look very attractive as the black band acts as a liner thereby, making the individual colours stand out.

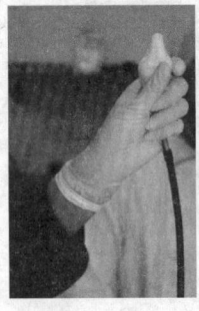

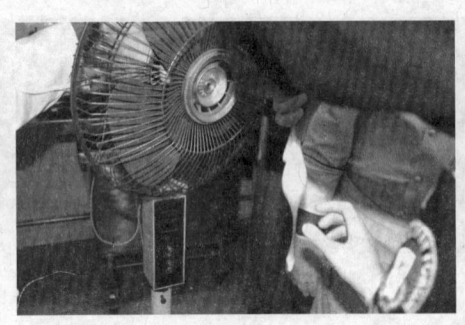

Step 1 Place the pulled sugar ball on the tube
Step 2 Blow and cool the figure at the same time
Step 3 Shape the figure and cool under the fan

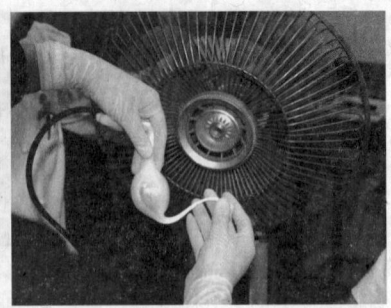

Fig. 10.8 Blowing sugar for duck figure

Now once you have learned the techniques go ahead and practice sugar work. After reading this chapter, the author expects you to see a demonstration of the sugar work from your professor or from YouTube and then use the technique and knowledge to create sugar showpieces. Start from a basic showpiece so that you can get motivated by achieving the desired results and then build on to make more complex sugar showpieces.

SUMMARY

In this chapter, we read about the range of sugar confections that are prepared in the pastry kitchen to be sold in pastry shops, restaurants, and even as decorative props in festive buffets. Pastry is a fairly busy department and during festive occasions it becomes even busier as it has to prepare a range of classical confections that are synonymous to that particular festivity. We read about sugar and types of sugar in Chapter 2, but in this chapter we have discussed how sugar is used in different ways to create a range of sugar confections.

When the sugar is heated it undergoes both chemical and textural changes. Each point of change in the property of sugar is termed as stage of sugar and we have discussed the various stages of sugar in this chapter. We have also seen the usage of each stage to make a particular sugar confection and read about the density of sugar syrup and how it is measured.

We also discussed the salient features of boiling sugar and what extra care needs to be taken whilst boiling as it is one of the most crucial stages of sugar cooking. Every rise of 1°C in sugar syrup can affect the texture of the sugar syrup and its intended usage.

We have also discussed basic products made with sugar along with their basic recipes for reference. Products such as basic sugar syrup and sugar confections such as marshmallows, caramel, fudge, toffee, candies, fondant, gum paste, nougatine, rock sugar, honeycomb, jam, and pate de fruits have been discussed with regards to their preparation, service, and storage as well.

In the later part of the chapter, we have discussed about the art of sugar work. In this section, we read how the sugar is boiled to create components for an artistic showpiece or even as a garnish for desserts and cakes. Basic equipment and ingredients required for basic sugar work have been discussed and explained in detail. Techniques such as spun sugar, casting, pulling, and blowing that are used to make some of the most intricate sugar showpieces have been explained with critical factors.

Using this knowledge, students will be able to create a range of sugar products. Though it takes months of practice to make artistic sugar showpieces, it is important to start with basic ones and then as you practice, you will start to achieve more complex ones. In the next chapter, we shall discuss about Indian sweets and how sugar is used in different ways to create a range of regional Indian specialties.

Sugar Confections 217

KEY TERMS

Baume Unit of measuring density of sugar syrup

Black jack Stage of sugar boiling, when the sugar burns to a black colour

Brix Another unit of measuring density of sugar syrup

Candy Sugar confection made in a variety of colours and flavours

Confiture French word for jam

Croquembouche Traditional French wedding cake made with choux pastry

Deco spray Also known as food varnish or food lacquer, is a lacquer that is sprayed over sugar structures to create a shiny film on top, to make the showpiece shiny and glittery

Dobos torte Classical cake from Hungary, where the top is glazed with caramelized sugar

Fondant An icing made by boiling sugar to 115°C and then cooling and kneading it into a white coloured mass

Gum tragacanth Kind of vegetable gum obtained from a plant and used as a thickening agent in pastry

Honeycomb Sugar confection made by addition of baking soda into boiled sugar syrup

Hygroscopic Property of sugar to absorb moisture from the environment

Invert sugar Type of sugar that does not crystalize easily

Isomalt Type of invert sugar

Macaroon French cookie made with egg whites and almond powder

Marshmallows Sugar confection made by whipping egg whites, sugar syrup, and gelatin

Nougatine Sugar confection made by boiling sugar to caramel stage and mixing with nuts

Pastillage French word for gum paste

Pate de fruit Jelly based confection made from a fruit rich in pectin

Pectin Natural enzyme present in a fruit or a vegetable, that helps in setting it to a jam/jelly consistency

Praline paste Nougatine grounded into paste form

Refractometer Equipment used for measuring density of sugar syrup

Rock sugar Type of a sugar confection made by combining sugar syrup and royal icing. Usually used for decorations and garnish

RTR Abbreviation for ready-to-roll fondant, is a readymade white coloured paste used for cake decorations

Silica gel Small granules of silica used for keeping the sugar structures free from moisture

Silpat Silicone mat used for baking and sugar work

Stick Jaws Kind of a toffee, which is cooked to higher degree and hence becomes chewy

Sugar pump Small apparatus with a metal tube and blow pump in the end, used for blowing air into sugar structure

OBJECTIVE TYPE QUESTIONS

1. What do you understand by the term sugar confections?
2. How old is the art of sugar confectionary?
3. What was used in sugar confectionary before sugar was produced by Chinese?
4. What is the unit of measuring the density of sugar syrup?
5. What is a saccharometer?
6. At what temperature should the density of sugar syrup be checked?
7. If the sugar syrup is at 118°C, then what is this stage called?
8. What is the temperature for the hard crack stage?
9. What would you do to protect your sugar syrup from being over cooked beyond its required temperature?
10. What should be the density of basic sugar syrup?
11. Why are marshmallows called by that name?
12. What is a stick jaw?
13. What do you understand by the word RTR?
14. What is invert sugar?

15. Why is pastillage also known as gum paste?
16. What is the difference between rock sugar and honeycomb?
17. What is the enzyme that helps in setting of a jam?
18. What is spun sugar?
19. Name at least two sugar confections that utilize gelatin.
20. What is the role of acid in boiling sugar syrup?
21. What equipment will you use for blowing sugar?
22. What kinds of pans should be used for boiling sugar?
23. What would you do to preserve sugar garnishes?
24. What is the wattage of bulb used on sugar work?
25. What is an isomalt?
26. At what stage should the acid be added in sugar syrup?
27. What is casting of sugar?
28. How is pulled sugar different from blown sugar?
29. Name the weakest acid used in sugar confections.
30. What would you do if you need a golden coloured pulled sugar?

ESSAY TYPE QUESTIONS

1. Working with sugar is both an art and science. Justify the statement.
2. Briefly describe the stages of sugar boiling and its uses.
3. Briefly describe the salient features that should be kept in mind whilst boiling sugar for confections.
4. Briefly describe the process of making marshmallows.
5. Briefly describe the process of making nougatine and its uses.
6. Briefly describe the process of making rock sugar.
7. What are anti-crystalizing agents and what role do they play? Explain in detail.
8. Differentiate between caramel, toffee, and fudge.
9. List down the ways in which the caramel can be used.
10. Briefly describe how would you make fondant.

ACTIVITY

1. In a group of 4 to 5 students, visit a pastry shop in a hotel and list down the products related to sugar confections, click pictures, and make a report of how they are decorated and presented.
2. In groups of 3-4, prepare a sugar structure using the various techniques mentioned in the chapter. Critique the showpiece from an artistic point of view.
3. In groups of 3-4, research about various garnishes made by utilizing sugar.

11 Indian Sweets

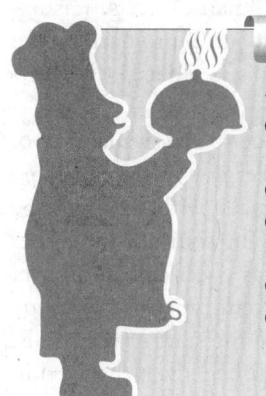

LEARNING OBJECTIVES

After reading this chapter, you should be able to
- understand the basic operations of a *halwai* section of any hotel or establishment
- appreciate the diversity in sweets from all the regions of India
- claim an insight into sweets and comfort food from north, east, west, and south of India with regards to ingredients and equipment used
- understand the importance of sweets in festivals and religious ceremonies
- judge the stages of sugar without using any equipment

INTRODUCTION

Indian *halwai* is a vast subject in itself. The sweets of India are not as simple as the Western desserts, because each dessert of India is a specialty in itself and has no particular standardized recipe like in case of the Western cuisine. This is because of many reasons. The desserts in India are made with a variety of ingredients that are different in each state and each of these require lots of experience and expertise as the Indian desserts are mostly based on the feel of texture and appearance rather than the standardized methods and procedure. The quality of the ingredients changes on a daily basis and hence, the recipes have to be altered accordingly.

Very few Indian desserts have gained popularity all over the world because Indian desserts tend to be very sweet and the concept of having Indian sweets has been restricted to special occasions and festivities. Diwali is one of the festivals that is associated with sweets. It is very common to see a number of sweet shops created along the road during Diwali that sell sweets. In the olden days, the sweet makers were known as *halwai* and even today each region and even each village has a *halwai* shop, no matter how small the shop or village is.

The making and eating of sweets is probably very old, but the recorded history from 7th century BC, which talks about the development of communities and social networking, stated that during this period elaborate rituals such as marriages, child birth, and even deaths came into existence and were related to family deities. Social religious functions such as moving to a new house, offerings in temples to Gods, and festivals became a part of Indian life. In all these festive and social occasions, one thing was common and that was the food and sweets. The sweets are offered to Gods as *naivaida* or *bhog*. The same is distributed amongst the people as *prashad*, which literally means blessings from the God. Lord Ganesha in the Hindu mythology is believed to have fascination for the sweet called *modak*. *Modak* is a very popular sweet made with rice flour and is still made on the festival of Ganesh Chaturthi.

ORIGIN AND HISTORY OF INDIAN SWEETS

Travellers and invaders from all over the world came to our country and some even settled here. Their food travelled with them and stayed here as well, though we did do some flavourful changes to it to suit our palettes and to have something that we could relate to. It would be quite surprising for many of us to learn that Indians got sugar from China and we still call it *cheeni* referring to China. Indian cuisine used jaggery and raw sugar known as *boora* that is still commonly used in Indian desserts. History reveals that the technology of making raw sugar by boiling down the sugar cane juice into dark brown crystals was developed in India around 500 BC. The tradition of Indian sweets is as old as 3,000 years and the same has been mentioned in the history books and epics as well.

Every culture has a typical sweet associated with it and this is probably due to the availability of ingredients, climatic conditions, and the cultural diversity of the people. The desserts in the north are made with reduced milk known as *khoya*, whereas in Bengal, the sweets are made with fresh cottage cheese known as *chenna*. There is hardly any usage of *khoya* in Bengali sweets. The south of India uses rice, jaggery, and coconut in their desserts and so on. Indian cuisine is known as sweet cuisine all over the world. It is so because many of its foods are sweet in taste and many different types of sweets are also made here. Sweets in some cultures/regions such as Gujarat are had before the start of the meals. Guajarati food also has a sweet taste as sugar is added to many of its savoury dishes. Even the food in Bengal has a slight touch of sugar in savoury dishes.

The preparation of the Indian sweets and savouries is an art developed over many centuries. The Portuguese, Mughals, and British have all influenced the desserts of India in one way or the other. The sweets of Goa have a strong influence of the Portuguese while Puducherry in Southern region of India has French influence as it was a French colony for a long period of time. The Iranians brought their subtle ways of sweets through the Parsi community and so on. In spite of being diverse, there is a common culture that runs from Kashmir to Kanyakumari and in ancient texts this has been referred to as *manav sanskriti* or human behaviour. The strength of being adaptable and open to all cultures has always been very prevalent in India.

INGREDIENTS USED IN INDIAN SWEETS

Before we read about the various sweets made in India, we need to understand the type of ingredients used in making the same. A range of commodities is used along with sweeteners to create the delicacies that have become famous around the world. Most of the sweets are made from dairy products, grains, or beans/lentils. Dried fruits such as raisins and nuts (especially pistachios and almonds) are used for garnishing and texture. Savoury spices such as cardamom seeds, fennel seeds, nutmeg, and cinnamon are used for aroma. Flowery scent is added from sandalwood, *khas* (vetiver), *kewra* (screw pine), and rose water.

Let us now read about these ingredients in detail.

Cereal Many types of cereals are used for preparation of sweets. Rice, wheat, and pulses are a few of the common cereals that are used in various forms to prepare Indian sweets. The availability of these cereals in various regions results in them finding their way into the production of sweets. Few of the most common cereals used in Indian sweets are mentioned in Table 11.1.

Table 11.1 Cereals used in Indian sweets

Item	Description	Examples
Rice	Rice is commonly used in Indian desserts in almost all the states of India. The most common dessert is *kheer* that is cooked by cooking rice and milk with sugar and flavourings. Rice can also be ground to a coarse powder to make *phirnee* or into a fine powder for making *modaks*.	Rice: *Payesh, kheer, ada pradaman* Rice flour: *Modak, phirnee*
Lentils	Lentils are commonly used in South India and in Maharashtra to make desserts. *Channa* lentil is the most common lentil used for making Indian sweets. In South, *channa* lentils are combined with coconut milk and jaggery to make *parupu paysam* and in Maharashtra boiled channa lentils and jaggery mixture is stuffed in wholewheat dough to make *puran poli*. Lentil powder such as *besan* made by grinding *channa* dal is also used for making famous Indian sweets such as *besan ladoo*, Mysore pak from South India. *Besan* is also added to *jalebis* to add a crisp texture to the final product. *Besan* batter is also forced through a perforated spoon to create *boondis*, which are soaked in sugar syrup to make *boondi ladoo* or *motichoor ladoo*. *Moong* lentils are also ground to a paste, which is commonly known as *pithi* and cooked in ghee, sugar, and milk to form a pudding called *moong dal halwa*. *Urad* lentils in South are ground into a paste and made into a dessert called *imarti*.	*Parupu paysam, puran poli, besan ladoo, Mysore pak, sohan halwa, motichoor ladoo, moong dal halwa, imarti*
Flour and by-products	Both refined flour and wholewheat flour are commonly used for making Indian sweets. Flour is used in many forms. Some desserts are made by batters made from flour as in case of *jalebi* and some are made from the dough of the flour. In some cases, the flour is roasted in ghee and combined with sugar and ghee to make *ladoos*. Other by-products of flour such as semolina and broken wheat are also used in making of *halwas* and other Indian sweets.	*Jalebi, balushahi, panjiri, pinni, suji halwa, kharak halwa*

Sweeteners Sweeteners are the most important ingredient in sweets or desserts. Refined sugar came to India from China and that is the reason it is called *cheeni* which is a common slang for China in India. Many types of sweeteners are used in Indian desserts. This ranges from raw sugar to refined sugar, to honey, jaggery and various other types that are indigenous to a particular region and culture. The desserts down south are mostly sweetened with jaggery whereas the Mughals brought the touch of honey.

Let us discuss a few of the commonly used sweeteners in Indian desserts in Table 11.2.

Table 11.2 Sweeteners used in Indian desserts

Sweetener	Description
Sugar	Granulated sugar is the most commonly used sugar in Indian desserts. It is combined with water to make syrup that is commonly known as *chashni*. The technology has evolved from using raw sugars to refined sugars; however, the method to check sugar density has remained constant.
Honey	Honey is a natural sugar obtained from bee hives. The colour and flavour of honey will vary with its source. Honey is used in those Indian desserts that have been influenced by Mughals and Arabs. Honey is used in *khubani ka meetha* that is a popular dessert from Hyderabad, where the apricots are stewed in honey.
Jaggery	Jaggery is a product made in India, Africa, and South America. It is produced from sugar cane and is healthy and nutritious as the whole sugar cane juice is cooked with molasses. The colour of the jaggery or *gur* as commonly known in India, can be light to dark depending upon the degree of cooking. Though also known as jaggery, it is not only made from sugar cane juice. Palm sugar jaggery is traditionally made from the sap of Palmyra palm or the date palm. It is extensively used in Asian cooking, especially Thai. In Bengali cuisine, a special kind of jaggery is obtained from palm tree known as *nolen gur* and is available in winters only. This is used to create many delectable sweets.
Boora	Boora is powdered raw sugar. It is usually unrefined sugar and is commonly used in Indian desserts and even *chaats*. The sugar needs to be clarified in some cases, where the dessert would be served with the accompanying syrup as in case of *gulab jamun*. In such cases where sugar is to be clarified, granulated or refined sugar is used.

Sugar and its Stages Since candy thermometers never found a way into Indian sweet making, the Indian sweet makers mastered the art of checking the density of the sugar by a method known as *Taar*. The *taar* or thread method is used to determine the stages of the sugar boiling. While making *chashni* (refer to Table 11.2), a drop of the mixture is pinched between the thumb and the index finger and released to see how many threads are made. *Chashni* is made using refined sugar and water without any acids (fruit juices or lime).

At room temperature, one can dissolve sugar to 50% of its weight in water. The extra sugar would get dissolved in water only if the temperature is raised and the water is allowed to boil. After the solution comes to a boil eventually, you cannot dissolve any more sugar. But continued heat evaporates water, making the syrup more concentrated. The sugar concentration determines the eventual texture and consistency of the product. Table 11.3 lists the various stages of sugar boiling and the relevant *taar* consistency used in Indian cooking.

Table 11.3 Stages of sugar boiling and corresponding *taar*

Temperature	Sugar density	Candy making stage	Taar stage	Application
212°F	0%	Water boiling point	No thread	Rasgulla
220°F-222°F	70%	Pearl	Single thread	Absorption
235°F-240°F	85%	Soft ball	Two threads	Burfi, gajak, gulab jamun
242°F-248°F	87%	Firm ball	Two and half threads	Sohan papdi
250°F-268°F	92%	Hard ball	Three threads	Icing
270°F-290°F	95%	Soft crack	Three and half threads	Brittle, *chikki*
300°F-310°F	99%	Hard crack	Not commonly used in Indian desserts except for a few candies such as *chikki*	Chikki
320°F	100%	Melting point	Not used in Indian desserts	Caramelize
350°F	100%	Burnt	Not used in Indian desserts	Black jack

Indian Sweets

Dairy products Indian desserts use two commodities in abundance—dairy products and sugar. These two are the most commonly used ingredients in almost every sweet of India. Apart from milk, ghee, cream, and curd, various forms of reduced milk are used in sweet making. Milk is also curdled into cheese and commonly used in Indian sweets. Let us discuss some of the common dairy products used in sweet making in Table 11.4.

Table 11.4 Dairy products used in Indian sweets

Dairy product	Description
Milk	In Indian sweets, usually cow milk is the most preferred. Generally, loose cow milk which is not homogenised is referred to as sweet milk. Buffalo milk has a peculiar smell and also the fat content is high, it is due to this reason that it is used for making *khoya* or *rabri*.
Khoya	*Khoya* or *mawa* is a dairy product. It is used in making many sweet dishes and gravies as well. In India, *khoya* is rarely made at home and is procured from stores that sell dairy products. However, outside India, *khoya* is perpetually unheard of as it is a perishable commodity and one has to master the art of preparing it. It can be made at home, though the method is a little tedious. It is prepared by boiling and reducing milk to a semi-solid stage. There are different types of *khoya* depending on the use of ingredients and moisture content. *Batti ka khoya*: This is solid and moulded *khoya*. It is made out of full cream buffalo milk. A litre of milk will yield 200 g of *khoya*. It is used in burfis and ladoos and in many other desserts of North India. *Daab ka (or chikna) khoya*: This is made with low fat buffalo milk. It is loose and sticky in consistency with higher moisture content. It is suitable for making *gulab jamun* and *gajar ka halwa*. *Daanedaar (or granulated) khoya*: This is made out of full cream buffalo milk. The difference is that khoya is curdled slightly by adding a little tartaric acid in powder form. The milk curdles slightly hence the khoya is soft textured. Care should be taken not to spoil the texture while stirring. The water content is more than *batti ka khoya* but less than *chikna khoya*. This type is used in making *kalakand* and ladoo.
Chenna	It is mostly used in desserts from Bengal. This is the main difference between the sweets of North and Bengal. Northern India uses more of *khoya* in desserts whereas Bengalis use only *chenna* or fresh cottage cheese. Ideally, *chenna* is made by curdling cow milk with previous day's whey, but it can also be made by boiling and curdling milk by tartaric acid.
Curd	Curd is also used in some of the Indian sweets. Fresh curd is hung and mixed with powdered sugar to make *shirikhand*, which is a very popular dessert from Gujarat.
Rabri	Milk is heated in a fairly shallow pan over an open fire and is allowed to simmer. The milk is neither stirred nor allowed to boil. The surface of the milk may be gently fanned to help the process of skin formation. A portion of this skin, about 3–4 sq cm, is continuously broken with a thick wooden stick (or bamboo/cane splints) and pushed to the side of the pan which is cooler and where the skin dries up. This operation requires considerable skill and constant attention. The preparation time is about 25–40 minutes depending on the rate of boiling. As the slow evaporation reduces the milk to about 1/5–1/8th of its original volume, good quality ground sugar (5–6 percent by weight of the original milk) is added to the milk concentrate and dissolved in it. The layers of skin collected on the sides of the pan are then immersed in the mixture and the final product is obtained by heating the whole mass for another brief period. The finished product consists of non-homogeneous skin flakes partly covered by and partly floating in sweetened condensed milk. By heating the concentrated mass slightly at the end, a more homogeneous chewy texture mass is obtained. The product can be packed and sold in any of the modern types of containers. Following two types of rabri are available in the market. *Lachedar rabri*: This *rabri* is like thick flakes and in the process of making it the milk is reduced with flakes intact. *Danedaar rabri*: This involves the normal cooking process of *rabri*, where the entire mass is stirred together in the end to yield a curdled mass called *danedaar rabri*.

Chemicals Various kinds of edible natural or artificial chemicals are used in making Indian sweets. Tartaric acid, citric acid, etc., are few of the commonly used chemicals in desserts. Many of these chemicals are used for the purpose of providing aeration or lamination to the product. Baking soda/powder is used for leavening (introducing air) into the product to make it seem light. Let us discuss some of the commonly used chemicals in Indian sweets in Table 11.5.

Fats and oils The choice of oil or fat used for cooking, gives an instant recognition to the origin of the dish and the social and economic status of the people. Ghee is the most commonly used fat in Indian sweets and the usage of ghee in Indian desserts is a matter of pride. Many sweet shops use this as a marketing punchline that all their desserts are made only in pure ghee. Connoisseurs are easily able to distinguish whether a *gulab jamun* is made in oil or ghee. Table 11.6 describes the basic fats and oils used in *halwai*.

Table 11.5 Chemicals used in Indian *halwai*

Chemical	Description
Tartaric acid	It is also known as *tantri* or *nimbu ka sat* in Hindi. It is a white coloured salt that is used as a preservative and also to add sourness to certain products. It is a natural organic acid that is extracted from fruits such as grapes, bananas, and tamarind. It is also known as *cream of tartar*. It is also used in the production of an Indian sweet called *milk cake*.
Citric acid	As the name suggests, these are organic salts extracted from citrus fruits especially lemon and lime.
Soda bicarbonate	Also known as baking soda or bicarbonate of soda or cooking soda, it is used in a variety of Indian desserts and savouries such as *nimkis* and *jalebis*. It can be mixed with cream of tartar to produce baking powder. It usually reacts in the presence of any acidic medium such as sour milk, buttermilk, or orange juice, which causes carbon dioxide gas to get released leading to the desired result in the sweets. It is commonly known as *meetha soda* in Hindi.
Ammonia bicarbonate	This salt is typically used in providing aeration and flavour. It is commonly used in a North Indian sweet called *balushahi*. The dough is leavened with ammonia bicarbonate and deep fried in ghee. The fried dumpling is then poached in sugar syrup.

Table 11.6 Fats and oils used in Indian *halwai*

Fats and Oils	Description
Desi ghee	Desi ghee refers to the ghee obtained from cow's milk. The fat collected from the milk is heated until all the moisture evaporates leaving behind burnt milk solids and clarified fat which is siphoned off and used as ghee. Ghee can be used as shortening in savoury as well as sweet doughs and can also be used for frying desserts and savouries.
Refined oil	Any kind of vegetable oil such as corn oil, groundnut oil, sunflower seed oil, or cottonseed oil can be used in Indian *halwai*. Not everything in savoury can be fried in ghee and hence, refined oil is used to fry many savoury dishes such as *mathis* and samosas. With an exception of mustard, various kinds of vegetable oils are used in Indian *halwai* section.
Vanaspati	This is an emulsion of water and oil. It is mainly vegetable oils that are saturated by addition of hydrogen, which makes it more stable and increases its melting point. The handling of this fat becomes very easy in warmer conditions and it can cream very well to give more structure and short texture to the final product. Vanaspati is also used for deep frying savoury items such as *nimkis* and *mathi*.

Fruits and vegetables It might come as a surprise to many of us that even vegetables are used in making Indian desserts. This trend is not only seen in India, but is quite common in Western bakeries as well where one can see vegetable based desserts such as carrot cake. Vegetables and fruits are used in one or many ways whilst making desserts. Some vegetables are poached in sugar syrups to make them soft, whilst some are treated with chemicals to get the crunch and the texture. Fruits are very commonly used in Indian sweets and the most common of them is mango. It can be used as puree, chopped, or simply mashed. In South India, bananas and coconut are combined with jaggery and steamed. Table 11.7 lists down some fruits and vegetables used in Indian *halwai*.

Nuts Nuts are commonly used in Indian desserts. Mostly they are used for garnishing and sometimes they are added to the soft pudding to give a bite and texture to the dessert. Still in some cases, the nut is made into a paste and cooked along with sugar to make *burfis*. In some cases, the whole fruit is crushed and fried with ghee and milk to make *halwas*. Let us discuss some of the common nuts used in Indian *halwai* in Table 11.8.

Table 11.7 Fruits and vegetables used in Indian *halwai*

Vegetables	Description
Ash gourd	Also called *petha*, it is also the name of the dessert which comes from Agra. *Petha* is cut into cubes and is soaked in *calcium hydroxide* for a couple of minutes and then drained well. Then *alum water* is sprinkled over it and the entire *petha* is coated well with it. Then it is drained off and boiled till it is soft. Finally, it is soaked in sugar syrup of 2 and ½ thread consistency and left overnight to macerate.
Oval gourd	Also known as *parwal* in Hindi, it is used extensively in Bengali sweets. The oval gourd is peeled and stewed in thick sugar syrup. It is then stuffed with a mixture of *chenna* and raisins.
Carrots	Carrots are grated and braised along with milk and sugar to make a pudding called *gajar ka halwa*, which is a very popular dessert of North India and is usually made in winters when carrots are found in abundance.
Garlic	It would come as a surprise to many of us, but garlic is also used in *Awadhi* cuisine to make a pudding known as *benami kheer*. The garlic cloves are boiled in water several times and then boiled with alum to get rid of their garlic flavour. The garlic is then cooked with milk and sugar to make this dessert.
Fruits	Many kinds of fruits are used in Indian *halwai* section. The usage of fruit depends upon the region. In north, apples, mangoes, etc., are commonly used in desserts whereas in south of India, bananas are combined with jaggery and steamed to make some desserts. Fruits are also used in a frozen dessert called *kulfi*.

Table 11.8 Nuts used in Indian *halwai*

Nuts	Description
Almonds	Usually a variety called *mamra*, which has high fat content is used for *halwas* such as *badam ka halwa*. *Mamra* is expensive, but whilst packing and processing some almonds get chipped and nibbled, which are sold at comparatively less price and are known as *taanch mamra*. Almonds are deskinned and grounded into a paste, which is then combined with *khoya* to prepare *badam burfis* and other desserts.
Pistachio	Usually, bright green coloured pistachios are used in Indian desserts. Mostly these are used for garnishing Indian sweets, but sometimes crushed pistachios can be combined with sugar to create *pista burfi* as well.

(Contd)

Table 11.8 (Contd)

Nuts	Description
Cashew nuts	Cashew nuts are very commonly used for garnishing and are also grounded into a paste to make *burfis* known as *kaju katli*.
Coconut	Coconut can be used in various forms depending upon the region of India. It is used as freshly desiccated or even dried, known as *copra*, in Indian sweets. Coconut milk is also used in south and west of India in Goa and Maharashtra.
Raisins	Raisins are dried fruit commonly used as an ingredient and garnish in an Indian pudding. It can be cooked along with milk and rice to make kheer or it can be quickly fried in ghee until it swells and then it can be added to the puddings.
Charaoli	These nuts, also known as cudapa nuts in English are commonly used for garnishing *shrikhand*.
Dates	Dates or *khajoor* can be used for making *halwa*, popular in Hyderabad and Lucknow during the period of Ramzaan.

Flavourings and spices Flavourings and spices play a major role in Indian *halwai*. The combination of spices is mostly used in *chaats* section. In desserts, fragrant spices are commonly used to flavour them. The most common ones are green cardamom and cinnamon. These spices have a sweet smell that goes very well with sweets. Let us discuss some of the commonly used spices in Table 11.9.

Table 11.9 Spices used in Indian *halwai*

Spices	Description
Cardamom	Green cardamom is commonly used in Indian desserts. It can be used whole to flavour the milk or can be used in the ground form. One has to be careful in using it in ground form as the flavour is much stronger when crushed. Black cardamom seeds are also used in many desserts around Bengal. They are combined with *chenna* and stuffed inside a *gulab jamun*.
Saffron	Saffron depicts purity and richness. It is used as flavouring but mostly it is also used to add garnish and colour to the dessert. The saffron water at times is sprinkled over puddings and desserts to add colour and flavour to them. In absence of saffron, lots of *halwai* use yellow colour that resembles saffron.
Kewra	This is the essence obtained from screw pine leaves and is used in various desserts that have Mughal influence. Kewra gives an aromatic sweet flavour to puddings.
Gulab jal	Rose water is the essence obtained from rose flowers. The subtle flavour of rose is used to add perfume to the Indian sweets. It is commonly used in Mughlai desserts.
Gulkand	Rose does not need any description. In Indian cooking, rose has been closely associated with Mughlai cuisine. The fresh petals are used to garnish desserts and sometimes these are ground and mixed with honey and flavourings to make *gulkand*.
Cloves	Cloves give a very pleasant aroma to the desserts. A very common dessert from Bengal known as *lavang latika*, utilizes cloves as its major flavouring spice.
Cinnamon	Cinnamon is another spice that is associated with sweets because of its sweet flavour and smell. Cinnamon can be used whole or in powdered form. When using whole, it needs to be taken out before the dessert is served to the guest.

Another commonly used ingredient in Indian desserts is *chandi ka warq*. A small piece of silver is beaten between two sheets of leather until it resembles a thin leaf. This is used as a covering on top of almost every dessert in India. The *burfis* are completely covered with silver *warq* before they are cut into shapes. In some places, the usage of this ingredient is banned due to leather being used for producing it. It is due to this reason that a few vegetarian communities do not consume desserts with *chandi ka warq*.

REGIONAL INFLUENCE ON INDIAN SWEETS

India is one country in the world that incorporates a saga of flavours and sensory stimulation in its meals. India presents a range of flavours, diverse culinary techniques, and eating habits. The variety of food in India is very vast and so are the types of sweets. Though there are also some common desserts made in India, we would divide the Indian sweets into four major regions namely North, East, West, and South.

North The north of India includes regions of Kashmir, Punjab, Himachal, and Uttar Pradesh. The abundance of milk in these regions has led to creation of delectable desserts that have spread far and wide to other states of India. Since North India is rich in its dairy products, the usage of ghee also finds its way into the sweets. The influence of Mughals in this region has also added dishes like halwas and other kinds of pudding.

Let us discuss a few common sweets of North India in Table 11.10.

Table 11.10 Common sweets from North India

Sweet	Description
Gulab jamun	The name literally translates to rose berries as *gulab* means rose and *jamun* means berries; it is a popular Indian sweet dish. The deep fried dumplings of *khoya* and flour depict the *jamun* and the rose, honey, and saffron flavoured syrup represents *gulab*, hence the name. It is traditionally made of *chikna khoya* and *maida* which gives the dough the correct consistency and prevents it from cracking while being fried. Sugar is added to the dough which helps to acquire the desired colour and the dumplings are soaked in rose flavoured sugar syrup.
Kala jamun	It is same like *gulab jamun*, the only difference is that it is fried until a deep colour is obtained and it is not served along with syrup. It is served after the *kala jam* has absorbed the sugar syrup.
Zauq-e-shahi	This is yet another variation of *gulab jamun* from Awadh. In this case, the *gulab jamun* is made into marble size and is served garnished with *lachedaar rabri* and chopped pistachios and saffron.
Jalebi	It is a common belief that Mughals brought *jalebis* to India from Arab countries. The *jalebis* are made by making a batter of flour, water, and baking powder. The same is kept in a hot place to ferment and then the consistency is adjusted with more water, if needed. The batter is poured in a thick cloth called *ratna*, which has a hole in the centre. The cloth is folded into a pouch and squeezed to drop the mixture onto hot ghee. The batter is poured in circles to form the peculiar *jalebi* shape. Once crisp fried, it is dipped into saffron flavoured sugar syrup and served hot with *rabri*.
Peda	The most famous *peda* comes from Mathura and Kanpur in Uttar Pradesh. This dessert is made by reducing milk and sugar to a caramelized texture. It is often flavoured with green cardamom powder.
Sohan papdi	*Sohan papdi* as known in Uttar Pradesh or even *pateesa* as known in Jammu, is a dessert made with a mixture of refined flour and *besan*. The mixture is roasted with ghee until fragrant. Then sugar syrup of 2 and 1\2 thread consistency is poured and stirred with a large fork or until thin strands form. The dessert is then flavoured with green cardamom powder, slivers of pistachio, and melon seeds.

(Contd)

Table 11.10 (Contd)

Sweet	Description
Gajar ka halwa	*Gajar ka halwa* is mostly eaten in winters owing to the availability of its ingredients. Bright red carrots are selected for this as this *halwa* is associated with a deep red colour and is garnished with dry fruits and *khoya*. Grated carrots are first allowed to braise in milk and cooked until the milk reduces to the consistency of a *rabri* and the carrots get cooked. Sugar is now added and cooked until it caramelizes. This also helps to deepen the colour. Fried cashew nuts, raisins, and slivers of pistachio are mixed to add richness to the *halwa*. *Daanedaar khoya* is then added to the *gajar ka halwa* and served hot. It is common to see that all *halwas* are served hot in India and probably this is the reason that most of the *halwas* are eaten during winters.
Phirnee	This is a perfect dessert for summers in India. The milk is boiled along with sugar and coarse paste of soaked rice is added to the milk and cooked until it thickens. It is then flavoured with cardamom powder and rose water and immediately poured into earthenware bowls known as *sakora*. The clay pots help to absorb the extra moisture from *phirnee* and allow it to become firm and yet stay creamy. The dessert is then garnished with slivers of pistachios and sprinkle of saffron water. This dessert is eaten chilled. It is made in Punjab and also in Kashmir. The only difference is that in Kashmir, semolina is used instead of rice and is known as *kong phiren*.
Motichoor key ladoo	*Ladoo* in India is referred to almost anything which is hand shaped, round, and sweet. *Motichoor key ladoo* are prepared throughout India and especially, in the areas around Rajasthan, Madhya Pradesh, and North India. A special type of *besan* known as *mota besan* is used for preparing the batter. The batter is then dropped into hot ghee through a slotted spoon which has very small perforations. The dropped pearls are then removed with a slotted spoon and immersed in sugar syrup of 2 and 1/2 thread consistency. The sugar syrup is flavoured with saffron to impart the golden colour to these *ladoos* that is synonymous with them. Chopped almonds and pistachios are added for crunch and taste. When the fried pearls are added to warm sugar syrup, they soak the syrup and swell. These are then shaped into rounds or *ladoos* and garnished with *chandi ka warq*.
Kheer	*Kheer* has been associated with Indian cuisine for more than 5000 years. It was also used as an offering to Gods and then served as *prashad*. It is part of many religious ceremonies as well. Ancient texts mention that rice equal to 1/8th the amount of milk is rubbed with little ghee and cooked in milk until soft and reduced to half. At this stage, it was known as *kshir*. Small amount of ghee and sugar was then added and cooked until thick. This then became *kheer* and was also known as *payas*. Till date *kheer* is made in the same manner and is also known as *payas* in many parts of India.
Kalakand	This dessert is very popular in North India. It is made from cow's milk and sugar. The milk is reduced on a slow flame and a drop of tartaric acid is added at frequent intervals to achieve a granular texture in the milk without curdling it fully. Sugar is then added along with green cardamom powder. It is then set onto a slab and cut into square shapes once cold. The same dessert when cooked for longer duration of time allows the milk solids to attain a caramelized texture and is then known as *milk cake*.
Pinni	*Pinnis* are commonly made in households and it is very common to see households boasting about their grandmother's recipe of the same. *Pinni* is made by roasting wholewheat flour with ghee until fragrant. The crushed dried fruits are then added along with ghee and the mixture is allowed to cool down before shaping it into *ladoos*. *Pinnis* are usually made for pregnant women as it gives strength and vitality required during that stage.

Table 11.10 (Contd)

Sweet	Description
Besan key ladoo	*Besan key ladoo* is another sweet made in North India. *Besan* is roasted in ghee until fragrant. Ghee and sugar are added along with *pindi khoya* and flavoured with green cardamom powder and melon seeds. The *ladoos* are shaped round and served.
Balushahi	*Balushahi* is a famous sweet that comes from Uttar Pradesh. This is made by rubbing flour with ghee and then kneading it into dough with curd and ammonia bicarbonate. The dough is not kneaded until smooth. After resting the dough for an hour, it is then shaped into balls and a dent is made in the centre with the help of the thumb. These are then fried in ghee until golden brown. They are removed from the ghee and dipped into sugar syrup of 2 thread consistency. Once they have soaked the sugar syrup, they are removed and served by garnishing with silver *warq*.
Moong dal halwa	*Moong dal halwa* is made in Uttar Pradesh and Punjab. The green *moong dal* is soaked in water and rubbed to remove the husk. The lentil is then made into a paste known as *pithi*. The *pithi* is cooked in ghee until golden brown. Milk and water cooked with sugar are then added to the *halwa* and cooked until the ghee floats on top. The *halwa* is then flavoured with saffron, green cardamom powder, dried fruits, and *daanedaar khoya*. *Moong dal halwa* is also served hot.
Kulfi falooda	It can be said that *kulfi* is an Indian ice cream. It is made by reducing milk to almost half. Sugar and flavourings are added and the mixture is then packed into special conical moulds that are closed with a cap and sealed with dough. The moulds are then placed in a large clay pot filled with ice and salt. The pot is then shaken until the *kulfi* sets in the mould. The sealing with dough prevents salt to get into the *kulfi*.
	Kulfi is served chilled along with thin noodles made of cornflour paste known as *falooda*. The basic *kulfi* is flavoured with saffron and chopped pistachios, but these days it is common to see a range of *kulfis* from mango to chickoo. Some people make *kulfi* in clay pots and freeze it in the same manner.
Shahi tukra	This dessert is commonly eaten in Uttar Pradesh and also in Hyderabad. This dessert is also an influence of the Mughals. Plain white bread is deep fried in ghee until golden brown and soaked in saffron flavoured *rabri*. It is served chilled garnished with *lachedaar rabri* and chopped pistachios. *Shahi* refers to royal and as the name suggests it was a delicacy eaten in royal courts of Mughal kings.
Ghevar	Ghevar is a very ancient dessert that is also featured in the ancient Hindu epic *Mahabharata*. It is made by combining flour, ghee, and ice cold water into a thin batter. The batter is poured in a thin stream in a tall ring that is placed inside the pan containing hot ghee. The moisture present in the batter turns to steam when poured in hot ghee and it evaporates leaving large holes in the resulting flat disc like structure that has raised edges. The *ghevar* is then removed and placed on a wire rack and flavoured syrup is poured over it. *Ghevar* can be garnished with *rabri*, nuts, and saffron.
Burfi	*Burfi* in India is synonymous to any sweet that is made with *khoya* as a base and then set into slabs and cut into different shapes. The two most common shapes are lozenge and squares.
	There can be various flavours and combinations of *burfis*, but the common ingredient is *khoya*. *Daab khoya* is cooked along with sugar on a very slow fire until the mixture stops sticking to hands. It is poured onto a greased surface and the *burfi* is cut into squares or lozenges and served covered with silver *warq*.

Gulab jamun

Kala jamun

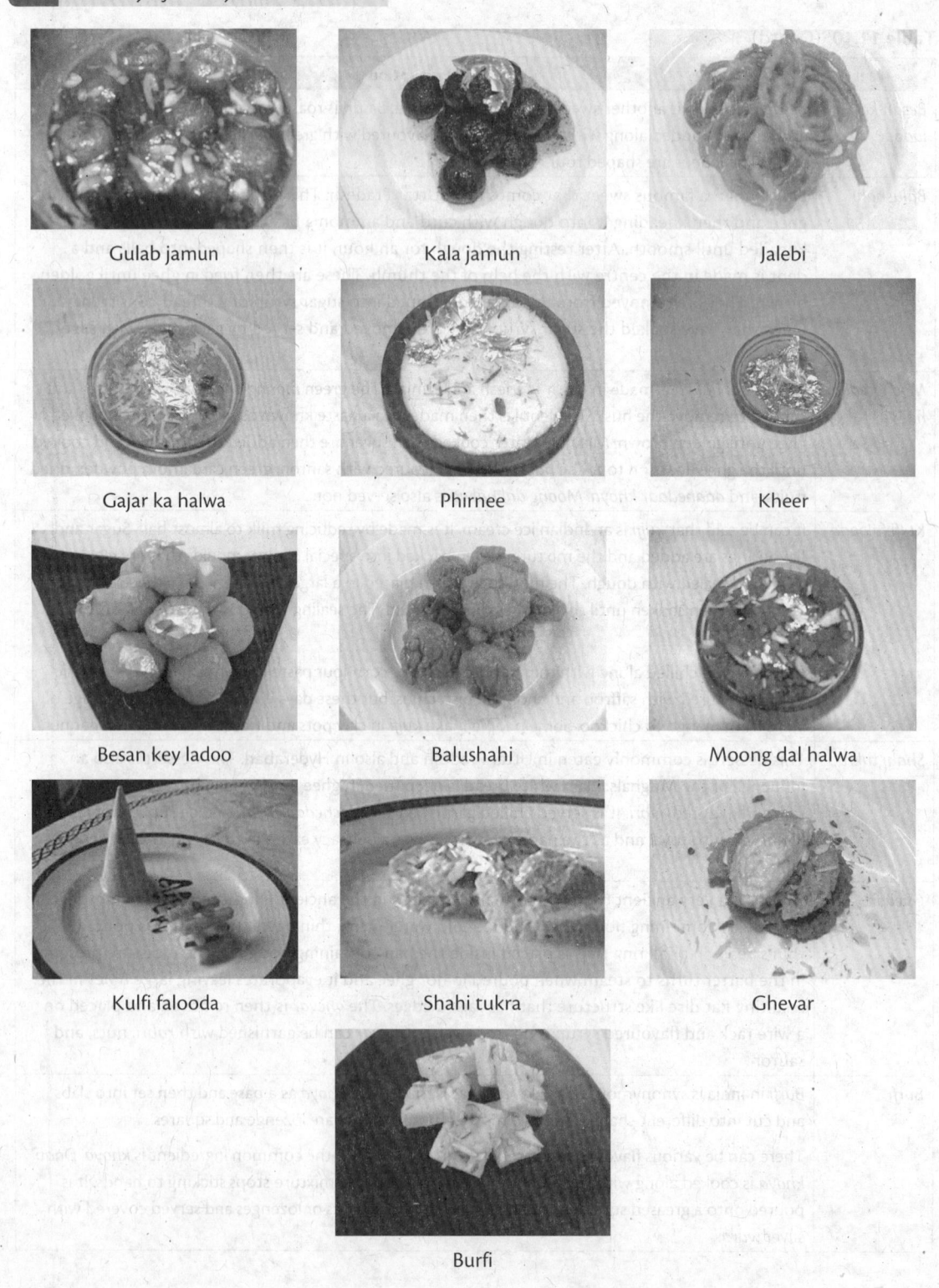

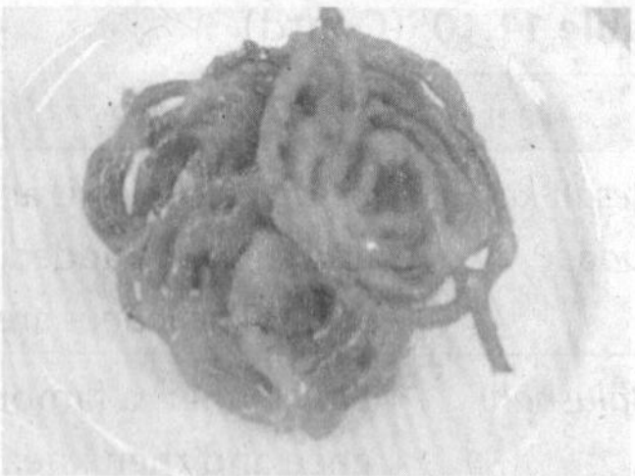

Jalebi

Gajar ka halwa

Phirnee

Kheer

Besan key ladoo

Balushahi

Moong dal halwa

Kulfi falooda

Shahi tukra

Ghevar

Burfi

Fig. 11.1 Common sweets from North India

Indian Sweets

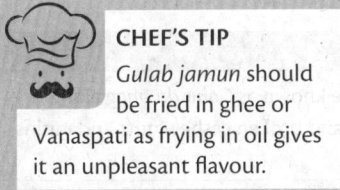

> **CHEF'S TIP**
> *Gulab jamun* should be fried in ghee or Vanaspati as frying in oil gives it an unpleasant flavour.

East In the eastern region of the country, there is a tradition of consuming sweets very frequently at the end of meals, or as a mini meal or snack. This behaviour can be observed in Bengal more often. Giving and consuming sweets has always been a very important gesture in any kind of East Indian festival be it Durga Puja or a happy occasion for family. Actually, it is from this gesture the word *sandesh* has originated that a person who used to carry a message (*sandesh*) also used to carry sweets as a gesture. This tradition is also closely followed in the other adjoining states such as Bihar and Odisha.

Bengalis have a great affinity towards sweet meats. They will have sweets not only at the end of their meals, but sweets also form a part of snacks in Bengali culture. Also different sweets are associated with different festivals, which are considered to be very important. Moreover, there are specific places in Bengal, which specialize in specific sweets. For example, *rasgulla* from Calcutta, *mihidana* and *sita bhog* from Burdwan, *pantua* from Ranaghat, *shor bhaja* from Krishnanagar, and *mowa* from Jaynagar.

Let us discuss some of the famous sweets that come from east of India in Table 11.11.

Table 11.11 Common sweets from east of India

Sweet	Description
Rasgulla	It is prepared from cottage cheese (*chenna*), which is kneaded first and then rolled into small balls. These balls are again cooked in thin, clear sugar syrup. The rasgulla did not reach its fame until K.C. Das popularized the same by canning and marketing it all over the world. Today, this is one of the sweets which is so popular that it is canned and exported to foreign countries. Rasgullas are made in various sizes and flavours and are named differently. Some of the most common ones are: *Nolen gurer rasgulla*: The *rasgullas* are poached in *nolen gur* and this is the only *rasgulla* that is served hot otherwise *rasgullas* are served chilled. *Raj bhog*: This *rasgulla* is large in size and the diameter can be between 3–4 inches. *Kamala bhog*: This is a large *rasgulla*, which is coloured yellow and is flavoured with oranges.
Rasmalai	This is a variation of *rasgulla*, as it is prepared like a *rasgulla* but the *chenna* dumplings are flattened and poached in syrup until cooked. These are then soaked in saffron flavoured sweetened *rabri* or reduced milk (refer to Table 11.4) and served chilled with chopped pistachios.
Patishapta	This is a dessert which is made to celebrate the end of the Bengali year called *poush sankranti*. It is made like a pancake from the batter of refined flour and milk and then it is stuffed with a cooked mixture of grated coconut, sugar or jaggery, and cardamom powder. While being stuffed, these pancakes are rolled with the stuffing in the middle.
Misti doi	This delicacy is prepared like a regular curd but with the addition of jaggery to it. Only palm jaggery is to be used to get that particular colour and taste. It is quite an art to make *misti doi* and the creamy texture of the curd with a layer of fat on top is a skill that is handed down from one generation to another.
Sandesh	It is one of the most famous Bengali desserts made with palm jaggery, reduced milk, and *chenna*. The ingredients are cooked in a thick bottom pan until they stop sticking. They are then pressed into moulds of various shapes to give them the characteristic shape. Variations of *sandesh* are prepared by altering its shape and flavour.

(Contd)

Table 11.11 (Contd)

Sweet	Description
Payesh	*Payesh* is commonly made at home by cooking short grain rice known as *Gobinda bhog* along with milk until creamy. Jaggery is used for sweetening *payesh* and broken cashew nuts and raisins are added for texture.
Lady Kenny	This sweet was made to honour Lady Canning, wife of Lord Canning, the Viceroy of India. She apparently liked the *gulab jamun* of north so much that she packed a few to be taken to Calcutta and requested the Bengali sweet makers to make this dessert. Since the usage of *khoya* was very less in Bengal, this dessert was achieved by using *chenna*. This particular sweet was much appreciated by the Lady and finally came to be known as Lady Canning, which over a period of time has been shortened to Lady Kenny. Various shapes and sizes using the same dough are prepared for making various other desserts such as: *Pantua*: Flat disc shaped, it is fried in ghee and poached in sugar syrup. *Lengcha*: It is 2 inches long and rod shaped. It is fried in ghee and poached in sugar syrup. *Chenaar jalepi*: Dough is shaped into a spiral, fried in ghee and poached in sugar syrup.
Khaja	This dessert comes from Bihar and it is prepared by kneading wheat flour that is rolled into circular shape in which *mawa* (cottage cheese, *khoya*, and dried fruits) is stuffed. It is then deep fried till crisp and then soaked in sugar syrup known as *pak*, till it absorbs the syrup. The most famous *khaja* comes from Gaya, it is also prepared as *prashad* in most of the famous temples of this region, and no wedding ceremony is considered complete without it.
Thekua	Another famous dessert from Bihar is made by mixing wholewheat flour, jaggery, ghee, and cardamom powder or coconut powder, then shaping the mixture in a *sancha* (mould) and deep frying it in ghee till reddish brown. It is then cooled and served or can be stored for quite a long time.
Kakara	This dessert comes from Odisha. It is a sweet prepared from dough of rice flour, refined flour, jaggery, and salt. It is stuffed with a mixture of grated coconut, black pepper, and jaggery. These dumplings are then deep fried until crisp.
Chenna poda	This is a very famous dessert from Odisha and is made in an interesting manner. It is baked and probably it has been influenced by the baked cheesecake of the West. To make this sweet, one has to make the paste of soaked rice and *urad* lentil. Water is added to this paste and it is made into a pouring consistency. Usually, crushed aniseed is used for flavouring the batter. Another mixture is made by cooking grated coconut and jaggery until the jaggery melts. *Chenna* or fresh cottage cheese is added and the mixture is cooked until it begins to leave the sides of the pan. Raisins, crushed aniseed, and ginger powder are added to it for flavouring. Then, a mould is prepared by lining it with banana leaves and alternatively the rice and lentil batter and cooked cottage cheese mixture is poured into the mould and baked until it is cooked and slightly brown.
Kancha gola	This is a soft *sandesh* from Bengal. It is made by cooking fresh curd, milk, and condensed milk. The boiling of curd along with milk results in a curdled texture that is cooked until it becomes sticky. At this stage, it is removed from fire and green cardamom powder is added to it. It is then shaped into round dumplings and served. This *sandesh* is slightly granular in texture.

Rasgulla 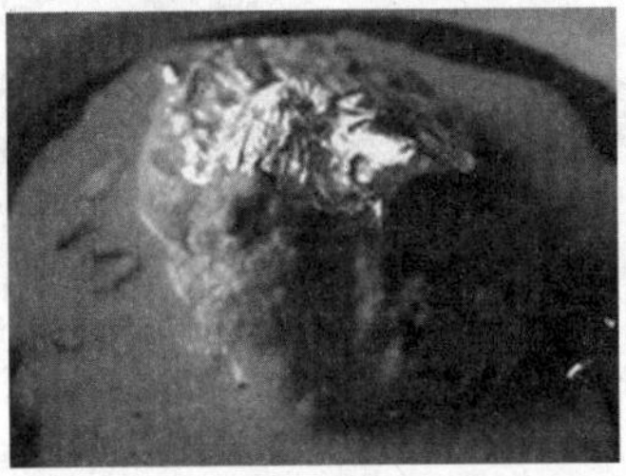　　　　Rasmalai　　　　Patishapta

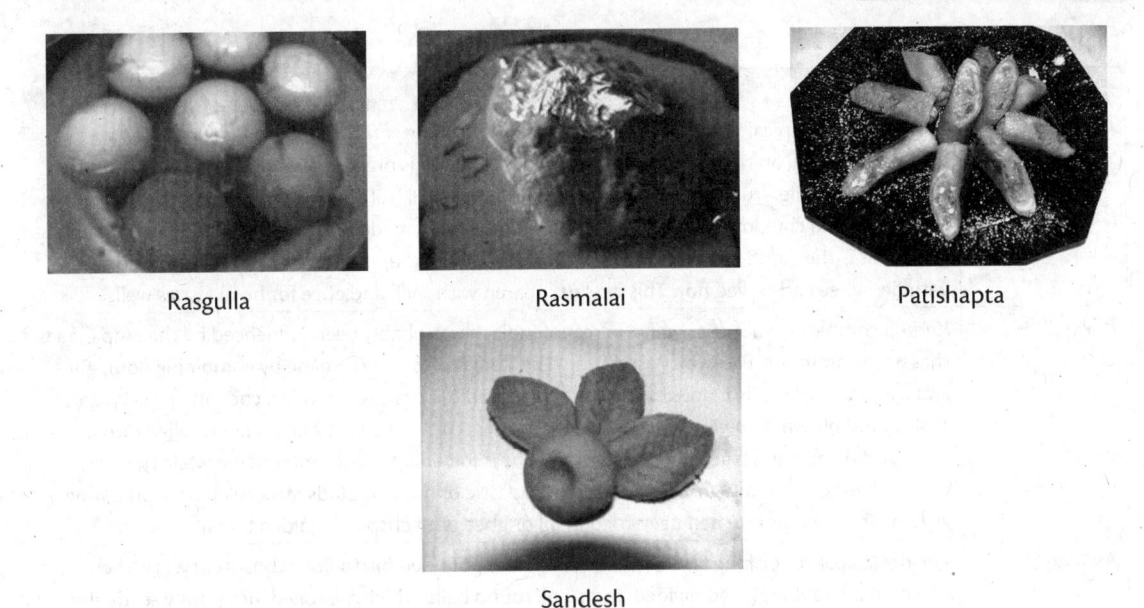

Sandesh

Fig. 11.2 Common sweets from east of India

West Western India comprises of Goa, Maharashtra, and Gujarat. Goan sweets have their origin both in Portugal and the local Konkani region. On Christmas, trays of delicacies are produced and consumed. After the Christmas midnight mass, families visit each other and share a slice of the Christmas cake and a glass of wine. The next morning there is an exchange of sweets, with each tray covered with a homemade Christmas crib and a Christmas star. Each locality usually has a competition to judge the best star and crib.

Coconut, rice, jaggery, and ghee are commonly used ingredients in western Indian sweets. Some of the sweets from Maharashtra are famous all around India. Gujaratis have such love for sweets that even their food is also slightly on the sweeter side. Let us discuss some of the famous sweets from western India in Table 11.12.

Table 11.12 Common sweets from west of India

Sweet	Description
Shrikhand	This is a yoghurt based dessert from Gujarat and is also made in Maharashtra. The dish is prepared by placing hung yoghurt and powdered sugar in a deep bowl and mixing them thoroughly. Cardamom powder and saffron are then added and mixed. This dessert is then strained through a fine muslin cloth a few times. This gives it a shiny texture. It is then stored in earthenware pots, so that it absorbs extra moisture and yields a thick and creamy dessert. The dish is served chilled. It is known as *amrakhand* if pureed mangos are added to it.
Modak	Rice flour is prepared into dough by adding hot water. The dough is rolled and a stuffing of jaggery, coconut, and dry fruits is placed in the centre. It is made into the shape of a *potli* that resembles the shape of a fig fruit and is then steamed. This dessert is prepared on Ganesh Chaturthi as it was the favourite dessert of Lord Ganesha. In some places, *modaks* are also deep fried until crisp.

(Contd)

Table 11.12 (Contd)

Sweet	Description
Puran poli	This is another typical sweet from Maharashtra that can be eaten as breakfast or simply as a dessert, especially on the occasion of Holi. The soft dough is prepared with ghee and water and left to rest. Meanwhile, stuffing is prepared by boiling *channa* lentil along with whole spices such as cardamom and cinnamon. Once cooked the *channa* dal is made into a paste by adding sugar and ghee. This is then stuffed in the dough and rolled out like *chappatis*. *Puran polis* are griddle fried with desi ghee and served hot. This dessert is eaten with milk and ghee for breakfast as well.
Karanji	*Karanji* commonly known as *gujiya* in rest of India, has probably been influenced by the empanadas that were commonly eaten by Portuguese. The dough of *karanji* is made by combining flour, ghee, and water to make a firm dough. Stuffing is prepared by roasting semolina, coconut, jaggery, and raisins until brown. *Khoya* is added to give moistness to the stuffing. The dough is rolled into a circle and the filling is placed in its centre, then it is folded into half-moon shape while the sides are pinched to give a design. These days many plastic or metal moulds are available for preparing *gujiyas*. The *karanjis* are then deep fried in oil or ghee until crisp and golden brown.
Anarsa	The rice is soaked for four days and then dried and pounded into a flour consistency. It is then prepared into a dough and divided into small round balls, which are rolled into poppy seeds and shaped into a *poorie*, then deep fried in ghee. It is also known as *shali poop* in Maharashtra as *shali* means rice.
Bibinca	The most famous Goan sweet meat is the many layered *bibinca*. It is prepared by adding extract of coconut milk to flour, sugar, and other flavourings. Each layer is baked before adding the next one and the traditional version has 16 layers.
Laganu custer	No Parsi wedding is complete without *laganu custer* being on the menu. To make *laganu custer*, milk is boiled along with sugar and reduced until half in size. Powdered nutmeg is added for flavour and when the mixture is cool enough, eggs are beaten into the mixture along with dried fruits. This is then baked in a moderate oven until the top surface is golden brown and the custard is firm.
Dodol	*Dodol* is another famous dessert from Goa and this has been influenced by the Portuguese. Fresh coconut milk is boiled along with rice flour and cooked on a slow flame until it thickens. Towards the end, jaggery and dried fruits are added and the mixture is cooked until it leaves the sides of the pan. It is poured onto a greased tray and then cut into squares after it has cooled down.
Bolinas	These are small cakes also known as coconut cookies in Goa. They are made with grated coconut, sugar, semolina, egg yolks, and butter; they are flavoured with cardamom and are shaped round with markings on top and baked gently. They taste great when served with a hot cup of tea/coffee or on the side of a scoop of ice cream as a dessert.
Baath	This is a famous dessert from Goa. It is a moist rich coconut tart baked in a large round shape with pastry lattice work on top and flavoured with cardamom and currants. Once baked, it is cut into pieces and served surrounded with other sweets on the festive sweet tray. It is served warm with scoops of melting ice cream or crème anglaise (egg custard) on top.
Kharak halwa	This is a famous dessert of the Bohri community in Gujarat. This dessert is a *halwa* made from a paste of dates that are roasted in ghee and cooked with milk and sugar. This is a very heavy dessert and is consumed in small quantities.
Sheer kurma	This is also from the Bohri community and is made on the occasion of Ramadan and Id. The milk is boiled along with sugar and reduced to half. In a separate pan, vermicelli is fried in ghee and reduced milk is added to the vermicelli along with raisins and dried fruits. The pudding is cooked until it becomes thick. It is served hot or cold garnished with silver *warq*.

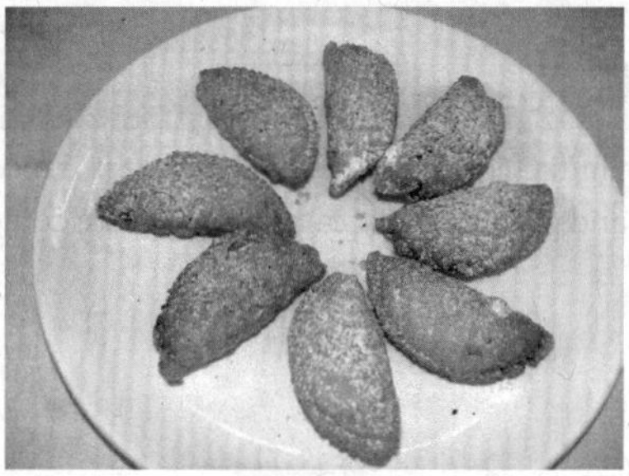

Karanji 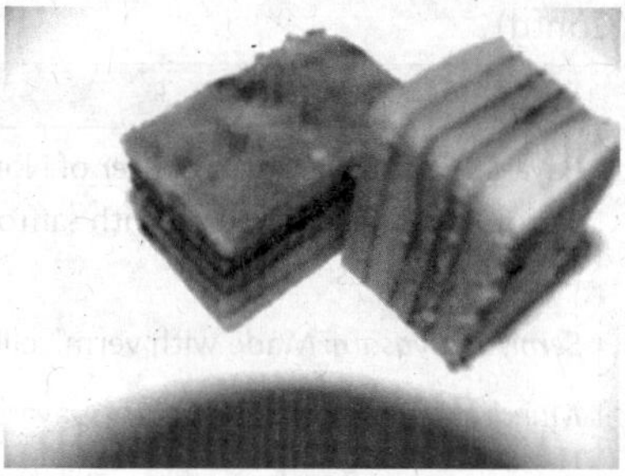   Bibinca

Fig. 11.3 Common sweets from west of India

South The most common sweet from South India is *payasam*. However, the popularity of the sweets from South India has not shown positive signs in north and other parts of the country as compared to their other foods such as *idli*, *dosa*, and *vadas*. *Payasam* is a milk based pudding often made with rice, milk, and sugar. The word *payasam* is derived from the Sanskrit word *peeyusham* which means nectar. *Payasam* is generally served as an offering to the Gods. South Indian people often have an affinity towards this dish and it is prepared during most festivals in south. It is also hard to find a South Indian wedding feast without *payasam*. In the state of Kerala, *payasam* is often made with coconut milk and jaggery.

The desserts made in south are made by cooking methods such as frying and steaming, and they are also made using the locally available ingredients such as coconut, jaggery, bananas, rice, and milk. Kerala, Andhra Pradesh, Chennai, and Karnataka largely form the states of South India. Let us discuss some of the common desserts from South India in Table 11.13.

Table 11.13 Common sweets from South India

Sweet	Description
Ada pradaman	This dessert is made with pressed rice also known as *poha*. The *poha* is soaked in water for 30 minutes and then drained. Jaggery is melted with water and soaked rice is added along with the thin extract of coconut milk. It is cooked till the mixture thickens. Thick coconut milk is now added and it is removed as soon as the mixture comes to a boil. This dish is garnished with fried flakes of coconut, cashew nuts, and raisins. This can be served hot or cold.
Pongal	The most important festival in Tamil Nadu is *Pongal*. It is the harvest festival and is celebrated at the beginning of the Tamil new year. *Pongal* literally translates to boiled rice and various types of *pongals* including savoury ones are prepared and eaten on this festive occasion. The sweet *pongal* is known as *sarkari pongal* or *chakkera pongal*.
	This dessert is made by boiling rice in combination of water and milk. Powder of roasted *moong dal* and Bengal gram is also added to the rice and cooked. Once the rice is boiled, mixture of jaggery and ghee is added to the rice and the mixture is allowed to cook on slow fire. The *pongal* is then garnished with cashew nuts and raisins, and flavoured with green cardamom.
Mysore pak	Mysore pak is one of the most famous sweets of South India. It originated from the city of Mysore in Karnataka. It is made with a generous amount of ghee, sugar syrup, and gram flour (*besan*). It was invented by a chef named Kakasura Madappa in the kitchens of the Mysore palace.

(Contd)

Table 11.13 (Contd)

Sweet	Description
Payasam	Payasam is usually like the *kheer* of North India. The only difference is that it is mostly served warm. Payasam is flavoured with saffron and ground green cardamom. There could be variations of payasam such as: *Semiya payasam*: Made with vermicelli *Mundriparupu payasam*: Carrot payasam *Ada payasam*: Rice flour paste and jaggery cooked with milk *Parupu payasam*: Milk, jaggery, and paste of *channa* lentil
Kaya porichattu	This is one of the simplest desserts commonly made in every household. Sliced bananas are shallow fried in ghee and sprinkled with sugar and rosewater.
Kalathappam	These are sweet rice cakes made by soaking rice in water and grinding it into a very fine powder. It is then cooked along with jaggery and flavoured with green cardamom powder in an *urli* on very low heat with some burning charcoals on top of the lid. This way the dessert gets baked and is served hot. It can also be baked in an oven.
Mutta mala	This is an egg based dessert from Kerala. Egg yolks are whisked and passed through muslin cloth. Water and sugar are boiled to one string consistency and clarified with small amount of egg whites. The egg yolk mixture is poured on to hot sugar syrup through a coconut shell which has a hole in the centre. It is poured in a circular motion to form rings in the syrup. The egg strings are removed without breaking them and put on top of wire rack to drain off the excess sugar syrup.
Basundi	*Basundi* is a creamy milk pudding, prepared by boiling milk until it reduces to one third of its volume. It is sweetened with sugar and flavoured with green cardamom and saffron, and is garnished with chopped pistachios. *Basundi* is served chilled.
Unni appam	One of the most famous sweets of Kerala, it is usually served as an offering to Lord Ganapati. *Unni appam* is small round shaped rice cakes made from a batter of rice, jaggery, and banana, which is fried in ghee. A special brass vessel which looks similar to a *paniharam* dish is used to make this sweet.
Pootharekulu	A sweet dish from the state of Andhra Pradesh developed by the Brahmin families of Rajahmundry. It consists of wafer thin rice sheets brushed with ghee and sprinkled with fine powdered sugar. It is rolled, cut and eaten. In Telugu, *pootha* means coating and *reku* means foil, it is considered one of the most difficult Indian sweet preparations. In traditional Telugu weddings, the bridegroom is fed this sweet by his bride.
Ariselu	*Ariselu*, a Dravidian word which means of rice, originated in the town of Guntur in Andhra Pradesh. It is made by making dough with equal proportions of rice flour, ghee, and jaggery; then it is rolled like a *poorie* which is then deep fried. It is served during the festivals of *Ugadi* and *Sankranti*.
Khubani ka meetha	*Khubani* is an Urdu term for apricots. It is a popular dessert of Hyderabad and is a common feature of Hyderabadi weddings. It is usually accompanied with cream. It is made by stewing apricots in sugar and then flavouring them with honey.
Double ka meetha	The word *double ka meetha* comes from the Hindi word *double roti*, referred to a loaf of bread. The bread is cut into small pieces and deep fried in ghee, then it is soaked in boiling milk to which sugar and *khoya* are added. It is garnished with slivers of almond and pistachios. This dessert is served hot.
Imarti	*Imarti*, also known as *jhangri*, is commonly made in Chennai. It is made with a paste of *urad dal*, which is forced through a bag into hot ghee as done in case of *jalebis*. The batter is poured in a flower shape and once fried crisp, it is soaked in saffron flavoured sugar syrup.

EQUIPMENT USED IN HALWAI

Every cuisine requires some kind of specialized equipment to produce its dishes. The equipment required in making Indian sweets are not as varied as the ones required in Western cuisines. However, the two most important things regarding utensils used for making Indian desserts are—the choice of metal and the thickness of the same. The metal chosen should be non-corrosive and should be such that it does not react with dairy products. A large iron *kadhai* that is always washed and kept clean is used for most of the desserts. However, certain typical kinds of tools and equipment are required for making Indian sweets and these are different from one region to another based on the kind of dish to be made. Let us discuss some of the commonly used equipment and tools in making Indian sweets in Table 11.14.

Table 11.14 Equipment and tools used in making Indian sweets

Equipment	Description
Kadhai/Karahi	This is also known as *halwai karahi*. It is made of cast iron and the surface is always clean and polished. There can be many varieties of *karahi* but they have one thing in common—the base. The base of *karahi* is thick bottomed and sometimes an extra piece of metal is sandwiched to the bottom of the *karahi*. The heavy base allows cooking on slow fire for longer duration of time without burning the product. The karahi for making *rabri* is shallow and has a larger surface area to allow the evaporation of liquid whilst boiling the milk.
Nounko	These are metal tubs used for storage of sweets in syrup. This equipment is commonly used in Bengal and the term *nounko* is also Bengali.
Milk cans	Large metallic drums are used for storage of milk in *halwai* shops. They are made of thick steel or aluminium.
Khoncha	It is the equipment for stirring milk; it has a very thin and sharp ending, just to scrap off the *kadhai* while reducing milk. It also helps in preventing the milk from sticking to the base.
Jhaara	It is basically a strainer used for straining excessive oil or ghee from *boondi* or any other sweet such as *jalebi*. It can be available in many sizes and the size of the perforations can vary as per its usage. As gram flour batter is dropped into hot ghee or fat to make *boondis*, the size of the *boondi* depends upon the size of the perforations in a *jhaara*. Jhaara for making *boondis* is numbered as 000, 001, 002 and so on. The 000 number is used for making the smallest *boondi*, which is used in preparing *motichoor key ladoo*.
Jalebi tawa	This utensil is made of cast iron and is only 3 inches deep and wide. The ghee is filled up to half of the utensil and the batter is dropped through a cloth pouch in circular rings.
Ratna	*Ratna* is a thick square piece of cloth that has a hole in its centre. It is also known as *jalebi* cloth. The batter is poured into the centre and the corners are lifted to form a pouch. This is then squeezed between the fists to drop the batter into hot fat for making *jalebis*. A similar kind of cloth is also used for making *imarti*.
Chalanee	This equipment is used to sift flour to remove impurities from it before using it as an ingredient. Sifting also helps to incorporate air in the flour and at the same time it helps to thoroughly mix the ingredients.
Lagan	*Lagan* is a shallow copper utensil with thick bottom. It is commonly used in Mughlai cooking, but it is also used very frequently to make *halwas*. The copper utensil should be tinned before it can be used for cooking.
Uniappam chatti	*Unniappam* is small round shaped rice cakes made from a batter of rice, jaggery, and banana and is fried in ghee. A special brass vessel which looks similar to a *paniharam* dish is used to make this sweet.

(Contd)

Table 11.14 (Contd)

Equipment	Description
Modak patra	This is a copper vessel used for making modak.
Gujiya sancha	This is a small equipment used for making gujiya. The designed edges help to crimp the edges of the dough and also give a design to the gujiya.
Sandesh moulds	These moulds are made with wood and are available in various shapes and sizes. Some of the shapes are symbolic to the type of sandesh. These are used in Bengal to make sandesh.
Gheevar ring	This is a tall metallic ring usually 12 inches high. The diameter of the ring would govern the diameter of the gheevar. This tube is placed inside a pot full of fat and the batter is dropped in thin stream in the centre of the tube to make gheevar.

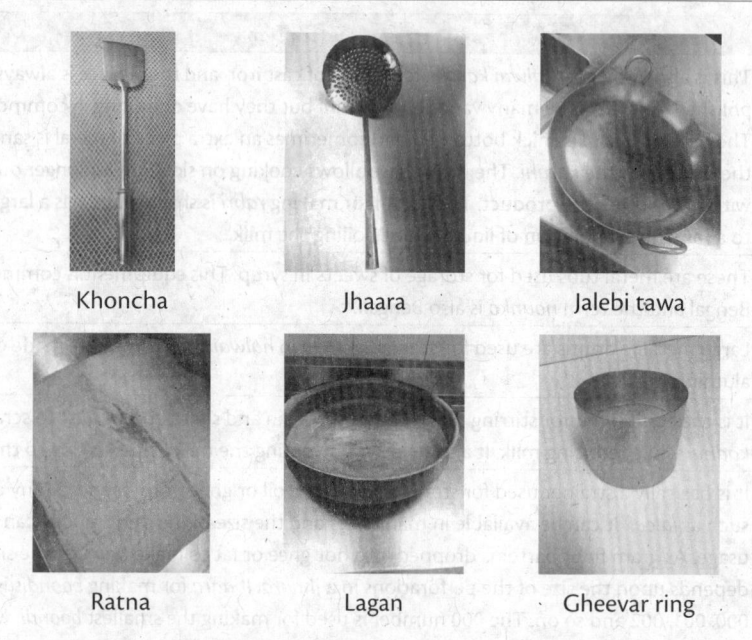

Khoncha   Jhaara   Jalebi tawa

Ratna   Lagan   Gheevar ring

Fig. 11.5 Equipment used in making Indian sweets

RELIGIOUS IMPORTANCE OF SWEETS

Indian sweets are synonymous with festive occasions. No festival or even a happy ceremony is complete without a sweet attached with it. Diwali is one of the festivals in India which is synonymous with sweets. Small road side shops mushroom up in every nook and corner and people buy sweets for themselves and their family and friends. On occasions such as marriages, it is customary to give sweet boxes in figures of 11, 21, 51, or 101 as a ritual that is known as *shagun*. Sweets are sold in kilos, but it is also common to see some sweets being sold per piece. Some sweets are offered as *prashad*, whilst some are relished as it is.

There is no particular time of having a sweet. Unlike Western countries, where desserts form a course after the meals, in India sweets can be eaten almost any time of the day. Any good news is accompanied with sweet and it is common to hear people ask for sweets, when good news is shared with them. India is a land of festivals and festivals mean celebrations. Families and friends get together to celebrate a festival and when people are together, sharing food and sweets becomes the norm. Different festivals fall on certain times of the year and the climate and the availability of ingredients during that time of the year has given birth to sweets that are now associated with those festivals. Some sweets are customary in a particular festival and it could be governed by many factors such as God's favourite sweet—*modak*, commonly made on Ganesh Chaturthi in Maharashtra.

SUMMARY

In the previous chapters, we discussed about the various products made in bakery and pastry and this chapter again unfolds the mystery of the Indian cuisine with a focus on Indian *halwai*—a vast subject in itself. The name *halwai* is coined from the word *halwa*, which means pudding, but in broader sense, *halwai* is the one who prepares sweets as well as snacks and things such as *chaats* and other savoury products. The desserts of India are simple and use very simple ingredients, yet the art of making them is quite complicated due to lack of standard recipes. The entire process is carried out on the feel of the product with hands at every stage and this can be only monitored when the person has been long enough in the trade of Indian sweets.

Very few of the Indian desserts have been popular all over the world, because of high content of sugar in them. Yet some of them are eaten quite commonly around the world. Desserts such as *kulfi*, *rasgulla*, *jalebi*, and *gulab jamun* have been popularized by the Indian restaurants abroad and the international traveller is aware of these dishes. The desserts in India have a very special place in the hearts of the people as they are related to happy memories and festive occasions. Any good news is accompanied with sweets and no festivity or celebration is complete without a sweet or two.

In this chapter, we discussed about various kinds of sweets that have been influenced by travellers and rulers who came to India in the past. We also discussed about ingredients commonly used by the *halwais* for making Indian desserts. Though most of the spices and ingredients are common to other foods of India, some specialized ingredients such as *khoya* and that too, types of *khoya*, spices such as cardamom and cloves are also usually used in Indian sweets. We read in this chapter about the various kinds of cereals, sweeteners, dairy products, and chemicals used by *halwais*. We also discussed the stages of sugar and the terminologies used by the sweet makers in India. The concept of *taar* is shown with relation to the Western stages of sugar such as soft ball and hard crack. This chapter describes the special tools and utensils used in making Indian sweets and last but not the least, it emphasizes on the importance of sweets in religion and during festivities.

KEY TERMS

Benami kheer Pudding made by cooking semolina or rice with garlic flakes and sugar

Bhog An offering made to God, also known as *naivaida*, and after that it is distributed as *prashad* amongst the devotees

Black jack The last stage of sugar boiling when it turns to black and emits smoke

Boora Raw sugar used in *chaats* and Indian sweets

Calcium hydroxide Chemical used as an alkaline base to add crunch to certain desserts

Chashni Sugar syrup of various consistencies used in Indian desserts

Chenna Fresh cottage cheese that is not pressed into a cake. The whey from the *chenna* is used for curdling the milk for more *chenna*

Chikki A candy made of caramelized sugar, nuts, and flavourings such as rose

Copra Dried coconut kernel used in Indian cuisine

Empanadas Sweet or savoury crisp fried pastries usually made in half-moon shapes and served in South America

Galettes Small round patties of minced meat or vegetables

Gulkand A kind of thick chutney made with rose, honey, and sugar

Gur Hindi name for jaggery

Halwai Person who makes sweets and savoury snacks

Kaju katli Another name for *Kaju burfi*

Khoya Reduced milk solids obtained by reducing milk on slow heat

Kong phiren Dessert made in Kashmir by boiling milk, sugar, and semolina and setting in earthenware bowls

Kulfi Frozen Indian dessert made by reducing milk with sugar and flavourings until it thickens

Ladoo A round dumpling of sweet commodity usually served as a dessert

Mamra Variety of almonds used for making almond *halwa*

Mawa Refer to *khoya*

Nolen gur New *gur* or *gur* from Palm tree usually available in winters in Bengal

Pithi Soaked white *urad* lentils that are ground to a paste without addition of water

Prashad A pudding usually a sweet that is distributed to the devotees as a blessing from God

Ratna Square shaped cloth made of thick cotton with a hole in centre to make *jalebis*

Sakora An earthenware bowl used for serving desserts such as *shrikhand* and *phirnee*

Sancha Hindi terminology for a mould

Taar The strings formed when the sugar is pulled between thumb and finger. The number of threads depicts the density and stages of sugar boiling

Vanaspati Vegetable oils that are saturated with hydrogen atoms to make them more stable and appear like fats at room temperature

OBJECTIVE TYPE QUESTIONS

1. What is the importance of sweets in India and how are these different from Western desserts?
2. What do you understand by comfort food?
3. What is the major difference between the desserts made in north and east India?
4. Which communities around the world have influenced the sweets of India?
5. Name at least three cereals that are used in sweet making and give three examples of each.
6. In what form are lentils used in making Indian sweets?
7. What are the two types of *besan* used in Indian sweets and what are their roles?
8. Name three types of sweeteners used in Indian sweets.
9. What is sweet milk and what is its usage in Indian *halwai*?
10. What is *rabri* and describe two types of *rabri*?
11. What role do chemicals play in making of Indian sweets? Name any three and their usage.
12. Name at least three vegetables that are used for making Indian sweets and give one example of each.
13. What is *gulkand*? Name at least three spices that are commonly used for flavouring Indian sweets.
14. Write a short note on sweets of North India.
15. Name two other sweets that are based on the concept of *gulab jamun*.
16. What is a *phirnee* and what is the process of making it?
17. Describe *gheevar* and its festive importance.
18. Write a short note on sweets from Bengal.
19. List at least three varieties of *rasgulla*.
20. What is the significance of *sandesh* in Indian sweets?
21. List at least two sweets from Bihar.
22. Why *shrikhand* is always served in an earthenware pot?
23. What is the difference between *karanji* and *gujiya*?
24. What is sweet *pongal* known as and what is its importance?
25. What is *basundi* and what is the process of making it?
26. How is the *halwai karahi* different from the regular *karahi*?
27. Explain *jhaara* and how does the selection of one impact the final product.
28. Describe *ratna* and its usage.

ESSAY TYPE QUESTIONS

1. Describe the word *payasam* and list at least three kinds of *payasam*.
2. Name at least three Goan desserts and write a brief note on any one.
3. What is the peculiarity of desserts of South India?
4. Why is the *gulab jamun* from Bengal known as Lady Kenny?
5. Write a short note on *motichoor key ladoo*.
6. Describe the process of making a *jalebi*.
7. What is the concept of checking the *taar* and how does it correspond to the stages of sugar boiling?
8. What is *khoya* and list three types of *khoya* with their characteristics?
9. What is the difference between *bhog* and *prashad* and how are they interrelated to sweets?

ACTIVITY

1. In a group of five, do a market survey of Indian sweet shops and list down the sweets that they sell. Make your observation in the following table as per the example given.
2. In groups of five, research about at least three desserts from each state of India, and write the unique process, ingredients, and equipment used in making of the same. Record your observations and make a presentation to the rest of the team.
3. In groups of four to five, visit the places that are famous for their product. Sample the food and record your observations with regards to what makes them so special. Present the findings to the team. This project would enable you to know more about the product and also recommend the place to your friends.

Sweet	Base	Region	Typical ingredients used	Festive influence	Flavour
Gulab jamun	*Khoya*	North	*Khoya*, paneer, flour	All year around	Saffron, rose

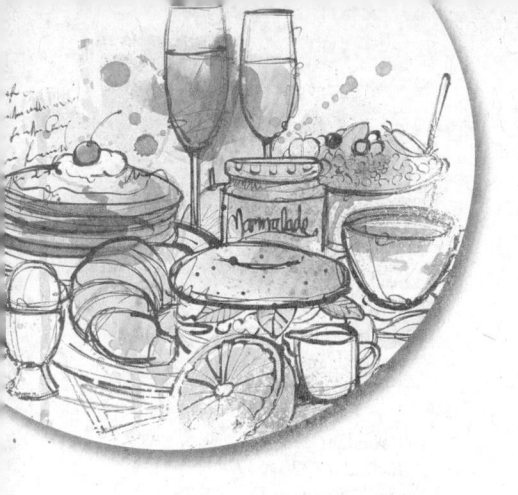

Index

A

Anti-crystalizing agents 209
  cream of tartar 210
  fondant 210
  glucose 209
  lemon juice 210
  tartaric acid solution 209

B

Bakery produces 1
  breads 1
  cakes 1
  chocolate 1
  cookies 1
  desserts 1
  pastries 1
Basic sponges 131
  angel food cake 132
  butter cake sponge 134
  chiffon cake 131
  dacquoise sponge 135
  devil's food cake 133
  eggless sponge 135
  genoese 131
  japonaise 135
  joconde sponge 134
  madeira sponge 133
  swiss roll sponge 133
  Victoria sponge 132
Bread making methods 67
  baking 71
  collecting the mise en place 67
  dividing and scaling 70
  final proof 70
  knock back 70
  mixing of the ingredients 67
    ferment/sponge method 68
    no time dough method 68
    salt delayed method 69
    straight dough method 68
  proving 69
  scoring 71
  shaping/panning 70
Breads of America 86
  banana bread 86
  burger bun 86
  hot dog bun 86
Breads of France 79
  baguette also known as french bread 79
  cereale 80
  epi 80
  fougasse 80
  pain de campagne 79
Breads of Germany 82
  kastenbrots 82
  kugelhopf 82
  landbrot 82
  pretzels 82
  pumpernickel 82
  stollen 82
  zopf 82
Breads of Great Britain 83
  bloomer 83
  cob 83
  Danish 83
  English muffins 83
  hot cross buns 83
  hovis 83
  pikelets 84
  stotie 84
Breads of Italy 80
  ciabatta 80
  focaccia 81
  grissini 81
  pagnotta 81
  panettone 81
  pugliese 81
Breads of Middle East 85
  khoubiz 85
  lavash 85
  pita 85

C

Cereals used in Indian sweets 221
  flour and by-products 221
    balushahi 221
    jalebi 221
    kharak halwa 221
    panjiri 221
    pinni 221
    suji halwa 221
  lentils 221
    besan ladoo 221
    imarti 221
    moong dal halwa 221
    motichoor ladoo 221
    Mysore pak 221
    parupu paysam 221
    puran poli 221
    sohan halwa 221
  rice 221
    ada pradaman 221
    kheer 221
    payesh 221
  rice flour 221
    modak 221
    phirnee 221
Cheese 30
  mascarpone 31
  philadelphia 31
  quark 31
  ricotta 31
  yoghurt 31
Classical and contemporary sauces 119
  apricot jam 121
  butterscotch 120

caramel 120
chocolate 120
crepe suzette 120
melba 120
sabayon 121
strawberry coulis 121
tropical fruit salsa 121
vanilla 119
Classical cakes and pastries 137
  baked cheesecake 140
  battenberg 138
  black forest gateaux 138
  Charlotte russe 139
  chilled cheesecake 141
  christmas cake 142
  croquembouche 141
  devil's food cake 140
  dobos torte 137
  gateau pithivier 142
  gateau St Honore 139
  linzer torte 138
  malakoff torte 138
  mud cake 140
  Napoleon gateau 139
  opera gateau 139
  Sacher torte 137
  walnut brownie 140
  yule log 141
Classical frozen desserts 189
  baked Alaska 190
  cassata 190
  fried ice cream 190
  sundaes and coupes 190
    arlesienne 190
    banana split 190
    black forest 190
    jacques 190
    marie louise 190
    peach melba 190
    pears belle helene 190
Classification of pastry sauces 113
  chocolate based 113
  cream based 113
  custard based 113
  miscellaneous 113
  puree based 113
  syrup based 113
Cold desserts 173
  cold puddings 173
    blancmange 174
    flummery 174
    fruit custard 174
    rice conde 174
  custard and cream-based desserts 175
    bavarois 175
    Charlotte 176

fools 176
mousse 176
soufflé 176
fruit-based cold desserts 173
  compotes or poached fruits 174
  fruit platter 174
  fruit salad 174
jellies 177
sponges and yeast-leavened desserts 177
  baba au rhum 178
  fruit trifle 178
  tiramisu 178
  zuccotto 178
tarts, pies, and flans 175
  baked custard flan 177
  bakewell tart 177
  cherry clafouti 177
  chocolate tart 177
  fruit tart 177
  lemon tart 177
Common bread shapes 78
  decorative 78
  knot 78
  logs 78
  moulded 79
  oval 78
  plaits 78
  round 78
  sticks 78
Common faults in bread making 73
  crumbly bread 74
  flaked crust also known as flying tops 73
  lack of colour on crust 74
  lack of flavour and aroma 74
  lack of shine on the crust 74
  lack of volume 74
  rapidly stales 74
  raw inside 74
  uneven texture, showing large irregular holes 74
Common faults in making cookies 162
  cookie does not get proper colour 163
  cookie does not spread 163
  cookie is very brittle and hard 163
  cookie spreads too fast 163
  cookies stick to pans 162
  too crumbly 162
Components of sauce 115
  flavouring agents 116
  liquid 115
  seasoning 117
  thickening agents 116

D

Dairy products 223
  chenna 223
  curd 223
  khoya 223
    batti ka 223
    daab ka 223
    daanedaar 223
  milk 223
  rabri 223
    danedaar 223
    lachedar 223
Diseases caused in breads 75
  moulds 75
  rope 75

E

Eggs 31
  air cell 32
  chalazae 32
  coagulation 33
  emulsification 36
  leavening 33
  lecithin 31
  shell 31
  shell membranes 32
  thick albumen 32
  thin albumen 32
  vitelline 31
  yolk 31

F

Fats and oils 27
  butter 27
  emulsified 27
  fatty acids 27
  glycerol 27
  hydrogenation 27
  lard 27
  lipid 27
  margarine 27
  mufa 27
  pufa 27
  saturation 27
  suet 27
  trans fats 27
Faults in cake making 143
  cake does not have good volume 144
  cracked top 144
  curdling of batter 144
  m fault 143
  sinking of fruits 144
  sugary top 144
  x fault 143

Frozen desserts 181
  bombe 188
    africaine 189
    aida 189
    alhambra 189
    bresilienne 189
    cardinale 189
    ceylon 189
    copella 189
    diplomat 189
    florentine 189
    formosa 189
    zamora 189
  churn-frozen desserts 182
    American ice cream 183
    basic ice creams 182
    French ice cream 183
    frozen yoghurt 183
    gelato 183
    ice milk 183
    sorbet 183
  frozen mousse and
      soufflé 189
  iced charlotte (charlotte
      glace) 189
  iced gateaux (torte glace) 189
  still-frozen desserts 187
    granita 187
    kulfi 187
    parfait 187

H

Hot desserts 167
  crêpes and pancakes 172
  deep-fried desserts 170
    beignets 170
    choux fritters 170
    helado frito 170
    oriental desserts 170
  fruit-based hot desserts 173
    baked 173
    compote 173
    flambéed fruit 173
  laminated pastries 172
    eccles 172
    lebanese baklava 172
    strudel 172
    tarte tatin 172
    turnovers 172
  puddings 167
    baked egg custards 168
    milk puddings 168
    sponge puddings 168
  soufflés 168
    cold 169
    hot 169
  tarts and pies 171

J

Jewish breads 85
  bagel 85
  challah 85
  matzo 85

M

Meringue 33
  floating islands 34
  French macaroons 34
  French meringue 33
  Italian meringue 34
  marshmallows 34
  pavlova 34
  Swiss meringue 34
  vacherin 34
Methods of making
    cookies 151
  creaming 151
  sanding 151
  sponge 151
  straight 151
Milling of flour 23
  acquatron 23
  cockle cylinder 23
  combinator 23
  emery scorer 23
  horizontal scorer 24
  main cleaning 23
  pre-cleaning 23
  tempering 23

N

Nuts used in Indian halwai 225
  almonds 225
  cashew nuts 226
  charaoli 226
  coconut 226
  dates 226
  pistachio 225
  raisins 226

P

Parameters for selecting quality
    flour 24
  ash content 25
  colour grading 24
  diastatic quality of flour 25
  gluten content 24
  moisture 24
  pH 24
  water absorption 25
Pastes 95
  almond paste 101

choux paste 98
  chocolate éclairs 100
  croquembouche 100
  gateau St Honore 100
  paris brest 100
  profiteroles 100
  swans 100
pate à brise 101
pate à sucre 102
puff pastry 101
short crust paste 95
  pinning method 95
  rubbing-in method 95
sweet paste 97
  creaming method 98
  rubbing-in method 98
Processing of chocolate 41
  conching 42
  drying in sun 42
  grinding 42
  harvesting 41
  ripening and fermentation 42
  roasting and crushing the
      beans 42
  selection and blending 42
  tempering 43
Products made with enriched
    dough 87
  berliner 87
  brioche 87
  doughnut 87

R

Raising agents 36
  ammonia bicarbonate 39
  baking powder 39
  bicarbonate of soda 39
  compressed yeast 40
  cream of tartar 40
  dry yeast 40
  fresh yeast 40
  instant yeast 40
  yeasts 39

S

Spices used in Indian halwai 226
  cardamom 226
  cinnamon 226
  cloves 226
  gulab jal 226
  gulkand 226
  kewra 226
  saffron 226
Stages of sugar 200
  107°C, thread 200
  112°C, strong thread 200

Index

118°C, soft ball 200
125°C, hard ball 200
140°C, soft crack 201
150°C, crack 201
155°C, hard crack 201
Sugar confections 198
  candies 203
  caramelitos 203
  caramels 202
  fondant 203
  fudges 202
  gum paste 204
  honeycomb 206
  jam 206
  lollypops 203
  marshmallows 201
  nougatine 204
  pastillage 204
  pate de fruits 207
  praline paste 204
  rock sugar 205
  spun sugar 206
  sugar syrup 201
  toffee 202
Sugar work 209
  pulled sugar 212
  pulled sugar flower 213
  pulled sugar ribbons 213
  sugar for casting 211
Sweeteners 221
  boora 222
  honey 222
  jaggery 222
  sugar 222
Sweets from east of India 231
  chenna poda 232
  kakara 232
  kancha gola 232
  khaja 232
  lady Kenny 232
    chenaar jalepi 232
    lengcha 232
    pantua 232
  misti doi 231
  patishapta 231
  payesh 232
  rasgulla 231
    Kamala bhog 231
    nolen gurer 231
    raj bhog 231
  rasmalai 231
  sandesh 231
  thekua 232
Sweets from South India 235
  ada pradaman 235
  ariselu 236
  basundi 236
  double ka meetha 236
  imarti 236
  kalathappam 236
  kaya porichattu 236
  khubani ka meetha 236
  mutta mala 236
  Mysore pak 235
  payasam 236
    ada 236
    mundriparupu 236
    parupu 236
    semiya 236
  pongal 235
  pootharekulu 236
  unni appam 236
Sweets from west of India 233
  anarsa 234
  baath 234
  bibinca 234
  bolinas 234
  dodol 234
  karanji 234
  kharak halwa 234
  laganu custer 234
  modak 233
  puran poli 234
  sheer kurma 234
  shrikhand 233
Sweets of North India 227
  balushahi 229
  besan key ladoo 229
  burfi 229
  gajar ka halwa 228
  ghevar 229
  gulab jamun 227
  jalebi 227
  kala jamun 227
  kalakand 228
  kheer 228
  kulfi falooda 229
  moong dal halwa 229
  motichoor key ladoo 228
  pateesa 227
  peda 227
  phirnee 228
  pinni 228
  shahi tukra 229
  sohan papdi 227
  zauq-e-shahi 227

T

Techniques of preparing bread 50
  autolysis 50
  baking 53
  kneading 50
    improved kneading method 51
    intense kneading method 51
    short kneading method 50
  prooving 51
    final proving 51
    first proving 51
    intermediate proving 51
    knock back 51
    proving 51
  scoring 54
  shaping 51
  sifting 50
Techniques related to pastry making 55
  blind baking 57
  creaming 55
  docking 56
  folding-in 56
  icing 58
  laminating 58
  pinning or rolling 57
  piping 57
  rubbing-in 55
  whisking 55
Tempering 43
  grafting method 44
  injection method 44
  machine method 45
  microwave method 45
  seeding method 44
  tabling method 44
Tools used in making Indian sweets 237
  chalanee 237
  gheevar ring 238
  gujiya sancha 238
  jalebi tawa 237
  jhaara 237
  kadhai/karahi 237
  khoncha 237
  lagan 237
  milk cans 237
  modak patra 238
  nounko 237
  ratna 237
  sandesh moulds 238
  uniappam chatti 237
Types of chocolate 43
  compound 43
  couverture 43
  dark chocolate 44
  milk chocolate 44
  white chocolate 44
Types of cookies 152
  bar cookies 157
    biscotti 158
    raisin spice bars 158
  cutter-cut cookies 156

Index

bull's eye 157
nice biscuit 157
shortbread 157
shrewsbury biscuit 157
drop cookies 152
  chocolate chip cookie 153
  crunchy drop 153
  florentine 153
  macaroon 153
  oatmeal raisin cookie 153
festive cookies 159
  basler läckerli 160
  brunsli 161
  cinnamon stars 161
  gingerbread 161
  pertikus 161
  pizzelle 160
  spekulaas 161
frozen and cut cookies 159
  chequered 160
  pinwheel 160
  sable 160
hand-rolled cookies 155
  crescents 156
  ginger snap 156
  melting moments 156
  nankhatai 156
  sweet paste cookies 155
piped cookies 154
  anisette 154
  butter cookie 154
  langues de chat 155
  savoiardi 155
sheet cookies 158
  almond bars 159
  bee sting 158
  brownie 159
  honey bee 159
Types of creams 30, 104
  buttercream 109
  caprice 109
  chantilly 108
  crème anglaise 114
  crème bavarois 112
  crème chiboust 107
  custard 104

double 30
frangipani 105
imitation 30
lemon curd 110
pastry 107
single 30
St Honore 107
whipping 30
Types of Danish 89
  bear's claw 89
  cinnamon roll 89
  custard 89
  flower 89
  pin wheels 89
Types of flour 25
  all-purpose flour 26
  brown flour 26
  buckwheat flour 26
  cake flour 26
  cornflour 26
  gluten-free flour 27
  maize flour 26
  pastry flour 26
  rice flour 26
  rye flour 26
  self-rising flour 26
  strong flour 26
  weak flour 26
  wholemeal flour 26
Types of milk 29
  buttermilk 29
  condensed milk 29
  dehydrated milk 29
  homogenised milk 29
  skimmed milk 29
  whole milk 29
Types of sweeteners 37
  brown sugar 37
  castor sugar/breakfast sugar 37
  corn syrup 37
  cyclamates 38
  demerara sugar 37
  fructose 37
  golden syrup 37
  granulated sugar 37
  honey 37

icing sugar 37
invert sugars 37
isomalt 38
liquid glucose 38
molasses 37
saccharin 38
sucrose 37
sugar substitutes 38
treacle 37
Types of touille paste 106
  almond touille 106
  basic touille 106
  brandy snaps 106
  july pan 106

V

Various glazes and toppings for breads 72
  cereals as toppings 72
  egg wash glaze 72
  flour as topping 72
  herbs as toppings 72
  honey glazes 72
  nuts as toppings 72
  salt water glaze 72
  seeds as toppings 72
  starch glazes 72
  vegetables as toppings 72
Various kinds of hi tea cakes 142
  banana bread 143
  carrot cake 143
  dundee cake 143
  fruit loaf 143
  madeira cake 142
  marbled cake 143
  tea cake 142
  Victoria sponge 142
Various kinds of icings 145
  buttercream 145
  chocolate icing 146
  foam type icings 146
  fondants 146
  glazed icings 146
  royal icing 146

Photo acknowledgements

p.100 (Profiteroles): Oxford University Press ANZ / Brent Parker Jones; **p.100** (Croquembouche): Elena Shashkina / Shutterstock; **p.154** (Oatmeal raisin cookie): CKP1001 / Shutterstock; **p.153** (Chocolate chip cookie): Moving Moment / Shutterstock; **p.35**, **p.154** (Macaroon): gresei / Shutterstock; **p.156** (Sweet paste cookies): A_Lein / Shutterstock; **p.157** (Bull's eye): Gareth Boden / Oxford University Press; **p.159** (Brownie): Lindsay Edwards / Oxford Univsrsity Press ANZ, MBI / Alamy; **p.161** (Gingerbread): Roman Prishenko / Shutterstock; **p.161** (Cinnamon stars): Shebeko / Shutterstock; **p.168** (Milk puddings): Monkey Business Images / Shutterstock; **p.168** (Christmas pudding): bonchan / Shutterstock; **p.171** (Choux fritters): cokemomo © 123RF.com; **p.171** (Toffee apples): Gareth Boden / Oxford University Press; **p.175** (Fruit salad): margouillat photo / Shutterstock; **p.175** (Compotes or poached fruits): R&R PhotoStudio / Brent Parker Jones / Oxford University Press ANZ; **p.176** (Mousse): R&R PhotoStudio / Brent Parker Jones / Oxford University Press ANZ; **p.176** (Soufflé): Brent Parker Jones / Oxford University Press ANZ; **p.177** (Lemon tart): Brent Parker Jones / Oxford University Press ANZ; **p.178** (Fruit trifle): Brent Parker Jones / Oxford University Press ANZ; **p.178** (Tiramisu): cobraphotography / Shutterstock; **p.35** (Pavlova): Brent Parker Jones / Oxford University Press ANZ; **p.35** (Marshmallows): Tiger Images / Shutterstock; **p.189** (Cross-section of an ice cream cake): saddako / Shutterstock.

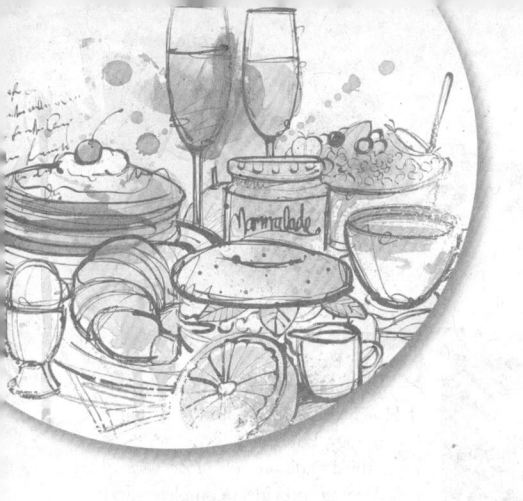

About the Author

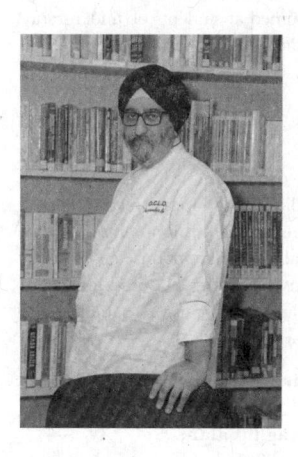

Chef Parvinder Singh Bali is Corporate Chef, Learning and Development, at The Oberoi Centre of Learning and Development (OCLD), New Delhi. He is a certified hospitality educator from the American Hotel and Lodging Association (AHLA), a certified professional chef from the Culinary Institute of America, and also a certified chef de cuisine from the American Culinary Federation. He has written three books with Oxford University Press which are very popular among students—*Food Production Operations*, now in its second edition, *Quantity Food Production Operations and Indian Cuisine*, and *International Cuisine and Food Production Management*. His books have received many awards as well, such as the prestigious Gourmand World Cookbook Award held in Spain and Excellence in Book Production 2012, awarded by The Federation of Indian Publishers.

Related Titles

Hotel Front Office, Second Edition [9780199464692]
Jatashankar R. Tewari,
Assistant Professor, Department of Hotel Management, School of Tourism, Hospitality, and Hotel Management, Uttarakhand Open University, Haldwani, Uttarakhand

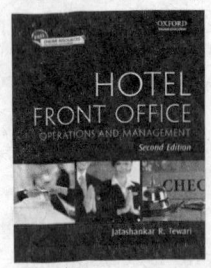

The second edition of *Hotel Front Office* is specifically tailored to meet the requirements of the students of hotel management courses. It aims to explore all the relevant aspects and issues related to front office operations and management with the help of numerous industry-related examples, cases, and project assignments.

Key Features
- Discusses the functions of front office operations, and suggests ways and means to make them more effective
- Includes well-illustrated chapters with numerous photographs, flowcharts, illustrations, tables, and examples

Food and Beverage Services, Second Edition [9780199464685]
R. Singaravelavan,
Principal, State Institute of Hotel Management & Catering Technology, Thuvakkudi, Trichy

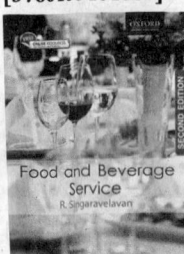

The second edition of the title is specifically tailored to meet the requirements of the students of hotel management courses. Each of the six sections—introduction to food and beverage service, menu knowledge and planning, food service, beverages and tobacco, bar operations and control, and ancillary functions—have been thoroughly updated to cover all the aspects of the food service industry.

Key Features
- New chapters on Menu Knowledge, Costs, Sales, and Profit, and Food Cost Control
- New sections on EU wine regulations and labelling laws, and pairing wine with Asian food

Food Science and Nutrition 3e [9780199489084]
Sunetra Roday,
Principal, Maharashtra State Institute of Hotel Management and Catering Technology, Pune

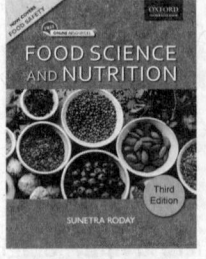

The third edition of *Food Science and Nutrition* provides complete and exhaustive coverage of topics related to food science, food safety, and nutrition. It is aimed at students of undergraduate, diploma, or certificate courses in hotel management, hospitality studies, and catering technology.

Key Features
- New chapters on *Food Safety and Food Standards, Regulations, and Quality Management*
- An appendix on *First Aid*
- Extended material including the latest 'recommended dietary allowances' table; new topic on non-communicable diseases (NCDs); additional information on new packaging options, safety concerns regarding plastics, and smart packaging; dietary guidelines for cancer patients and Naturopathy, and many more

Hotel Housekeeping, Third Edition (With DVD) [9780199451746]
G. Raghubalan,
Hospitality Consultant and Trainer
Smritee Raghubalan, *Associate Professor,* Department of Hotel Management, Garden City College, Bengaluru

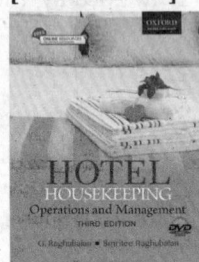

The third edition of *Hotel Housekeeping: Operations and Management* continues its endeavour to provide a comprehensive text to students of diploma, undergraduate, and postgraduate courses in hotel management.

Key Features
- Provides a good balance between theory and practice by presenting important elements of housekeeping in the companion DVD
- Includes case studies that discuss the challenges faced by housekeeping personnel

Other Related Titles

9780198084006 Seal: *Computers in Hotels*
9780198062912 Ghosal: *Hotel Engineering*
9780198064633 Bansal: *Hotel Facility Planning*
9780199458844 Devendra: *Soft Skills in Hospitality*
9780198069850 Biswas: *Human Resource Management in Hospitality*
9780198084013 Devendra: *Hotel Law*

Books by the same author

9780199450510
Bali: *Food Production Operations 2e*

9780198073895
Bali: *International Cuisine and Food Production Management*

9780198068495
Bali: *Quantity Food Production Operations and Indian Cuisine*